ADVANCED IMAGING IN CORONARY ARTERY DISEASE

PET, SPECT, MRI, IVUS, EBCT

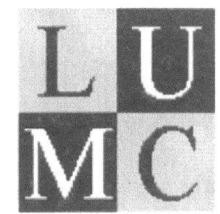

Developments in Cardiovascular Medicine

VOLUME 202

The titles published in this series are listed at the end of this volume.

Advanced Imaging In Coronary Artery Disease

PET, SPECT, MRI, IVUS, EBCT

Edited by

ERNST E. VAN DER WALL
Department of Cardiology,
Leiden University Medical Center Leiden,
Leiden, The Netherlands

PAUL K. BLANKSMA
Department of Cardiology,
University Hospital Groningen,
Groningen, The Netherlands

MENCO G. NIEMEYER
Department of Cardiology,
Martini Hospital,
Groningen, The Netherlands

WILLEM VAALBURG
PET-center,
University Hospital Groningen,
Groningen, The Netherlands

and

HARRY J.G.M. CRIJNS
Department of Cardiology,
University Hospital Groningen,
Groningen, The Netherlands

This publication has been made possible with an educational grant from Byk Nederland BV, Zwanenburg, The Netherlands

SPRINGER SCIENCE+BUSINESS MEDIA, LLC

Library of Congress Cataloging-in-Publication Data

ISBN 978-94-010-3746-4 ISBN 978-94-007-0866-2 (eBook)
DOI 10.1007/978-94-007-0866-2

Printed on acid-free paper

TABLE OF CONTENTS

Part two : MYOCARDIAL ISCHEMIA

Part three: MYOCARDIAL VIABILITY

Part four: HEART FAILURE

FOREWORD

Conventional myocardial imaging techniques provide a clear means of evaluating the anatomy and function of the heart. However, these methods show limitations in answering questions regarding the physiologic significance of a given anatomy or concerning myocardial viability. Whereas planar imaging and single photon emission tomography (SPECT) have considerable practical advantages and can be applied in almost any hospital with current commercially available nuclear medicine equipment and radiopharmaceuticals, positron emission tomography (PET) theoretically offers major advantages in its potential to quantitatively study regional myocardial metabolism and blood flow because of its ability to correct for attenuation. In cardiac studies, PET can be used for the detection of myocardial ischemia, identification of tissue viability, and the pathophysiological assessment of various myocardial diseases such as coronary artery disease, hypertrophic cardiomyopathy, and heart failure. Also neuronal control assessment of the myocardium by receptor imaging by PET can be evaluated.

PET has great clinical potential. To understand the present and future role of PET, the main advantages and limitations should be considered. The advantages of PET are 1) its noninvasive character, 2) the availability of many radionuclides, 3) its excellent temporal and spatial resolution, and 4) the ability to quantify myocardial perfusion and metabolism in absolute terms using physiologically appropriate mathematical models. Major limitations of PET are 1) the cost of providing PET imaging, 2) the technical and logistic complexities, all resulting in a limited availability of PET facilities.

At present almost 80 PET facilities have been installed within Europe. In order to compete favorably with the more conventionally applied techniques, such as echocardiography, SPECT or magnetic resonance imaging (MRI), the inherent weaknesses and strengths of PET should be weighed against the advantages and limitations of these techniques. In the era of cost-benefit assessment, health care departments require the development of adequate diagnostic and therapeutic strategies with the emphasis on cost/effectiveness for different imaging modalities. The algorithm of using PET as an initial test, which seems highly justified by its superior diagnostic accuracy over other noninvasive techniques, would shorten the diagnostic procedure and thereby reduce costs. PET has an important role in showing the way and direction for conventional imaging techniques. The recent modification of the thallium-201 protocols is an example of cross-fertilization by PET. When the limitations of the conventional exercise/3-4 hour delayed thallium-201 imaging for complete visualization of viable myocardium were recognized, PET provided a benchmark for differentiation between viable and non-viable tissue.

Advanced Imaging in Coronary Artery Disease is a bibliographical reflection of the second European Conference on Cardiac PET Research held on May 14 and 15, 1998, Groningen, The Netherlands. At this symposium all major issues considering Cardiac PET are addressed. The role of imaging techniques in diagnosing atherosclerosis, assessment of myocardial ischemia, myocardial viability, and heart failure are broadly discussed. The issues from cardiac PET are also presented in relation to the conventional techniques, such as echocardiography, SPECT and MRI. In addition, newer imaging techniques such as angioscopy, intracoronary ultrasound, electron beam computed tomography, and Raman spectroscopy are given wide attention. Also the effect of drug treatment, such as anti-ischemic and lipid-lowering drugs, are being evaluated.

We would like to acknowledge all individuals, societies and institutions who have had a contribution to our Symposium and, hence, to the appearance of ***Advanced Imaging in Coronary Artery Disease.*** We thank the (co)-authors, as experts in the field of Cardiac PET or related imaging modalities, for their excellent contributions. We are very honored that this year the *Wenckebach lecture* will be presented by Prof. dr H.R. Schelbert, one of the first outstanding pioneers in PET imaging.

We would also like to thank our sponsors i.e. the Working Group on Nuclear Cardiology and MRI of the Dutch Society of Cardiology, the Dutch Society of Nuclear Medicine (chairman: dr. P.P. van Rijk), the Interuniversity

Cardiology Institute of the Netherlands (chairmen: Prof. dr. H.J.J. Wellens and Prof. dr. N. Bom), and the Working Group on Nuclear Cardiology and MRI of the European Society of Cardiology (chairman: Prof. dr. S.R. Underwood), all of which tremendously contributed to the success of our Symposium. We acknowledge the indispensable assistance offered by the Board of Directors of the University Hospital Groningen, who laid to the basis for the Symposium. This book would not have been possible without an educational grant supplied from Byk Nederland BV. We are most grateful for the support by Ria van der Poel (secretary Department of Cardiology) and Nettie Dekker (Kluwer Academic Publishers) for carefully preparing and editing this book. We hope that this book will assist the clinical cardiologist, the nuclear medicine physician, the fellows in cardiology and nuclear medicine, the radiochemist, the basis research fellow and the technician in understanding the new advances in clinical cardiac PET.

Ernst E van der Wall
Paul K Blanksma
Menco G Niemeyer
Willem Vaalburg
Harry JGM Crijns

LIST OF CONTRIBUTORS

Bax, Jeroen J.
Department of Cardiology, Leiden University Medical Centre, Albinusdreef 2, 2333 AA Leiden, The Netherlands
Co-authors: Frans C. Visser, Jan H. Cornel, Paolo M. Fioretti, Arthur van Lingen and Cees A. Visser

Brouwer, René M.H.J.
Division of Thoracic Surgery, Academic Hospital Groningen, Hanzeplein 1, 9700 RB Groningen, The Netherlands
Co-authors: Maarten P. van den Berg and Eduard L. Mooyaard

Camici, Paolo G.
MRC Cyclotron Unit, Imperial College School of Medicine, Hammersmith Hospital, London, United Kingdom
Co-author: Ornella Rimoldi

Elsinga, Philip H.
PET-center, Groningen University Hospital, P.O. Box 30001, 9700 RB Groningen, The Netherlands
Co-authors: Aren van Waarde, Ton J. Visser and Willem Vaalburg

Germano, Guido
Nuclear Medicine Physics, Cedars-Sinai Medical Center, 8700 Beverly Blvd., A047N, Los Angeles, CA 90048, USA

Heijer, Peter den
Department of Cardiology, University Hospital Groningen, Oostersingel 59, 9713 EZ Groningen, The Netherlands

Horst, Gert J. ter
Department of Biological Psychiatry, University of Groningen, P.O. Box 30001, 9700 RB Groningen, The Netherlands

Monnink, Stefan H.J.
Department of Cardiology, University Hospital Groningen, P.O. Box 30001, 9700 RB Groningen, The Netherlands
Co-authors: Hendrik Buikema, Ad J. van Boven and Wiek H. van Gilst

Mulder, Han J.G.H.
Department of Cardiology, Leiden University Medical Centre, Albinusdreef 2, 2333 AA Leiden, The Netherlands
Co-authors: Albert V.G. Bruschke, Martin J. Schalij and Ernst E. van der Wall

Römer, Tjeerd J.
Department of Cardiology, Leiden University Medical Centre, Albinusdreef 2, 2333 AA Leiden, The Netherlands
Co-authors: James F. Brennan III and Hendrik P.J. Buschman

Rosen, Stuart D.
MRC Cyclotron Unit and Imperial College, School of Medicine, Hammersmith Hospital, Du Cane road, London W12 0NN, United Kingdom

Rossum, Albert C. van
Department of Cardiology, Free University Hospital, De Boelelaan 1117, 1081 HV Amsterdam, The Netherlands

Ruigrok, Tom J.C.
Department of Cardiology, Heart Lung Institute, University Hospital Utrecht, The Netherlands
Co-authors: Xavier A. van Binsbergen and Cees J.A. van Echteld

Schelbert, Heinrich R.
Department of Molecular and Medical Pharmacology, UCLA School of Medicine, P.O. Box 951735, Los Angeles, CA 90095, USA

Siebelink, Hans-Marc J.
Department of Cardiology, University Hospital Groningen, Oostersingel 59, 9713 EZ Groningen, The Netherlands
Co-author: Ad J. van Boven, Ad J. van Boven and Paul K. Blanksma

Gunning, Mark
Royal Brompton Hospital, Sydney Street, London SW3 6NP, United Kingdom
Co-author: Richard Underwood

Vanoverschelde, Jean-Louis J.
Department of Cardiology, Cliniques Universitaires St. Luc, Avenue Hippocrate 10, B-1200 Brussel, Belgium
Co-authors: Bernhard L. Gerber and Jacques A. Melin

Veldhuisen, Dirk J. van
Division of Cardiology, University Hospital Groningen, P.O. Box 30001, 9700 RB Groningen, The Netherlands
Co-authors: Ad F.M. van den Heuvel and Maarten P. van den Berg

Visser, Frans C.
Department of Cardiology, Free University of Amsterdam, De Boelelaan 1117, 1081 HV Amsterdam, The Netherlands
Co-authors: Jeroen J. Bax, Lucas J. Klein, William Wijns and Cees A. Visser

Wal, Allard C. van der
Department of Cardiovasculair Pathology, Amsterdam Medical Centre, University Hospital Amsterdam, Meibergdreef 9, 1105 AZ Amsterdam, The Netherlands
Co-author: Anton E. Becker

CLINICAL IMPACT OF CARDIAC PET

Heinrich R. Schelbert

Introduction

An assessment of the virtues of positron emission tomography (PET) and its current and future role in the diagnosis and management of cardiovascular disorders must include an examination of the technical features that are unique to this sophisticated medical imaging technology. One feature unique to PET is the quantitative, autoradiography-like ability to generate cross-sectional images of the true radiotracer concentrations in organs or the entire body. The second feature, entails the use of physiologic tracer substances that are labeled with radioactive isotopes of elements that constitute living matter and are abound in nature. With these tracers, biochemical processes in organ regions are now accessible to noninvasive visualization. Finally, the high temporal resolution capability measures dynamic changes of these radioactively tagged compounds in tissue so that a broad range of physiologic and biochemical processes can be determined in an almost entirely noninvasive fashion. Not only does this methodologic approach represent a transfer of assays used widely in the life sciences from the in vitro to the in vivo and in situ environments, it also affords the demonstration of physiologic processes explored, defined and established over centuries and culminating in fundamental insights into the biochemistry of living matter directly in the human body. Fick's early and Kety and Schmidt's subsequent studies on measuring regional organ blood flow, the pursuit of measurements of myocardial oxygen consumption through a series of often dramatic accomplishments and discoveries beginning with Dieffenbach in 1834 and culminating in the achievements by Forssmann,

Cournand and Richard Bing are now readily and conveniently accomplished with cardiac PET. Key steps and components of substrate metabolism discovered by Nobel laureates Sir Hans Krebs and Otto Warburg or, most recently, by Paul Moyer at University of California, Los Angeles in in-vitro experimental systems can now be readily assessed in the human organs. Indeed, many of these fundamental discoveries serve as underpinnings of procedures performed routinely with PET. It is fair to state that Warburg's discovery of anaerobic glycolysis in an oxygen rich environment has become fundamental for the PET based detection of malignant tumors. Krebs' central substrate cycle named after him, is now accessible to study directly in the human myocardium. Together with Pasteur's observation of enhanced glucose metabolism, these discoveries form the base for identifying and defining ischemia in human myocardium. It is thus that information generated in the research laboratory can now readily be applied to the study of physiologic and pathologic processes in the human body and emerges as an important means for recognizing and characterizing disease.

Positron Emission Tomography and Cardiovascular Disease

PET offers an incredibly broad scope of possibilities for probing human biochemistry and physiology. Yet, we must ask which ones have or are likely to impact health care. Clearly, there are several ones that can and already have decisively influenced patient management. There will be others that integrate emerging fundamental knowledge in order to explain novel aspects of cardiovascular function and, lastly, the merger of molecular biology with PET imaging technology promises new and exciting future applications.

PET's Role in Coronary Artery Disease

Detection and risk assessment of coronary artery disease continue to be mainstays of modern cardiology. They have gained in importance because of the broad range of therapeutic options that are now available to patients with coronary artery disease. These options range from mechanical revascularization to modern pharmacologic interventions and, likely in the near future, in gene therapy. PET's high diagnostic accuracy in identifying functionally significant coronary artery disease is now well established (Figure 1)[1-5.] Direct and indirect comparisons with the diagnostic performance of single photon emission computed tomography (SPECT) based perfusion imaging approaches confirmed PET's superiority; [3-6] even detecting only mild coronary artery disease seems now feasible. [7] Head to head comparisons in the same patient populations similarly established the high diagnostic accuracy of PET relative to that of conventional SPECT. Gains in specificity seem particularly important. Reports have been brought to our attention that this diagnostic gain reduced the need for coronary angiography [4,5,8]. This of course would lower risk to the patients and cost of the diagnostic work-up of patients suspected of having coronary artery disease. Yet, these reports have been anecdotal so that a true assessment of PET's cost effectiveness remains incomplete. In the absence of hard evidence the question then remains whether the about 10% gain in diagnostic accuracy over SPECT based approaches will justify the widespread use of PET for the diagnosis of coronary artery disease. It is also clear that PET must compete in this area with current developments and improvement in SPECT with for example gated image acquisition or possibilities of correction for photon attenuation. At the same time, one needs to acknowledge that the presence of coronary artery disease can be confirmed or excluded with a high level of certainty within less than one hour if PET is combined with Rubidium-82 rest and pharmacologic stress imaging. Thus, PET offers a possibility for high volume patient studies. Equally important is the use of PET in patients with suspected mild coronary artery disease or in patients with a low likelihood of coronary artery disease.

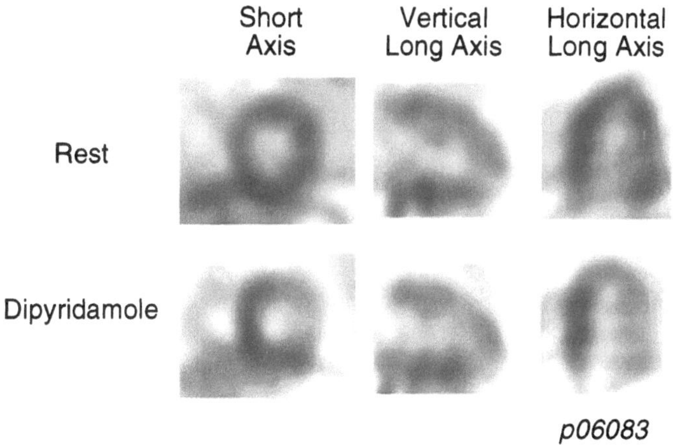

Figure 1. Detection of coronary artery disease by PET. Short axis and vertical and horizontal long axis myocardial images are shown at rest (upper panel) and during dipyridamole induced hyperemia (lower panel). Note the near normal distribution of myocardial blood flow throughout the entire left ventricular myocardium. Stress however induces marked defects in the anterior and posterolateral wall as seen in the lower panel.

PET for the Management of Ischemic Cardiomyopathy

Less ambiguity surrounds PET's clinical utility in the assessment of myocardial viability. Clearly, such assessment will increase in importance as the prevalence of ischemic cardiomyopathy rises. Successes in the treatment of myocardial infarction with lower mortalities and broad applications of mechanical revascularization increased the number of surviving patients with severe coronary artery disease and ischemic cardiomyopathy. At the same time, limited treatment options in such end-stage patients, the often staggering cost of management, and especially the risk of catastrophic cardiovascular events have accelerated PET's use in this particularly serious clinical situation. Numerous clinical studies attest to PET's high diagnostic accuracy for identifying reversibly dysfunctional myocardium that is viability and its separation from myocardium with irretrievable loss in contractile function (Figure 2) [9-20].

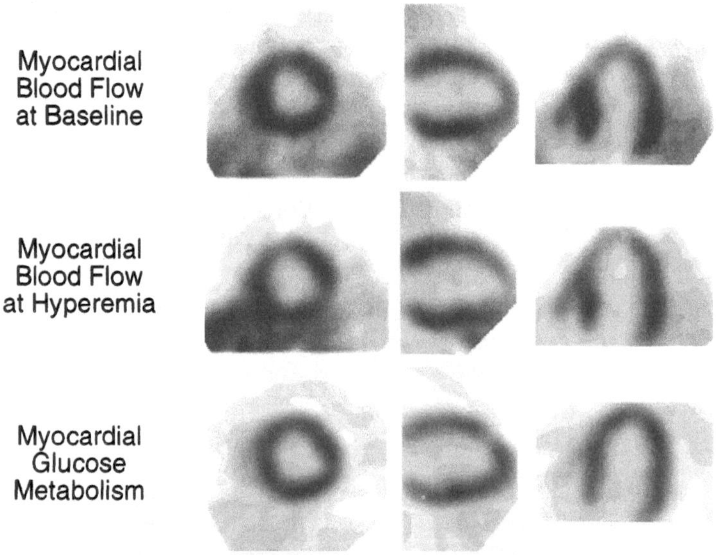

Figure 2*. Example of blood flow metabolism imaging in a patient with known coronary artery disease and impaired anterior wall motion. Again, short axis and vertical and horizontal long axis images are shown. The upper panel shows the myocardial perfusion at rest (baseline) indicating a moderate reduction in blood flow in the anteroseptal wall. A subsequent study using dipyridamole induced hyperemia demonstrates a marked increase in this moderate perfusion defect suggesting the presence of stunned myocardium that also accounted for the impaired wall motion of the anterolateral wall. In contrast, the myocardial substrate images (lower panel) demonstrate a near normal and homogeneous glucose metabolism.*

At the same time, blood flow metabolism imaging with PET identifies those patients with coronary artery disease who are at high risk for cardiac mortality and morbidity [21-24]. It thus guides clinicians to institute appropriate treatments to avert fateful cardiac events and prolong life. Beyond this, there is evidence of PET's role in predicting post-revascularization gains in global left ventricular function and relief from symptoms of congestive heart failure[25-27]. Besides these long term outcome predictors, recently reported information also implies a possible role of PET in the immediate management of ischemic cardiomyopathy patients [28]. Patients selected by PET for revascularization frequently experience a more uneventful post-surgical course with little if any peri-operative mortality. This markedly differs from that from that in unselected patients. The peri-operative mortality of PET selected patients approaches zero; their recovery from surgery is less complicated and frequently uneventful. In addition to the direct benefit to patients such PET selection is likely to translate also into reduction in cost. There are additional cost considerations. Given PET's ability of predicting which patient will or will not significantly benefit from surgical revascularization, PET has emerged as an important tool for stratifying patients who are initially thought of to benefit only from cardiac transplantation to surgical revascularization [29,30]. Obviously, this will result in substantial cost savings but also opens the door for alternative and equally effective treatment strategies for transplant candidates.

Cost Considerations in Clinical Cardiac PET

Undoubtedly, start-up and operational costs for PET are, at least at present, high or even excessive. Although the quality of the imaging product and its clinical implications appear to justify such cost per se, PET must in today's climate of limited resources compete with alternative, less costly or, conversely, more profitable diagnostic approaches, even though those competing approaches do not provide the same level of diagnostic accuracy. Research has therefore focused on improvements of now standard nuclear medicine approaches entailing PET and thallium-201 or technetium-99m perfusion imaging agents without however reaching a level of diagnostic accuracy that matches that of PET. Nevertheless, health care insurers and providers ask whether the diagnostic gain justifies the increased cost. On the other hand, to reduce costs or to provide adequate information with more widely available standard imaging instrumentation, hybrid approaches have emerged where myocardial blood flow at rest is evaluated with the thallium-201 or technetium-99m sestamibi SPECT approach followed by a PET based evaluation of glucose metabolism. A further expansion of this approach has resulted in the use of multi-purpose SPECT-like systems using either high energy photon collimators or coincidence detection.[31-33] These approaches seem to achieve diagnostic accuracies that approach those by the pure PET technology. Clearly, PET's spatial, temporal and contrast resolution remains unmatched by these emerging devices. If recovery of global left ventricular function or symptomatic improvement critically depend on accurate estimates of the amount of viable myocardium then future studies will need to define how well such outcomes can be predicted with less sophisticated and less expensive imaging instrumentation.

Alternatively, a substantial reduction of the cost of full fledged PET systems would be equally desirable to remain competitive not only with standard radionuclide approaches but also with magnetic resonance imaging, electron beam computed tomography (EBCT) or even stress echocardiography. The danger is that PET might price itself out of what today is economically feasible and acceptable. No less important for reducing the operational cost of PET will be the substantial shortening of imaging times so that cardiac examinations can be completed within minutes rather than hours and patient throughput be enhanced. Such efforts are in progress for imaging modalities like MRI and EBCT and again, will be essentially for PET's future clinical success.

Emerging Clinical Applications of Cardiac PET

If such full capacity but low cost PET systems will become available, it then is easy to envision a gamut of clinical applications in cardiovascular diseases. Likely among those are the identification of pre-clinical coronary artery disease, a procedure that clearly would compete successfully or even out-perform the assessment of coronary calcifications with EBCT. The conceptual framework for such PET approaches already exist. Initial studies are promising. Other applications include assessment of what constitutes myocardial ischemia in non-coronary artery cardiovascular diseases, characterization of the human heart's neuronal control and receptor activities, especially in view of the fact that much of the current pharmacologic armamentarium relies on receptor blocking or stimulation [34-38]. Lastly, the future importance of gene therapy to cardiovascular disease is unquestioned. It is likely that PET will participate in these current developments and their application to human cardiac disease. While these developments remain still undefined a second major role in the modern management of cardiovascular disease begins to emerge. They are predicated on PET's ability of measurements of absolute myocardial tissue blood flow.[39-47] It probably does not matter which of the currently available measurement approaches, that is 0-15 water, N-13 ammonia or rubidium-82, will be used. What will matter is how precisely, accurately and reproducibly blood flow can be measured.[48-49]

PET and Preclinical Coronary Artery Disease

The past years witnessed remarkable advances in vascular biology. Not only have these achievements unraveled mechanisms critical in the evolution of coronary artery disease but have established the fundaments for combating disease or, if already present, to halt its progression or even reverse it. Many investigations point to the development of endothelial dysfunction as a pivotal event in the development of atherogenesis. Other studies again have convincingly demonstrated that such dysfunction is indeed reversible. It is in this particular area where PET can and is likely to play an important clinical role. PET's advantage is based on the ability to measure regional myocardial blood flow. Initial findings have been promising. For example, PET based measurements of myocardial blood flow convincingly demonstrated an impairment in coronary vasodilator capacity in hypercholesteremic patients without apparent coronary artery disease.[50-54] The reduction in vascular smooth muscle mediated vasodilator capacity did, as expected from earlier invasive studies, correlate with lipid abnormalities but also with the duration of the hypercholesteremic disorder (Figure 3).[51]

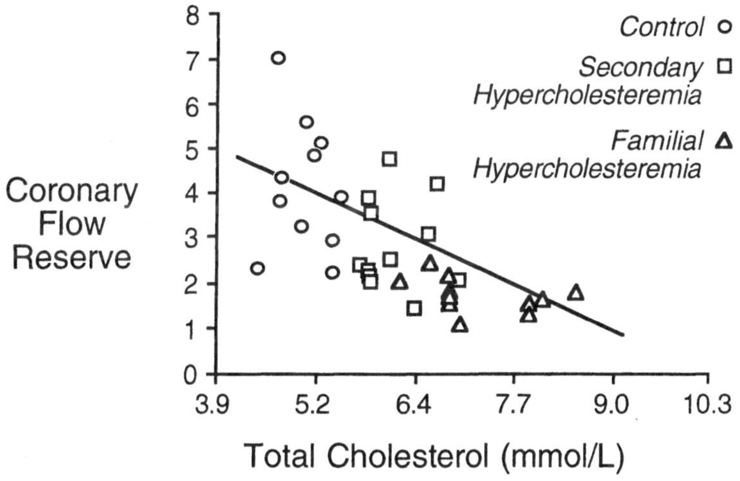

***Figure 3**. Correlation between PET measured myocardial flow reserve and total serum cholesterol levels. Note the inverse correlation. Data reproduced with permission from Yokoyama et al. J Nucl Med 1996;37:1937-1942.*

Similar abnormal vasodilator responses have also been demonstrated noninvasively with PET in patients with diabetes as another, well-established coronary risk factor. What these observations indicate is the possibility of exploring and defining integrated responses of the human coronary microcirculation to pharmacologic tests. Thus, a tool exists now for demonstrating disturbances in coronary vasomotion. At the same time, these observations are puzzling. While the endothelium has been implicated as the initial site of a defective microcirculatory system, these PET based investigations bypassed the endothelium by targeting primarily the direct smooth muscle mediated vasorelaxation. Opportunities however exist for targeting more specifically endothelial dependent vasomotor control of the human coronary circulation. Initial studies suggest altered flow responses to cold pressor testing as an approach that depends on a close interplay between vasoconstrictor and (mostly endothelial dependent) vasorelaxant effects. Such abnormal responses have been elicited in hypercholesteremia but also as a consequence of chronic cigarette smoking as another well established coronary risk factor.[55] Future research will be needed to more clearly and definitively define the significant and implications of such altered flow responses to cold. If confirmed, PET based measurements of myocardial blood flow then offer a means of probing coronary vasomotion and, even more importantly, a test of early, evolving but preclinical atherosclerosis.

Several reasons underscore and emphasize the importance of such test. One is the emergence of pharmacologic strategies to normalize human coronary vasomotion which is likely, as shown by several multicenter trials, to translate into dramatic improvements in primary and secondary prevention of coronary events.[56-57] Again, PET based flow measurements convincingly demonstrated improvements in coronary vasodilator function after only six weeks of cardiovascular conditioning including weight loss, low cholesterol diet and regular physical exercise.[58] Even more exciting and promising are preliminary findings on how PET based blood flow measurements can objectify responses to cholesterol lowering treatment. The current emphasis on coronary prevention or reversal through pharmacologic approaches, ranging from cholesterol lowering compounds to possibly anti-atherogenic agents, ACE inhibitors or angiotensin receptor blockers promises an open field for clinical PET. This field extends further to insulin sensitizers or, in the aging population, to the coronary effects of estrogen and progesterone. Thus, it is likely that PET based approaches will emerge which target specific aspects of coronary vascular function that can identify individuals at risk or with early coronary atherosclerosis as well as responses to dietary and lifestyle changes and to pharmacologic interventions. As another aspect of considerable clinical importance PET can play a potentially major role in the development of new anti-atherosclerotic drugs. Again, early observations are fascinating as for example the recently reported initial drug induced decline in serum cholesterol concentrations without a prompt normalization of coronary vasomotor function which however was noted after a six month delay.

Conclusion

What lies ahead in the long term future will be difficult to predict. Yet, it is important to recall the near unlimited potential and possibilities of PET, its technological advantages and the enormous number of radiotracers that are available. Established methodologies like receptor assays, analysis of adrenergic neuronal function and innervation of the human heart have remained largely unexplored or underutilized in the clinical arena. At the same time, development of new radiotracers is in progress. Molecular biology has and continues to dominate the biomedical sciences. It is thus likely that new insights gained into fundamental processes of disease will have substantial impact on management of disease. Initial accomplishments as for example a gene therapy based biologic bypass in coronary artery disease carry considerable promise. It is in this area where PET can monitor the consequences of gene therapy approaches on cardiovascular function as well as directly visualizing gene expression.

Acknowledgments

The author thanks Diane Martin for preparing the illustrations and Eileen Rosenfeld for her critical assistance in preparing this manuscript.

References

1. Schelbert HR, Wisenberg G, Phelps ME, et al. Noninvasive assessment of coronary stenoses by myocardial imaging during pharmacologic coronary vasodilation. VI. Detection of coronary artery disease in human beings with intravenous N-13 ammonia and positron computed tomography. Am J Cardiol 1982;49:1197-207.
2. Gould KL, Goldstein RA, Mullani NA, et al. Noninvasive assessment of coronary stenoses by myocardial perfusion imaging during pharmacologic coronary vasodilation. VIII. Clinical feasibility of positron cardiac imaging without a cyclotron using generator-produced rubidium-82. J Am Coll Cardiol 1986;7:775-89.
3. Demer LL, Gould KL, Goldstein RA, et al. Assessment of coronary artery disease severity by positron emission tomography. Comparison with quantitative arteriography in 193 patients. Circulation 1989;79:825-35.
4. Stewart RE, Schwaiger M, Molina E, et al. Comparison of rubidium-82 positron emission tomography and thallium-201 SPECT imaging for detection of coronary artery disease. Am J Cardiol 1991;67:1303-10.
5. Go RT, Marwick TH, MacIntyre WJ, et al. A prospective comparison of rubidium-82 PET and thallium-201 SPECT myocardial perfusion imaging utilizing a single dipyridamole stress in the diagnosis of coronary artery disease. J Nucl Med 1990;31:1899-905.
6. Tamaki N, Yonekura Y, Yamashita K, et al. SPECT thallium-201 tomography and positron tomography using N-13 ammonia and F-18 fluorodeoxyglucose in coronary heart disease. Am J Card Imaging 1989;3:3-9.
7. Gould KL, Schelbert HR, Phelps ME, Hoffman EJ. Noninvasive assessment of coronary stenoses with myocardial perfusion imaging during pharmacologic coronary vasodilation. V. Detection of 47 percent diameter coronary stenosis with intravenous nitrogen-13 ammonia and emission-computed transaxial tomography in intact dogs. Am J Cardiol 1979;43:200-8.
8. Tamaki N, Yonekura Y, Senda M, et al. Value and limitation of stress thallium-201 single photon emission computed tomography: comparison with nitrogen-13 ammonia positron tomography. J Nucl Med 1988;29:1181-8.
9. Marshall RC, Huang SC, Nash WW, Phelps ME. Assessment of the 18-fluorodeoxyglucose kinetic model in calculations of myocardial glucose metabolic rate during ischemia. J Nucl Med 1983;24:1060-4.
10. Tillisch J, Brunken R, Marshall R, et al. Reversibility of cardiac wall-motion abnormalities predicted by positron tomography. N Engl J Med 1986;314:884-8.
11. Tamaki N, Yonekura Y, Yamashita K, et al. Positron emission tomography using fluorine-18 deoxyglucose in evaluation of coronary artery bypass grafting. Am J Cardiol 1989;64:860-5.
12. Tamaki N, Ohtani H, Yamashita K, et al. Metabolic activity in the areas of new fill-in after thallium-201 reinjection: comparison with positron emission tomography using fluorine-18-deoxyglucose. J Nucl Med 1991;32:673-8.

13. Lucignani G, Paolini G, Landoni C, et al. Presurgical identification of hibernating myocardium by combined use of technetium-99m hexakis 2-methoxyisobutylisonitrile single photon emission tomography and fluorine-18 fluoro-2-deoxy-D-glucose positron emission tomography in patients with coronary artery disease. Eur J Nucl Med 1992;19:874-81.
14. Carrel T, Jenni R, Haubold-Reuter S, Von Schulthess G, Pasic M, Turina M. Improvement of severely reduced left ventricular function after surgical revascularization in patients with preoperative myocardial infarction. Eur J Cardiothorac Surg 1992;6:479-84.
15. Knuuti M, Saraste M, Nuutila P, et al. Myocardial viability: fluorine-18-deoxyglucose positron emission tomography in prediction of wall motion recovery after revascularization. Am Heart J 1994;127:785-96.
16. Vom Dahl J, Altehoefer C, Sheehan FH, et al. Recovery of regional left ventricular dysfunction after coronary revascularization. Impact of myocardial viability assessed by nuclear imaging and vessel patency at follow-up angiography. J Am Coll Cardiol 1996;28;948-58.
17. Depré C, Vanoverschelde JL, Melin J, et al. Structural and metabolic correlates of the reversibility of chronic left ventricular ischemic dysfunction in humans. Am J Physiol 1995;268:H1265-75.
18. Depré C, Vanoverschelde JL, Gerber B, Borgers M, Melin JA, Dion R. Correlation of functional recovery with myocardial blood flow, glucose uptake, and morphologic features in patients with chronic left ventricular ischemic dysfunction undergoing coronary artery bypass grafting. J Thorac Cardiovasc Surg 1997;113:371-8.
19. Maes A, Flameng W, Nuyts J, et al. Histological alterations in chronically hypoperfused rnyocardium. Correlation with PET findings. Circulation 1994,90:735-45.
20. Maes AF, Borgers M, Flameng W, et al Assessment of myocardial viability in chronic coronary artery disease using technetium-99m sestamibi SPECT. Correlation with histologic and positron emission tomographic studies and functional follow-up. J Am Coll Cardiol 1997;29:62-8.
21. Eitzman D, Al-Aouar Z, Kanter HL, et al. Clinical outcome of patients with advanced coronary artery disease after viability studies with positron emission tomography. J Am Coll Cardiol 1992;20:559-65.
22. Di Carli MF, Davidson M, Little R, et al. Value of metabolic imaging with positron emission tomography for evaluating prognosis in patients with coronary artery disease and left ventricular dysfunction. Am J Cardiol 1994;73:527-33.
23. Lee KS, Marwick TH, Cook SA, et al. Prognosis of patients with left ventricular dysfunction, with and without viable myocardium after myocardial infarction. Relative efficacy of medical therapy and revascularization. Circulation 1994;90:2687-94.
24. Tamaki N, Kawamoto M, Takahashi N, et al. Prognostic value of an increase in fluorine-18 deoxyglucose uptake in patients with myocardial infarction: comparison with stress thallium imaging. J Am Coll Cardiol 1993;22:1621-7.
25. Di Carli M, Sherman T, Khanna S, et al. Myocardial viability in asynergic regions subtended by occluded coronary arteries: relation to the status of collateral flow in patients with chronic coronary artery disease. J Am Coll Cardiol 1994;23:860-8.

26. Di Carli MF, Asgarzadie F, Schelbert H, et al. Quantitative relation between myocardial viability and improvement in heart failure symptoms after revascularization in patients with ischemic cardiomyopathy. Circulation 1995,92:3436-44.
27. Di Carli MF, Maddahi J, Rokhsar S, Schelbert HR, Brunken RC. Long-term survival of patients with coronary artery disease and left ventricular dysfunction: implications for the role of myocardial viability assessment in management decisions [abstract]. Circulation 1997;96 Suppl 1: I434.
28. Haas F, Haehnel CJ, Picker W, et al. Preoperative positron emission tomographic viability assessment and perioperative and postoperative risk in patients with advanced ischemic heart disease. J Am Coll Cardiol 1997;30:1693-700.
29. Beanlands R, deKemp R, Smith S, Johansen R, Ruddy TD. F-18-fluorodeoxyglucose PET imaging alters clinical decision making in patients with impaired ventricular function. Am J Cardiol 1997;79:1092-5.
30. Duong TH, Hendi P, Fonarow G, et al. Role of positron emission tomographic assessment of myocardial viability in the management of patients who are referred for cardiac transplantation [abstract]. Circulation 1995;92 Suppl 1:I123.
31. Burt RW, Perkins OW, Oppenheim BE, et al. Direct comparison of fluorine-18-FDG SPECT, fluorine-18-FDG PET and rest thallium-201 SPECT for detection of myocardial viability. J Nucl Med 1995;36:176-9.
32. Sandler MP, Patton JA. Fluorine 18-labeled fluorodeoxyglucose myocardial single-photon emission computed tomography: an alternative for determining myocardial viability. J Nucl Cardiol 1996;3:342-9.
33. Bax JJ, Visser FC, Blanksma PK, et al. Comparison of myocardial uptake of fluorine-18-fluorodeoxyglucose imaged with PET and SPECT in dyssynergic myocardium. J Nucl Med 1996;37:161-36.
34. Bax JJ, Jr Cornel JH, Visser FC, Fioretti PM, Visser CA. Prediction of improvement of global function after revascularization in patients with ischemic left ventricular dysfunction: detection by F18-fluorodeoxyglucose SPECT [abstract]. J Am Coll Cardiol 1997;29 Suppl A: 377A.
35. Merlet P, Delforge J, Syrota A, et al. Positron emission tomography with ^{11}C CGP-12177 to assess beta-adrenergic receptor concentration in idiopathic dilated cardiomyopathy. Circulation 1993;87:1169-78.
36. Schwaiger M, Kalff V, Rosenspire K, et al. Noninvasive evaluation of sympathetic nervous system in human heart by positron emission tomography. Circulation 1990;82:457-64.
37. Syrota A, Comar D, Paillotin G, et al. Muscarinic cholinergic receptor in the human heart evidenced under physiological conditions by positron emission tomography. Proc Natl Acad Sci USA 1985;82:584-8.
38. Syrota A. Receptor binding studies in the living heart. In: Pohost GM, Higgins CB, Morganroth J, Ritchie JL, Schelbert HR, editors. New concepts in cardiac imaging 1988. Chicago: Year Book Medical Publishers, Inc.; 1988: p.141-66.
39. Sun D, Nguyen N, DeGrado TR, Schwaiger M, Brosius F 3rd. Ischemia induces translocation of the insulin-responsive glucose transporter GLUT4 to the plasma membane of cardiac myocytes. Circulation 1994;89:793-8.
40. Krivokapich J, Smith GT, Huang SC, et al. 13N ammonia myocardial imaging at rest and with exercise in normal volunteers. Quantification of absolute myocardial perfusion with dynamic positron emission tomography. Circulation 1989;80:1328-37.

41. Hutchins GD, Schwaiger M, Rosenspire KC, Krivokapich J, Schelbert H, Kuhl DE. Noninvasive quantification of regional blood flow in the human heart using N-13 ammonia and dynamic positron emission tomographic imaging. J Am Coll Cardiol 1990;15:1032-42.
42. Kuhle WG, Porenta G, Huang SC, et al. Quantification of regional myocardial blood flow using 13N-ammonia and reoriented dynamic positron emission tomographic imaging. Circulation 1992;86:1004-17.
43. Muzik O, Beanlands RS, Hutchins GD, Mangner TJ, Nguyen N, Schwaiger M. Validation of nitrogen-13-ammonia tracer kinetic model for quantification of myocardial blood flow using PET. J Nucl Med 1993;34:83-91.
44. Merlet P, Mazoyer B, Hittinger L, et al. Assessment of coronary reserve in man: comparison between positron emission tomography with oxygen-15-labeled water and intracoronary Doppler technique. J Nucl Med 1993;34:1899-904.
45. Bergmann SR, Herrero P, Markham J, Weinheimer CJ, Walsh MN. Noninvasive quantitation of myocardial blood flow in human subjects with oxygen-15-labeled water and positron emission tomography. J Am Coll Cardiol 1989;14:639-52.
46. Iida H, Kanno I, Takahashi A, et al. Measurement of absolute myocardial blood flow with $H_2{}^{15}O$ and dynamic positron-emission tomography. Strategy for quantification in relation to the partial-volume effect [published erratum appears in Circulation 1998;78:1078]. Circulation 1988;78:104-15.
47. Herrero P, Markham J, Weinheimer CJ, et al. Quantification of regional myocardial perfusion with generator-produced 62Cu-PTSM and positron emission tomography. Circulation 1993;87:173-83.
48. Nagamachi S, Czernin J, Kim AS, et al. Reproducibility of measurements of regional resting and hyperemic myocardial blood flow assessed with PET. J Nucl Med 1996;37:1626-31.
49. DeGrado TR, Hanson MW, Turkington TG, et al. Estimation of myocardial blood flow for longitudinal studies with ^{13}N-labeled ammonia and positron emission tomography. J Nucl Cardiol 1996;3:494-507.
50. Dayanikli F, Grambow D, Muzik O, Mosca L, Rubenfire M, Schwaiger M. Early detection of abnormal coronary flow reserve in asymptomatic men at high risk for coronary artery disease using positron emission tomography. Circulation 1994,90:808-17.
51. Yokoyama I, Murakami T, Ohtake T, et al. Reduced coronary flow reserve in familial hypercholesterolemia. J of Nucl Med 1996;37:1937-42.
52. Yokoyama I, Ohtake T, Momomura S, Nishikawa J, Sasaki Y, Omata M. Reduced coronary flow reserve in hypercholesterolemic patients without overt coronary stenosis. Circulation 1996;94:3232-8.
53. Pitkanen OP, Raitakari OT, Niinikoski H, et al. Coronary flow reserve is impaired in young men with familial hypercholesterolemia. J Am Coll Cardiol 1996;28:1705-11.
54. Pitkanen OP, Raitakari OT, Ronnemaa T, et al. Influence of cardiovascular risk status on coronary flow reserve in healthy young men. Am J Cardiol 1997:79:1690-2.
55. Campisi R, Czerrun Jr, Schöder H, Schelbert HR. Abnormal coronary vasomotion in long-term smokers depends on duration and dose of smoking [abstract]. J Am Coll Cardiol 1997;29 Suppl A:70A.
56. Randomised trial of cholesterol lowering in 4444 patients with coronary heart disease: the Scandinavian Simvastatin Survival Study 48. Lancet 1994;344:1383-9.

57. Shepherd X, Cobbe SM, Ford I, et al. Prevention of coronary heart disease with pravastatin in men with hypercholesterolemia. West of Scotland Coronary Prevention Study Group. N Eng J Med 1995;333:1301-7.
58. Czernin J, Barnard RJ, Sun KT, et al. Effect of short-term cardiovascular conditioning and low-fat diet on myocardial blood flow and flow reserve. Circulation 1995;92:197-204.

Chapter 1

STABLE AND UNSTABLE ATHEROSCLEROTIC PLAQUES: PLAQUE BIOLOGY IN RELATION TO ACUTE EVENTS

Allard C. van der Wal and Anton E. Becker

Introduction

Most acute ischemic syndromes, with totally different clinical presentations such as myocardial infarction, stroke or acute limb ischemia, share a common pathogenetic feature: disruption of an atherosclerotic plaque followed by luminal thrombosis [1-3]. Plaque disruptions under these circumstances may vary greatly in extent: from focal erosions of the plaque surface, to deep ruptures throughout the fibrous cap reaching into the soft lipid core of lesions. Discontinuity of the endothelium allows a contact between the blood stream and highly thrombogenic plaque materials (collagen fibrils and lipid debris insulated with Tissue Factor), which initiates activation of the coagulation system with at least some degree of thrombus formation [4]. The differences in the type and extent of plaque laceration may have implications for the clinical outcome of the rupture event (figure 1). In coronary arteries, the arterial site where plaque rupture has been studied most extensively, a number of correlations have emerged between the morphology of the plaque, the degree of thrombus formation and the clinical syndrome of patients.

Mural, not occluding, thrombus can be detected in culprit lesions of many patients with (one of the various forms of) unstable angina [4,5]. Complete coronary obstructions are often seen during autopsies of patients with large transmural infarction. Infarct related plaques may be highly stenotic (often with complete thrombotic occlusion), but when large series of patients with

Van der Wall et al. (eds.),
Advanced Imaging in Coronary Artery Disease, 1-14.

acute myocardial infarction are evaluated, most of the underlying lesions appear to be only mildly or moderately stenotic [6].

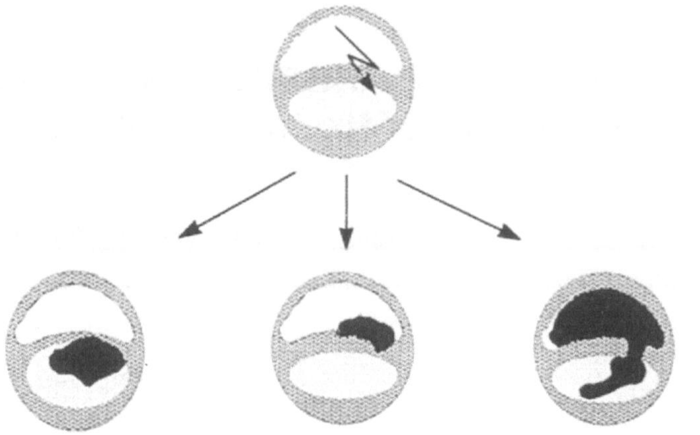

***Figure 1.** Three main types of thrombus formation following coronary plaque disruption. **Left:** intraplaque thrombus, without thrombus formation in the lumen of the artery (or early lysis of small amounts of mural thrombus).Substantial amounts of thrombus in the central lipid core of a plaque, with subsequent organization of the thrombus mass, may lead to an angiographically unexpec-ted increase in stenosis rate in a short period of time. **Middle:** mural not occluding thrombus, with preservation of an antegrade flow through the coronary vessel lumen is the prototype of thrombus formation in patients with unstable angina pectoris. **Right:** Complete thrombotic occlusion of the arterial vessel lumen.*

Coronary atherectomy specimens obtained from patients with different types of ischemic syndromes show that there is a relationship between the presence of thrombus and the clinical severity of the ischemic syndrome [7-9]. Minor plaque ruptures in coronary plaques of autopsied patients who died of non-cardiac disease are regularly seen, and indicate apparently clinically silent events. However, they may lead to episodes of sudden and unexpected plaque growth, due to rapid plaque expansion when blood has entered the soft lipid core [10]. All these notions fit nicely the concept of unstable atherosclerotic plaques: plaques with an unstable morphology give rise to the onset of unstable coronary artery disease. Over the past years many research efforts have been performed for the identification of features of plaques which increase their vulnerability and related risk of rupture and thrombosis.

The atherosclerotic plaque

Atherosclerotic plaque formation results from complex cellular interactions in the intima of arteries, which take place between the resident cells of the vessel wall (smooth muscle cells and endothelial cells) and cells of the immune system (macrophages and lymphocytes). Many cytokines and other growth factors have been identified which regulate the growth, the differentiation and the functional status of these cells, and it is presently widely accepted that this type of tissue reaction has many features of chronic inflammation [11].

The presence of lipids as a driving force seems to be obligatory in this process. Once an atherosclerotic plaque has formed, it shows the well known architecture of a fibrous cap encaging a central lipid-rich core, the "atheroma". Smooth muscle cells produce the extracellular matrix proteins of the fibrous cap, among them collagen I and III, which support the structural integrity of a plaque. On the other hand, the atheroma is soft and weak, rich in extracellular lipids and practically devoid of cells, but is bordered by a rim of lipid-laden macrophage (foam cells). Foam cell death, due to the cytotoxic effects of oxidized lipoproteins, plays an important role in the formation and growth of the atheroma, together with extracellular binding of lipids to collagen fibers and proteoglycans [12].

Less well known are the quantitative differences in these structural components: substantial variations may occur in the thickness of fibrous caps, in the size of atheromas, in the extent of its calcification and, as has been shown more recently, in the relative amounts of major cell types: smooth muscle cells and inflammatory cells [13,14.] This notion is of importance, since only specific types of lesions in this spectrum of morphologies appear to be associated with acute manifestations of atherosclerotic disease.

Stable and unstable plaques

Lipid content

The extremes at both ends of the spectrum appear to have a totally different clinical outcome. Essentially clinically stable are the fibrous plaques, composed of solid fibrous or fibrocellular tissue, and only small amounts of lipid or no lipid at all (figure 2A.) In coronary arteries most of these lesions remain clinically silent, or on the long term, may lead to stable angina pectoris. On the other hand, typically vulnerable plaques are characterized by large lipid pools and have a thin or virtually absent fibrous cap (figure 2B).

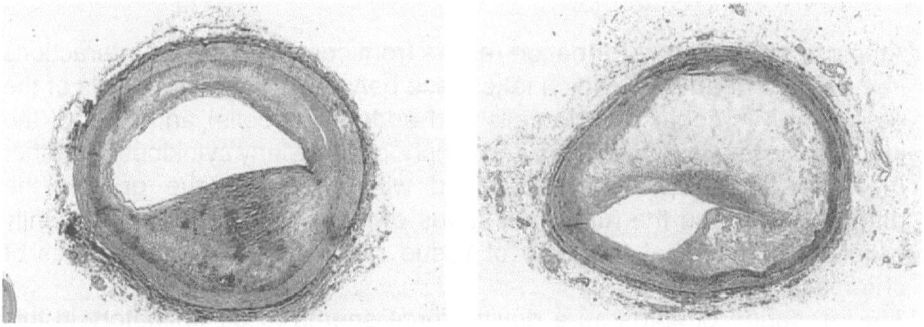

Figure 2A. *Eccentric coronary fibrous plaque completely composed of fibrous tissue.* ***Figure 2B.*** *Eccentric coronary lipid plaque with a large atheroma and a thin fibrous cap.Elastic von Gieson stain.*

These so-called lipid-rich plaques are frequently found underlying coronary thrombosis, and therefore considered as "rupture prone" [4,15]. Atherectomy specimens obtained from patients with unstable coronary artery disease are indeed more often lipid-rich than those of patients with stable angina [7-9]. Plaques derived from the aorta also show a clear relationship between the size of the lipid core and ruptures, Davies et al. established a critical threshold for plaque vulnerability in these lesions: more than 50% of lipids makes a plaque at high risk for rupture [13]. But, certainly not all the plaques in patients with stable coronary artery disease fulfill these criteria for stability. Thrombus, not related to the interventional procedure, can also be detected in atherectomy tissues of patients with chronic stable angina (table 1).

	stable angina (n=23)	unstable angina I (n=18)	unstable angina II (n=11)	AMI (n=19)
thrombus	6/23 (26%)	11/18 (61%)	9/11 (82%)	19/19 (100%)
atheroma	12/23 (52%)	14/18 (78%)	9/11 (82%)	18/19 (95%)

Numbers (and percentages of total number of lesions) of coronary atherectomy specimens containing thrombus or atheroma in 4 patient groups with different types of ischemic coronary syndromes. *Unstable angina I*: new onset, accelerated, or at rest but not within 48h (Braunwald class I,II). *Unstable angina II*: at rest within 48h (Braunwald class III). *AMI*: Acute Myocardial Infarction.

Table 1. *Pathologic analysis of coronary atherectomy specimens grouped according to specific types of coronary syndromes*

In coronary arteries of 54 patients with stable angina, Davies found that in only 15% patients all lesions were fibrous, and two-thirds of the patients had at least one plaque with a large lipid pool [16].On the other hand, in a study on 20 thrombosed coronary arteries in our laboratory, the classical lipid-rich morphology was found indeed in 10 of the underlying ruptured plaques (8 plaques with deep intimal tears, 2 plaques with superficial erosions), but 7 had a thick fibrocellular cap (4 deep intimal tears, 3 erosions), and 3 were completely fibrocellular (3 erosions) [17]. In other words, lipid content and thickness of the fibrous cap appear to be not the only determinant of plaque instability.

Biomechanical factors

The mechanical properties of complicated structures, like atherosclerotic plaque with their heterogenous tissue composition, can be studied with the use of finite element analysis. The complex structure is divided up into many small sections with a simple structure, "elements", and interactions between the elements are evaluated by computer analysis. Circumferential tensile stress on the fibrous cap came out of these investigations as the most important intrinsic mechanical stress factor involved in plaque rupture [18]. Most plaques rupture at sites of high calculated circumferential stress, which is usually at the periphery of eccentric plaques. These studies also showed the importance of the thickness of a fibrous cap (thickness in mm being inversely related to the peak stress in the cap), and the stenosis rate (the circumferential stresses in the plaques gradually decreased when stenosis severity increased) [19]; the latter provides at least one explanation for the fact that many plaques rupture at a stenosis rate of less than 50%.

Intrinsic mechanical forces clearly contribute to the process of plaque rupture, but of equal importance is the tissue composition of the fibrous cap. Lendon et al. tested the mechanical strength of human fibrous cap tissue and observed significantly reduced maximum stress at fracture when fibrous caps are infiltrated with macrophages [20]. Richardson showed that plaques rupture at sites of high circumferential stress, but that the site of rupture was influenced by variations in the mechanical strength due to macrophage accumulations [21]. These studies emphasize the importance of cellular infiltrations in the cap, particularly the presence of inflammatory cells.

Plaque inflammation

Adhesion of inflammatory cells to the arterial intima and migration into the intima is regarded as one of the earliest discernible events in atherogenesis. Immunohistochemical analysis of plaque cells, using cell specific antibodies, has identified macrophages,T-lymphocytes and mast cells, in ratios of approximately 100:10:1, as most prominent cellular components of the inflammatory infiltrate [22-24]. Fully developed plaques contain highly variable amounts of inflammatory cells, but largest concentrations can be found in lipid-rich lesions were they occupy the attenuated cap and the shoulder parts of the lesions [13,14]. The preference of these cells for lipid plaques suggests a relationship between lipids and inflammation. This relationship is more substantiated by several laboratory investigations indicating the existence of T-cell responses (in plaque tissue) and B-cell responses (circulating antibodies) to lipoproteins, particularly derivates of oxidized lipoproteins, in patients with atherosclerosis [see for review [25]].

In the atherosclerotic plaque, subpopulations of macrophages and T-lymphocytes express activation of antigens, and communicate through the release of various cytokines and other growth regulating factors. These cellular interactions are well-known features of a cell mediated immune response, probably initiated by lipid-related antigens localized in the plaque. The significance of this particular type of inflammatory response for the stability of plaques becomes evident when its tissue remodeling capacities are evaluated.

Cytokines, metalloproteinases and plaque remodeling

The various inflammatory mediators that have been detected in atherosclerotic plaque tissue are not unique for atherosclerosis. They are also active in other immune mediated inflammatory diseases with fibrosis and tissue lysis as key features, such as rheumatoid arthritis or leprosy. Presently, there is a great deal of evidence that these mediators may also have profound effects on the integrity of the connective tissue meshwork of plaques.

Transforming growth factor β (TGFβ), for example, is one of the most potent stimulators of connective tissue production by smooth muscle cells. Large amounts of this growth factor are detected in restenosis lesions after Percutaneous Transluminal Coronary Angiography (PTCA) [26], and it also participates in the repair process after natural plaque disruption. TGFβ and other growth factors, including platelet derived growth factor (PDGF), collagen growth factor (CGF) and basic fibroblast growth factor (bFGF), play an important role in wound healing and the reparative stage of many chronic inflammatory diseases; in atherosclerosis they have a stabilizing effect on the plaque structure.

In contrast, several other cytokines which are produced by activated T-lymphocytes and macrophages in plaques promote destabilizing effects, through inhibition of the production of collagens. They may act by either by inducing smooth muscle cell death (apoptosis) in the plaque (TNF-α IL-1) or by selectively inhibiting the growth of smooth muscle cells and their production of collagens (IFN-γ) [27]. In addition, during inflammation an even more powerful pathway of plaque disintegration is initiated by extracellular matrix degrading metalloproteinases. Metalloproteinases (MMPs) are proteolytic enzymes, which are normally involved in the physiologic process of connective tissue turnover.

In pathologic states such as chronic inflammation, their synthesis and activation can be markedly up regulated. Several types of MMPs have been identified in human plaques [28,29], and macrophages appear to be their most important cellular source of production. The secretion of these enzymes is stimulated by the cytokines TNF and IL-1, and in the extracellular space of the plaque they are activated by plasmin, or alternatively by mast cell products (tryptase and chymase). In the activated state they initiate a cascade of proteolytic activities with a very broad substrate specificity, which include all the extracellular matrix components of the fibrous cap (table 2).

Name	MMP	Main Substrates
Interstitial collagenase	1	Fibrillary collagens I, II,III,VII,X, Proteoglycans
Gelatinase A (72 kD)	2	Denaturated collagens (Gelatins), Collagen IV and V, Elastin, Proteoglycans
Stromelysin-1	3	Proteoglycans, Elastin, Laminin, Fibronectin Activates procollagenase
Matrilysin	7	Proteoglycans, Elastin, Gelatins, Fibronectin
Gelatinase B (92kD)	9	Gelatins, Collagen IV and V, Proteoglycan, Elastin

Table 2. *Matrix Metalloproteinases (MMP) in human atherosclerotic plaques*

Tissue Inhibitors of Metalloproteinases (TIMPs), also present in plaques, are able to keep the strong proteolytic activities of MMPs under control. But, the secretion of TIMPs is only marginally up regulated by inflammatory cytokines, which creates a situation in favor of the degrading activities of MMPs [18]. Evidence for this is gained by in situ zymographic studies of Galis et al. which showed localized lytic effects of frozen sections of human plaques on gelatin gels (gelatinase activity) and casein gels (stromelysin activity) [29]. Another observation of particular interest is that synthesis as well as lytic activity of these enzymes is most abundant in the lipid-laden macrophages and in the extracellular space around lipid cores of plaques. Studies on experimental atheromas have endorsed these observations: lipid loading of isolated macrophages augments the production of collagenases[30]. These observations provide another link between lipids and inflammation, and furthermore might explain why the lytic effects of inflammation are most prominent in lipid-rich plaques.

Inflammation and plaque rupture: pathologic evidence

Activated immune cells can be detected in all stages of atherosclerotic plaque development, which indicates that inflammation is a constitutive phenomenon of atherogenesis [23]. However, inflammation appears to be associated with the initiation of plaque rupture also. In a series of 20 of acute myocardial infarction related thrombosed coronary artery plaques we found abundant infiltration of activated T-cells and macrophages, and decreased densities of smooth muscle cells (SMC) and interstitial collagen at the immediate site of erosion or rupture [17]. This was in contrast to the overall morphology of the adjacent plaque tissue of the ruptured lesions, which was heterogenous both with respect to plaque architecture and inflammation (figure 3).

Kaartinen et al. extended these observations by identifying neutral proteases producing mastcells as participants in the inflammatory process, providing another indication for active inflammation at rupture sites [23]. In other words, postmortem observational studies on the inflammatory infiltrate at sites of rupture, supported by data from experimental studies, indicate that the tissue degrading effects of active inflammation induce weak areas in the plaque tissue, which in turn prepare the way for a rupture event. Pathologic analysis of coronary atherectomy specimens, obtained from living patients with different types of ischemic coronary syndromes have further supported this concept.

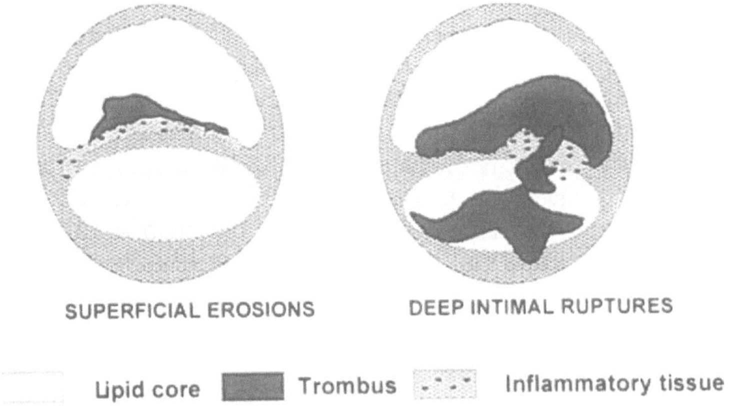

Figure 3. *The role of inflammation in coronary plaque rupture.* ***Left:*** *superficial plaque erosion underlies a mural thrombus. An inflammatory infiltrate has eroded the plaque surface with denudation of the endothelium.Tissue factor, produced by macrophages at these sites, facilitates thrombus formation.* ***Right:*** *deep intimal rupture with complete laceration of the fibrous cap, which allows blood to enter the atheroma. An inflammatory infiltrate composed of activated mononuclear cells at the immediate site of rupture is also a constant feature of this type of plaque disruption. The fibrous cap tissue adjacent to the inflammatory tissue has a variable tissue composition, but is completely fibrous in many cases. In both instances, the inflammatory infiltrates are similar to those observed at vulnerable sites in uncomplicated plaques.*

Several histopathological parameters of plaque destabilization were analyzed and quantified in tissue specimens of culprit lesions, and correlated with the clinical status of the patient. In most of these studies a comparison was made between the tissues derived from patients with chronic stable angina and patients with various types of acute coronary syndromes. In comparison with chronic stable angina, the lesions of patients with unstable syndromes show significantly larger amounts of inflammatory cells [9,32], including activated inflammatory cells, and a decrease in the amounts of SMC [9].

Other findings of interest in the culprit lesions of patients with unstable angina are significantly increased numbers of gelatinase B (MMP9) producing macrophages, expression of vasoactive substances (angiotensin[33] and endothelin [34]) and large amounts of the thrombosis initiator tissue factor.

Moreover, an interesting relationship was seen between the amounts of inflammatory cells in the lesions and the *severity* of unstable ischemic syndromes [9,32]. In our studies on markers for activation immune responses in coronary atherectomy tissues (measured by the expression of Interleukin-2 Receptors on T-cells), we found that lesions of patients with "refractory" unstable angina (Braunwald class III unstable angina [37]) showed an inflammatory activity close to that of the lesions of patients with acute myocardial infarction. Indeed, in this type of unstable angina a high percentage of interventional procedures and progression to myocardial infarction is reported [38]. Conversely, in patients with "stabilized" unstable angina (Braunwald class III unstable angina,) which have a much more favorable outcome, the inflammatory activity did not differ significantly from patients with stable angina [9].

An overall impression emerging from these investigations is that the biologic state of lesions must be considered of prime importance in determining the clinical outcome of patients with coronary atherosclerosis. Inflammation related tissue degradation, and (related) vasoreactivity and thrombogenecity, sets the scene for vasospasms or elevated blood pressures, so called rupture triggers [39], to induce a rupture event.

Risk factors and plaque instability

Although the major risk factors for clinical disease (age, gender, hypercholesterolemia, hypertension, smoking, diabetes) clearly correlate with the extent of plaque formation in coronary arteries [40], little is known about whether, and if so, how they influence the composition and vulnerability of plaques.

Recently, important data came up from investigations on large series of human plaques of patients with well documented coronary risk factors. Burke et al. compared morphologic plaque features with the profile of risk factors of corresponding patients [41]. Vulnerable plaques were defined as lesions with a fibrous cap of less than 65µm and infiltrated with >25 macrophages per high power field. Low serum levels of HDL and high LDL were associated with vulnerable plaques. Smoking did not influence the composition of the plaques with respect to features of vulnerability, but appeared to be highly thrombogenic. Moreover, 69% of deep plaque ruptures reaching into a lipid core were found in man, whereas in a previous study of the same group [42], 69% of superficial erosions was reported in women (in plaques composed of SMC and matrix proteins rather than lipids and macrophages), indicating sex related differences in the type of rupture, and probably also plaque composition. Studies on thrombosed coronary plaques in the laboratory of Davies father support the influence of risk factors on plaque composition. They found ruptured plaques in 84% of patients without diabetes, and only 34% ruptured plaques in patients with diabetes; remaining cases showed superficial erosions as underlying cause of thrombus formation in both patient groups [43].

Haemodynamic factors such as flow velocity and shear stress form another risk factor for plaque initiation and growth [44]. Recent studies in our laboratory on carotid artery bifurcation plaques have revealed flow dependent consistent variations in macrophage and SMC densities between different areas of one and the same plaque. Macrophages contents appeared to be significantly increased in the upstream parts of plaques, which are associated with high flow and high shear stress. These findings suggest that flow dynamics may influence plaque stability through alterations in the cellular composition of plaques (M. Dirksen et al, manuscript submitted for publication).

So, the molecular and cellular mechanisms that underlie these risk factor dependent differences in plaque composition, and related types of plaque disruption, are largely unknown. Nevertheless, it appears that the various risk factors may influence the balance between stabilizing and destabilizing mechanisms in the plaque each in their own way. This notion may illustrate the value of a proper understanding of atherosclerotic plaque biology in patients with acute coronary syndromes, which will certainly have implications for patient care.

References

1. Davies MJ, Thomas AC. Plaque fissuring -the cause of acute myocardial infarction, sudden ischemic death and crescendo angina. Br Heart J 1985;53:363-73.
2. Falk E. Morphologic features of unstable atherothrombotic plaques underlying acute coronary syndromes. Am J Cardiol 1989;63:114E-120E.
3. Eliasziw M, Streifler JY, Fox AJ Hachinski VC, Ferguson GG, Barnett HJ. Significance of plaque ulceration in symptomatic patients with high-grade carotid stenosis. North American Symptomatic Carotid Endarterectomy Trial. Stroke 1994;25:304-8.
4. Davies MJ. A macro and micro view of coronary vascular insult in ischemic heart disease. Circulation 1990;82 (3 Suppl.): II 38-46.
5. Levin DC, Fallon JT. Significance of the angiographic morphology of localized coronary stenoses: histopathologic correlations. Circulation 1982;66:316-20.
6. Alderman EL, Corley SD, Fisher LD, et al. Five-year angiographic follow-up of factors associated with progression of coronary artery disease in the Coronary Artery Surgery Study. "(CASS), CASS Participating Investigators and Staff."J Am Coll Cardiol 1993;22:1141-54.
7. Rosenschein U, Ellis SG, Haudenschild CC, et al. Comparing of histopathologic coronary lesions obtained from directional atherectomy in stable angina versus acute coronary syndromes. Am J Cardiol 1994;73:508-10.
8. Van der Wal AC, Becker AE, Koch KT, et al. Clinically stable angina pectoris is not necessarily associated with histologically stable atherosclerotic plaques. Heart. 1996;76:312-6.
9. Van der Wal AC, Piek JJ, de Boer OJ, et al. There is recent one activation of the plaque immune response in coronary lesions underlying acute coronary syndromes. Heart. In press 1998.
10. Davies MJ, Bland JM, Hangartner JR, Angelini A, Thomas AC. Factors influencing the presence or absence of acute coronary artery thrombi in sudden ischemic death . Eur Heart J 1989;10:203-8.
11. Ross R. The pathogenesis of atherosclerosis: a perspective for the 1990s. Nature. 1993; 362:801-9.
12. Ball RY, Stowers EC, Burton JH, Cay NR, Skepper JN, Mitchinson MJ. Evidence that the death of macrophage foam cells contributes to the lipid core of atheroma. Atherosclerosis 1995;114:45-54.
13. Davies MJ, Richardson P, Woolf N, Katz DR, Mann J. Risk of thrombosis in human atherosclerotic plaques: role of extracellular lipid, macrophage, and smooth muscle cell content. Br Heart J 1993;69:377-81.
14. Van der Wal AC, Becker AE, Van der Loos CM, Tigges AJ, Das PK. Fibrous and lipid-rich atherosclerotic plaques are part of interchangeable morphologies related to inflammation: a concept. Coron Artery Dis 1994;5:463-9.
15. Falk E. Why do plaques rupture? Circulation 1992;86(6 Suppl):III30-42.
16. Hangartner JR, Charlston AJ, Davies MJ, Thomas AC. Morphological characteristics of clinically significant coronary artery stenosis in stable angina. Br Heart J 1986;56:501-8.
17. Van der Wal AC, Becker AE, van der Loos CM, Das PK. Site of intimal rupture or erosion of thrombosed coronary atherosclerotic plaques is characterized by an inflammatory process irrespective of the dominant plaque morphology. Circulation 1994;89:36-44.

18. Lee RT, Libby P. Metalloproteinases and atherosclerotic plaque rupture. In: Schultheiss HP, Schwimmbeck P, editors. The role of immune mechanisms in cardiovscular disease. Berlin: Springer, 1997: 238-45.
19. Cheng GC, Loree HM, Kamm RD, Fishbein MC, Lee RT. Distribution of circumferential stress in ruptured and stable atherosclerotic lesions. A structural analysis with histopathological correlation Circulation 1993;87:1179-87.
20. Lendon CL, Davies MJ, Born GV, Richardson PD. Atherosclerotic plaque caps are locally weakened when macrophages density is increased. Atherosclerosis 1991;87:87-90.
21. Richardson PD, Davies MJ, Born GV. Influence of plaque configuration and stress distribution on fissuring of coronary atherosclerotic plaques. Lancet 1989;2:941-4.
22. Jonasson L, Holm J, Skalli O, Bondjers G, Hansson GK. Regional accumulations of T-cells, macrophages, and smooth muscle cells in the human atherosclerotic plaque. Arteriosclerosis 1986;6:131-8.
23. Van der Wal AC, Das PK, Bentz van de Berg D, Van der Loos CM, Becker AE. Atherosclerotic lesions in humans. In situ immunophenotypic analysis suggesting an immune mediated response. Lab Invest 1989;61:166-70.
24. Kaartinen M, Pentilla A, Kovanen PT. Accumulation of activated mast cells in the shoulder region of human coronary atheroma, the predilection site of atheromatous rupture. Circulation 1994;90:1669-78.
25. Hansson GK. Cell-mediated immunity in atherosclerosis. Curr Opin Lipidol 1997;8:301-11.
26. Nikol S, Isner JM, Pickering JG, Kearney M, Lecler G, Weir L. Expression of transforming growth factor beta 1 is increased in human vascular restenosis lesons. J Clin Invest 1992;90:1582-92.
27. Libby P. Molecular bases of the acute coronary syndromes. Circulation 1995;91:2844--50.
28. Henney AM, Wakeley PR, Davies MJ, et al. Localization of stromelysin gene expression in atherosclerotic plaques by in situ hybridization. Proc Natl Acad Sci USA 1991;88:8154-8.
29. Galis ZS, Sukhova GK, Lark MW, Libby P. Increased expression of matrix metalloproteinases and matrix degrading activity in vulnerable regions of human atherosclerotic plaques. J Clin Invest 1994;94:2493-503.
30. Galis ZS, Sukhova GK, Kranzhofer R,Clark S, Libby P. Macrophage foam cells from experimental atheroma constitutively produce matrix-degrading proteinases. Proc Nat Acad Sci USA 1995;92:402-6.
31. Kovanen PT, Kaartinen M, Paavonen T. Infiltrates of activated mast cells at the site of coronary atheromatous erosion or rupture in myocardial infarction. Circulation1995;92:1084-88.
32. Moreno PR, Falk E, Palacios IF, Newell JB, Fuster V, Fallon JT. Macrophage infiltration in acute coronary syndromes. Implications for plaque rupture. Circulation, 1994;90:775-8.
33. Brown DL, Hibbs MS, Keaney M, Loushin C, Isner JM. Identification of 92 kD gelatinase in human coronary atherosclerotic lesions: Association of active enzyme synthesis with unstable angina. Circulation 1995;91:2125-31.
34. Haberbosch W, Bohle RM, Franke FE, et al. The expression of angiotensin-I converting enzyme in human atherosclerotic plaques is not related to the deletion/inserton polymorphism but to the risk of restenosis after coronary interventions. Atherosclerosis 1997;130:203-13.

35. Zeiher AM, Gobel H, Schachinger V, Ihling C. Tissue endothelin-1 immunoreactivity in the active coronary atherosclerotic plaque. A clue to the mechanism of increased vasoreactivity of the culprit lesion in unstable angina. Circulation 1995;91:941-7.
36. Annex BH, Denning SM, Channon KM, et al. Differential expression of tissue factor protein in directional atherectomy specimens from patients with stable and unstable coronary syndromes. Circulation 1995;91:619-22.
37. Braunwald E. Unstable angina. A classification. Circulation 1989;80:410-4.
38. Van Miltenburg-van Zijl AJ, Simoons ML, Veerhoek RJ, Bossuyt PM. Incidence and follow up of Braunwald subgroups in unstable angina pectoris. J Am Coll Cardiol 1995;25:1286-92.
39. Falk E. Advanced lesions and acute coronary syndromes: a pathologist's view. In: Fuster V, editor. Syndromes of atherosclerosis. Armonk: Futura, 1996: 81-104.
40. Wissler RW. An overview of the quantitative influence of several risk factors on progression of atherosclerosis in young people in the United States. Pathobiological Determinants of Atherosclerosis in Yough (PDAY) Research Group. Am J Med Sci 1995;310:Suppl 1:529-36.
41. Burke AP,Farb A, Malcolm GT, Liang YH, Smialek J, Virmani R. Coronary risk factors and plaque morphology in men with coronary disease who died suddenly. N Engl J Med 1997;336:1276-82.
42. Farb A, Burke AP, Tang AL, et al. Coronary plaque erosion without rupture into a lipid core. A frequent cause of coronary thrombosis in sudden coronary death. Circulation 1996;93:1354-63.
43. Davies MJ. The composition of coronary artery plaques. N Engl J Med 1997;336:1312-14.
44. Zarins CK, Giddens DP, Bharaduaj BK, Sottiurai VS, Mabon RF, Glagov S. Carotid bifurcation atherosclerosis. Quantitative correlaton of plaque localization with flow velocity profiles and wall shear stress. Circ Res 1983;53:502-14.

Chapter 2

Atherosclerosis Viewed from the Inside

Peter den Heijer

Introduction

The clinical illness of coronary artery disease is the end-stage of silent long established arterial disease or the rapid consecutive events following injury to the vessel wall. The most common form of degenerative arterial disease is atherosclerosis, which is a complex process determined by endothelial cell injury, migration, thrombosis and monocytes infiltration. These factors are related to the two main mechanisms of smooth muscle cell proliferation and lipid infiltration. Warning signs are present and timely action can reduce the risk both of a first attack and a recurrence. Cardiovascular medicine has improved the understanding of the clinical responsibility. This has involved a change in role perception and then a new technology, which is still evolving. Physicians are learning to move beyond the stage of treating the single risk factor which is readily accessible and measurable such as raised blood pressure to the concept of multiple interventions such as the implementation of systemic or local drug treatment and biomedical device delivery. There is still much scope for clinical scientists and practitioners to treat cardiovascular disease. Proper guidance by newly developed diagnostic methods and strategies will improve the therapeutic prospects of coronary artery disease.

This chapter will help to understand and exploit the exciting use of intracoronary imaging. The underlying theme of this review is to illustrate some key issues of current intracoronary imaging, which may be complementary to standard diagnostic strategies.

Van der Wall et al. (eds.),
Advanced Imaging in Coronary Artery Disease, 15-27.

Intravascular ultrasound

Coronary interventional techniques have made dramatic advances over the last 20 years. More sophisticated interventional soft and hardware are now available for routine clinical practice. The need to assess coronary lesions and the response to various therapeutic interventions more accurately and in greater detail than is possible with coronary arteriography, has led to the development of new invasive imaging techniques. Morphological assessment of complex lesions and adequate deployment of intracoronary stents were closely related to the miniature design and implementation of intravascular ultrasound (IVUS) such as for the evaluation of barotrauma after balloon dilatation and the remodeling process of restenosis. IVUS imaging caused a dramatic change of the perception of the dynamic atherosclerotic process.

First, IVUS enables direct visualization of early intimal changes before angiographic detection. Secondly, trans-catheter mechanisms are better defined which may improve initial device choice and endpoint assessment. The quality of the stent deployment algorithm has improved.

IVUS versus angiography

Pathological examinations have always emphasized the difference between the aspect of the atherosclerotic process at autopsy and the findings from angiography.[1] Angiography provides a "cast" of the arterial lumen and does not demonstrate the direct relationship between the plaque and the arterial wall. IVUS discriminates several plaque types by differences in acoustic properties of plaque components. Luminal narrowing and the cross-sectional distribution and composition of the plaque are clearly established by IVUS.

The detection of mild to moderate plaque deposition in angiographically normal coronary arteries such as in heart transplant recipients [2, 3] or the irregularly shaped postintervention lumen by IVUS illustrates its diagnostic accuracy. Close correlations of IVUS and angiography are mostly encountered in vessel segments with little disease. Multiple view angiography can cope with eccentric lesions.[4]

In patients with atherosclerotic disease, IVUS demonstrates a larger disease burden of a coronary lesion compared to angiography. The reference segment contains 30-40% of plaque by area.[5] Angiography may underestimate the size of the plaque because it does not have the ability to depict the phenomenon of plaque remodeling, which is known as the expansion of the vessel segment in an area of plaque accumulation.[6] There is less encroachment on the lumen as would be seen in the absence of remodeling.

IVUS appears to have an important clinical impact, although it is unknown to which extent patient care and economic savings are improved. In several studies IVUS changed the revascularization strategy of 28-40% of interventional procedures.

IVUS and coronary interventions

Percutaneous transluminal coronary angioplasty
IVUS showed plaque dissections in 60-80% of percutaneous transluminal coronary angioplasty (PTCA) procedures. Only 50% of these cases were diagnosed by angiography.[7, 8] An apparent increase in acute lumen gain may be shown by angiography and is caused by contrast medium which gains access into crevices and beneath dissected tissue arms. Dissection occurs at a thin portion of the plaque or at the border of localized calcium deposits.[9] Several studies used IVUS as a tool to examine the clinical outcome of PTCA. These trials showed that the percentage of plaque area was a powerful predictor of 6-month outcome following PTCA such as the clinical presentation of restenosis.[10] However, these studies did not identify any qualitative variables such as dissection, calcification or eccentricity that correlated with the 6-month angiographic or clinical outcome.

IVUS has been used to examine the mechanism of lumen expansion with PTCA and the subsequent restenosis process. The primary mechanisms of increased luminal patency with PTCA were plaque compression and fracture.[11] Vessel stretching contributed less to the process. However, this was not confirmed by others which reported that vessel stretching and plaque tearing were the main causative mechanisms.[12] It is suggested that remodeling or changes of the overall caliber of the vessel probably due to tissue shrinkage contribute to restenosis following intervention. This process may be the result of subintimal trauma. Preliminary results show that IVUS measurements contribute to the use of significantly larger balloons than with angiographic guidance alone.[13] This has translated into larger post PTCA lumen areas.

Directional and rotational coronary atherectomy
IVUS shows a larger residual plaque burden than angiography, typically more than 50%. IVUS reveals the exact location of calcium within the

plaque.[14, 15] If calcium is localized in the superficial layers at the intimal surface, tissue retrieval is minimal by deflection of the atherectomy cutter. Deeper calcium deposits causes effective tissue excision since the soft plaque is removed on the intimal side of the calcium rim. Moreover, deep calcium reduces the chance of aggressive excision into the medial and adventitial layers.[16]

IVUS is very useful to guide rotational ablation because it enables the interventionalist to visualize the extent of superficial calcium and determine vessel size. Hereby improving appropriate burr-sizing strategy. In addition, IVUS demonstrated that dissections occur less after stand-alone rotational atherectomy than with PTCA. Smaller lumina may either be the cause of spasm or ineffective ablation.[17]

Intravascular stents

At present, conventional X-ray provides insufficient information to assess whether intracoronary stents are optimally deployed. However, intracoronary imaging provides direct visualization of the stent struts and its relation to the vessel wall.[18, 19] Therefore it is possible to evaluate stent expansion and tissue apposition accurately (figure 1).

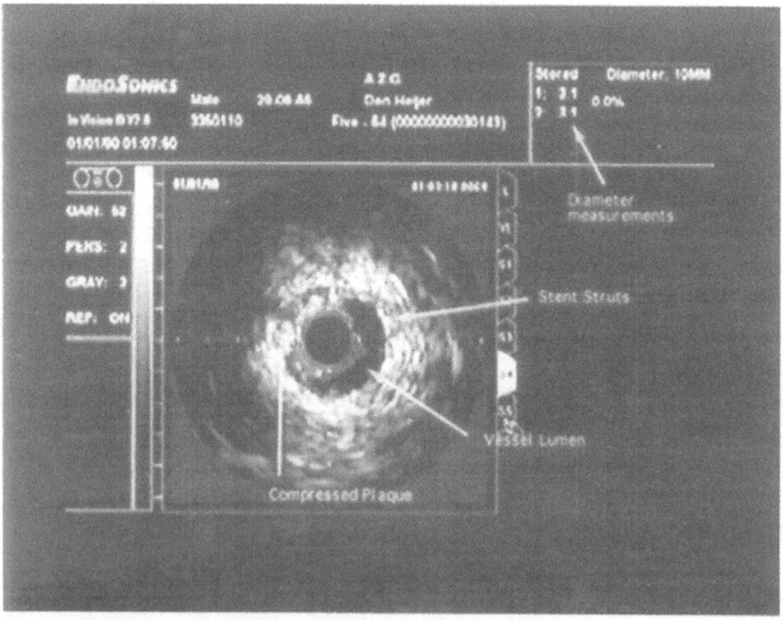

***Figure 1.** IVUS recording after stent implantation, showing adequate stent expansion and optimal apposition of the struts*

(See also Colour Plates, p. 337)

The aforementioned characteristics of stent deployment are related to plaque composition and compliance. Fibro-calcified lesions are less easily deformed. IVUS demonstrated that 80% of the intracoronary stents with an angiographic good result were incompletely deployed defined as incomplete expansion, apposition or asymmetry.[20] These findings resulted in higher inflation pressures for stent delivery and a subsequent reduction of the rate of suboptimal deployment to 30-40%. Another characteristic sonographic appearance is the tissue flap caused by tissue torn at the edges of the stent. Revision of the anticoagulation protocol after optimization of ultrasound guided stent deployment resulted in fewer bleeding events and a reduction of the length of hospital stays.

Coronary Angioscopy

Coronary angioscopy is well recognized as an important research tool, especially for studies addressing intracoronary thrombus formation. In contrast to IVUS, the clinical applicability of angioscopy is not so well defined, and has not led to routine use in the interventional catheterisation laboratory. Angioscopy has nevertheless contributed substantially to the understanding of the following clinical syndromes and interventional therapies.

Angioscopic assessment of lesions in stable and unstable angina
The clinical syndrome of unstable angina pectoris has been associated with platelet aggregation, intracoronary thrombosis, alterations in vasomotor tone, and complicated and ruptured atheromatous plaque.[21] In fact, angioscopy has identified a complex lesion morphology and a high incidence of thrombus in the culprit lesions of patients with unstable angina.[22, 23] In order to demonstrate whether culprit lesions in unstable angina could be angioscopically distinguished from stenotic lesions in stable angina by means of the modified Ermenonville classification, [24] we have analyzed 33 undisturbed native coronary stenoses in patients with unstable angina pectoris, and compared these lesions to those of a control group consisting of 19 patients with stable angina. Unstable angina pectoris was defined as the presence of one or more of the following 3 features:
1) crescendo angina superimposed on a pre-existing pattern of relatively stable, exertion-related angina pectoris; 2) angina at rest or with minimal exertion; 3) new onset angina pectoris, which is brought on by minimal exertion. The classification data were compared between the 2 groups using the Chi-Square test. There were no significant differences between the groups in the grading or shape of the narrowings. Although 13 of 33 (39.4%)

of patients with unstable angina proved to have lining red thrombus at angioscopy, versus 4 of 19 (21.1%) of the stable angina group, this difference was not significant with this sample size. There was however a significant difference in the incidence of white thrombus: eleven (33.3%) of the unstable angina patients had lining (n=5) or protruding (n=6) white thrombus, which could not be demonstrated in any of the stable angina patients. We found a highly significant difference in the distribution of the atheroma types. A so-called "complicated lesion" was identified in 25 of 33 (75.8%) patients of the unstable angina group, versus 2 of 19 (10.5%) patients of the stable angina group. The observation of a grade 5 ("complicated") lesion had a sensitivity of 85%, and a specificity of 83% for the clinical syndrome of angina pectoris. It is evident that unstable angina is associated with a specific angioscopic lesion morphology, and that the finding of such a morphology is highly predictive for an unstable lesion. Unstable angina is associated with less favorable PTCA results than stable angina Whether or not a specific plaque will become unstable appears to be related to its composition. Thieme et al. demonstrated by means of directional atherectomy that angioscopic yellow lesions had the histopathological substrate of atheroma or degenerated plaque.[25] Indeed, the risk of adverse PTCA outcome is increased if these lipid-rich, yellow lesions are observed by means of angioscopy.[26, 27] On the other hand, atherosclerotic disease has also been found by angioscopy at angiographically normal sites.[28]

Angioscopy – if it would be easier to perform and more readily available – could thus be applied to obtain an indication of the expected outcome and risk involved before angioplasty attempts. An alternative to PTCA might, in certain cases, be the stabilization of unstable plaques by cholesterol-lowering "statin"-therapy. Such a strategy can perhaps in the future be controlled by angioscopic and/or ultrasound imaging of the vessel wall.

Acute myocardial infarction

Although coronary angioscopy, with its potential for intracoronary thrombus detection, can be used to assess the occluding lesion in acute myocardial infarction, its clinical use for this indication is limited. In fact, red thrombus was found by angioscopy in almost all cases of acute myocardial infarction.[29] Lablanche et al have demonstrated that red thrombus can even be found up to 60 days after clinically and angiographically successful thrombolysis in a large majority of patients.[30] Of course, such findings generally have no bearing on the therapeutic options available. We have seen one exception in an unusual case of acute myocardial infarction caused by trauma. A 32-year old goalkeeper in amateur football was admitted with an acute anterior infarction after stopping a penalty ball with his sternum. Angiography showed abrupt closure of the left anterior descending coronary artery (LAD). Angioscopy was performed in order to prove the presence of occlusive red thrombus, excluding such causes as intramural or extravascular compression (figure 2). Vessel patency was restored by direct PTCA, and follow-up angioscopy confirmed absence of thrombus 10 days after intravenous heparin treatment. Recently, Ueda et al provided more insight into the pathogenesis of acute myocardial infarction by proving the hypothesis that white thrombus is overlying yellow plaque, in some cases followed by red thrombus after obstruction of the blood flow. [31]

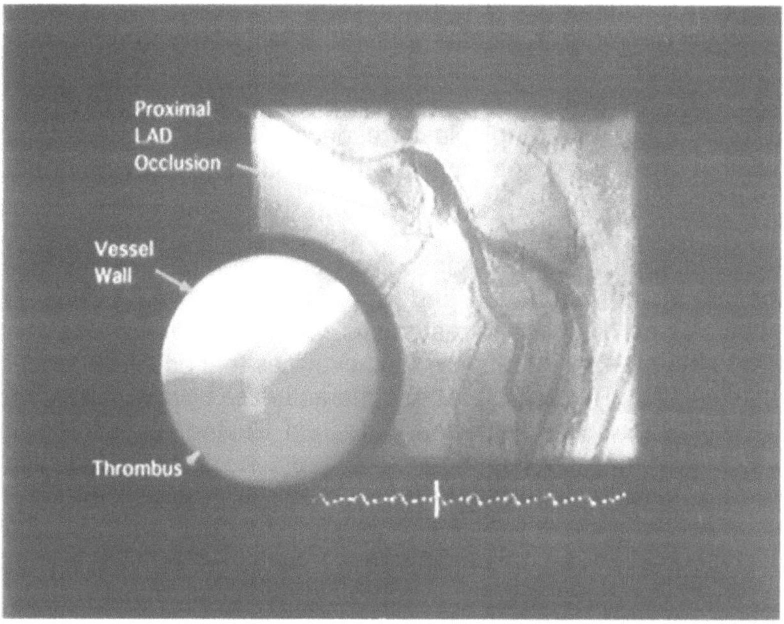

Figure 2. Coronary angiogram in cranial LAO view showing abrupt LAD occlusion caused by trauma. Angioscopy reveals a large, red, occluding thrombus
(See also Colour Plates, p. 337)

Angioscopy after PTCA: early observations and restenosis

Although coronary stenting has markedly reduced the interventional cardiologist's anxiety over angiographically suboptimal PTCA results, the pathophysiology behind such threatened occlusions after balloon dilatation is often unclear. Sassower et al. have carried out angioscopy in 2 cases of abrupt closure post PTCA, and found that in one patient the obstruction was caused by extruded plaque material, while the other patient had a large white thrombus at the occlusion site.[32] Jain et al. have reported a series of

10 patients with acute closure.[33] They observed that, although the primary cause of occlusion was a dissection in 8 of 10 patients, concomitant non-occlusive thrombus was present in 9 patients. We have attempted angioscopic imaging of threatened or frank occlusion in 18 patients. Successful angioscopy was possible in 17 of these patients. Acute occlusion was present in 5 patients, and impending occlusion or subtotal occlusion in 12 patients. Angioscopy confirmed large intimal dissection and absence of thrombus in 9 of these patients. Palmaz-Schatz™ coronary stents (Johnson & Johnson Interventional Systems Corp., Warren, NJ, USA) were implanted in 7 of these 9 patients. Obstructing thrombus, without evidence of dissection, was encountered in 2 of the 17 patients. The remaining 6 patients proved to have dissection as well as thrombus at angioscopy. The opinion seems justified that coronary angioscopy, by providing the ability to discern thrombus from dissection, could be a valuable tool to improve the management of abrupt or threatened occlusion during or after coronary angioplasty, especially since new potent platelet aggregation inhibiting drugs such as the IIb/IIIa inhibitors have become available.

On the assumption that angioscopy could demonstrate a possible relationship of the magnitude and amount of arterial wall damage and thrombus caused by PTCA to restenosis, we have undertaken a study, in which we documented the angioscopic changes that occur during the first hour after PTCA.[34] These changes are characterized by progressive red and white thrombus formation and intima disruption. Bauters and Lablanche and co-workers have published an angioscopic restenosis study, in which they confirmed a high angiographic restenosis rate in lesions that contained thrombus at the time of PTCA.[35] The next important question of course is, if this restenosis rate can be influenced by effective management of intracoronary thrombus, e.g. by glycoprotein IIb/IIIa inhibitors.

Coronary stenting

Angioscopy can be used to assess the correct deployment, adequate expansion, and possible presence of thrombotic material following stent implantation.[36] We have studied 11 patients with freshly implanted stents of several brands and types (figure 3). Imaging was successful in all patients. At angioscopy, all stents were found to be well expanded, although small intima flaps (grade 2 dissection) were seen to protrude through the gaps between the stent wires in 8 patients. Whereas intravascular ultrasound imaging is superior in assessing the optimal expansion of a stent,[18] angioscopy is useful to check for remaining thrombotic or intimal material that may remain undetected at angiography.[36, 37]

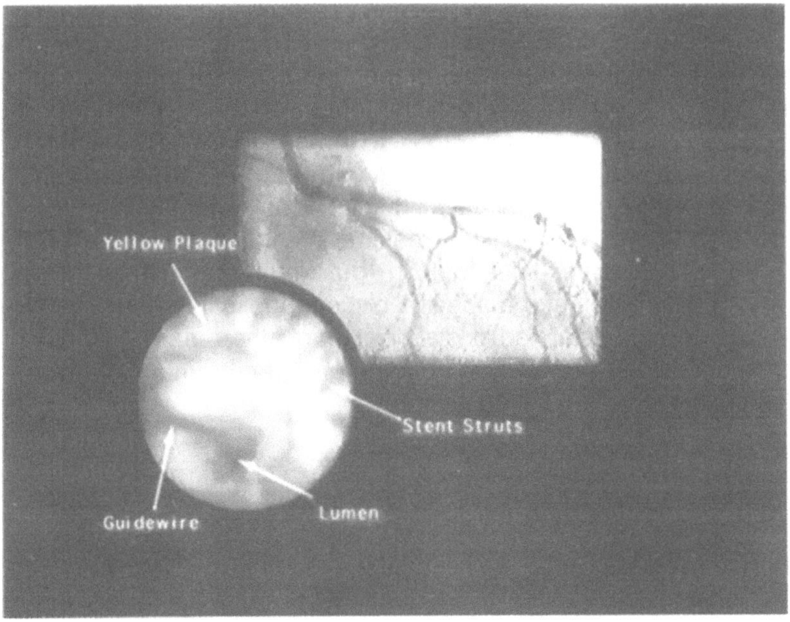

Figure 3. Angioscopy after stent implantation, same patient as in figure 1
(See also Colour Plates, p. 338)

Angioscopy can also be useful when adverse results are encountered during follow-up after stent implantation, again by providing the ability to discern thrombus from other intraluminal filling defects. Resar and Brinker have described a case where renarrowing inside a coronary stent, 6 weeks after its delivery, proved to consist of intimal hyperplasia, although thrombus was suspected angiographically.[38] Similarly, Strumpf et al. have reported 2 cases in which thrombolytic therapy was avoided because stent restenosis proved to exist of tissue instead of thrombus.[37] We have used angioscopy to determine the cause of subacute stent closure in 3 patients. Although subacute stent occlusion in the literature exclusively has been attributed to thrombosis,[39, 40] we discovered that the occlusion was caused by dissection rather than thrombus in 2 of these patients.[41] The third patient with subacute stent occlusion appeared to have an occluding mixed red and white thrombus within his stent, and was treated with PTCA and intracoronary thrombolytic therapy.

Discussion

It appears that the clinical utility of coronary angioscopy is related directly to its ability to visualize unstable lesions and especially to its high sensitivity for demonstrating intracoronary thrombus. There is no doubt about the superiority of angioscopy in this respect. In a comparative, retrospective study, we have found that 48% of angioscopically observed thrombi remained undetected at angiography.[42] Comparable results were published by Uretsky et al.[43] Nevertheless, at the current time angioscopy still has to be regarded mainly as a very useful research tool, rather than a method that has a large impact on decision making in interventional cardiology. To become an indispensable tool in the interventional catheterisation laboratory, it should have a specific clinical applicability. Research using angioscopy should be aimed at stabilization of atheromatous plaque by lipid lowering agents, and the effects on intracoronary thrombus of glycoprotein IIb/IIIa inhibitors.

References

1. Willard JE, Netto D, Demian SE, et al. Intravascular ultrasound imaging of saphenous vein grafts in vitro: comparison with histologic and quantitative angiographic findings. J Am Coll Cardiol 1992;19:759-64.
2. Rickenbacher PR, Pinto FJ, Chenzbraun A, et al. Incidence and severity of transplant coronary artery disease early and up to 15 years after transplantation as detected by intravascular ultrasound. J Am Coll Cardiol 1995;25:171-7.
3. St Goar FG, Pinto FJ, Alderman EL, Fitzgerald PJ, Stadius ML, Popp RL. Intravascular ultrasound imaging of angiographically normal coronary arteries: an in vivo comparison with quantitative angiography. J Am Coll Cardiol 1991;18:952-8.
4. Waller BF. Anatomy, histology, and pathology of the major epicardial coronary arteries relevant to echocardiographic imaging techniques. J Am Soc Echocardiogr 1989;2:232-52.
5. Mintz GS, Painter JA, Pichard AD, et al. Atherosclerosis in angiographically "normal" coronary artery reference segments: an intravascular ultrasound study with clinical correlations. J Am Coll Cardiol 1995;25:1479-85.
6. Glagov S, Weisenberg E, Zarins CK, Stankunavicius R, Kolettis GJ. Compensatory enlargement of human atherosclerotic coronary arteries. N Engl J Med 1987;316:1371-5.
7. Honye J, Mahon DJ, Jain A, et al. Morphological effects of coronary balloon angioplasty in vivo assessed by intravascular ultrasound imaging. Circulation 1992;85:1012-25.
8. Fitzgerald PJ, Yock PG. Mechanisms and outcomes of angioplasty and atherectomy assessed by intravascular ultrasound imaging. J Clin Ultrasound 1993;21:579-88.
9. Fitzgerald PJ, Ports TA, Yock PG. Contribution of localized calcium deposits to dissection after angioplasty. An observational study using intravascular ultrasound . Circulation 1992;86:64-70.
10. Mintz GS, Popma JJ, Pichard AD, et al. Intravascular ultrasound predictors of restenosis after percutaneous transcatheter coronary revascularization. J Am Coll Cardiol 1996;27:1678-87.
11. Losordo DW, Rosenfield K, Pieczek A, Baker K, Harding M, Isner JM. How does angioplasty work? Serial analysis of human iliac arteries using intravascular ultrasound. Circulation 1992;86:1845-58.
12. Mintz GS, Pichard AD, Kovach JA, et al. Impact of preintervention intravascular ultrasound imaging on transcatheter treatment strategies in coronary artery disease. Am J Cardiol 1994;73:423-30.
13. Hodgson JM, Stone GW, St Goar FG, Linnemeier T, Sheehan H. Can intracoronary ultrasound improve PTCA results? Preliminary core lab ultrasound analysis from the CLOUT pilot study [abstract]. J Am Coll Cardiol 1995;25 (Special Issue):143A.
14. Suarez de Lezo J, Romero M, Medina A, et al. Intracoronary ultrasound assessment of directional coronary atherectomy: immediate and follow-up findings. J Am Coll Cardiol 1993;21:298-307.
15. Tenaglia AN, Buller CE, Kisslo KB, Stack RS, Davidson CJ. Mechanisms of balloon angioplasty and directional coronary atherectomy as assessed by intracoronary ultrasound. J Am Coll Cardiol 1992;20:685-91.

16. Hinohara T, Rowe MH, Robertson GC, et al. Effect of lesion characteristics on outcome of directional coronary atherectomy. J Am Coll Cardiol 1991;17:1112-20.
17. Mintz GS, Potkin BN, Keren G, et al. Intravascular ultrasound evaluation of the effect of rotational atherectomy in obstructive atherosclerotic coronary artery disease. Circulation 1992;86:1383-93.
18. Nakamura S, Colombo A, Gaglione A, et al. Intracoronary ultrasound observations during stent implantation. Circulation 1994;89(5):2026-34.
19. Goldberg SL, Colombo A, Nakamura S, Almagor Y, Maiello L, Tobis JM. Benefit of intracoronary ultrasound in the deployment of Palmaz-Schatz stents. J Am Coll Cardiol 1994;24:996-1003.
20. Colombo A, Hall P, Nakamura S, et al. Intracoronary stenting without anticoagulation accomplished with intravascular ultrasound guidance. Circulation 1995;91:1676-88.
21. Ambrose JA, Winters SL, Stern A, et al. Angiographic morphology and the pathogenesis of unstable angina pectoris. J Am Coll Cardiol 1985;5:609-16.
22. Mizuno K, Miyamoto A, Isojima K, et al. A serial observation of coronary thrombi in vivo by a new percutaneous transluminal coronary angioscope. Angiology 1992;43:91-9.
23. De Feyter PJ, Escaned J, Di Mario C, et al. Combined intracoronary ultrasound and angioscopic imaging in patients with unstable angina: target-lesion characteristics [abstract]. Eur Heart J 1993;14:25 (Abstr Suppl):25
24. Den Heijer P, Foley DP, Hillege HL, et al. The "Ermenonville" classification of observations at coronary angioscopy - evaluation of intra- and inter-observer agreement. European Working Group on Coronary Angioscopy. Eur Heart J 1994;15:815-22.
25. Thieme T, Wernecke KD, Meyer R, et al. Angioscopic evaluation of atherosclerotic plaques: validation by histomorphologic analysis and association with stable and unstable coronary syndromes. J Am Coll Cardiol 1996;28:1-6.
26. Waxman S, Sassower MA, Mittleman MA, et al. Angioscopic predictors of early adverse outcome after coronary angioplasty in patients with unstable angina and non-Q-wave myocardial infarction. Circulation 1996;93:2106-13.
27. Feld S, Ganim M, Carell ES, et al. Comparison of angioscopy, intravascular ultrasound imaging and quantitative coronary angiography in predicting clinical outcome after coronary intervention in high risk patients. J Am Coll Cardiol 1996;28:97-105.
28. Alfonso F, Goicolea J, Hernandez R, et al. Findings of coronary angioscopy in angiographically normal coronary segments of patients with coronary artery disease. Am Heart J 1995;130:987-93.
29. Knopf WD, Cates CU, Doby B, Langlois K. Coronary angioscopy influences intervention in patients with unstable angina and recent myocardial infarction. Circulation 1992;86:(Suppl 1):I651.
30. Lablanche JM, Hamon M, McFadden EP, Bauters C, Quandalle P, Bertrand ME. Angiographically silent thrombus frequently persists after thrombolytic therapy for acute myocardial infarction: a prospective angioscopic study. Circulation 1993;88(Suppl):I595.
31. Ueda Y, Asakura M, Hirayama A, Komamura K, Hori M, Komada K. Intracoronary morphology of culprit lesions after reperfusion in acute myocardial infarction: serial angioscopic observations. J Am Coll Cardiol 1996;27:606-10.

32. Sassower MA, Abela GS, Koch JM, et al. Angioscopic evaluation of periprocedural and postprocedural abrupt closure after percutaneous coronary angioplasty. Am Heart J 1993;126:444-50.
33. Jain A, Ramee SR, Mesa J, Collins TJ, White CJ. Intracoronary thrombus: chronic urokinase infusion and evaluation with intravascular ultrasound. Cathet Cardiovasc Diagn 1992;26:212-4.
34. Den Heijer P, Van Dijk RB, Hillege HL, Pentinga ML, Serruys PW, Lie KI. Serial angioscopic and angiographic observations during the first hour after successful coronary angioplasty: a preamble to a multicenter trial addressing angioscopic markers for restenosis. Am Heart J 1994;128:656-63.
35. Bauters C, Lablanche JM, McFadden EP, Hamon M, Bertrand ME. Relation of coronary angioscopic findings at coronary angioplasty to angiographic restenosis. Circulation 1995;92:2473-9.
36. Teirstein PS, Schatz RA, Wong SC, Rocha-Singh KJ. Coronary stenting with angioscopic guidance. Am J Cardiol 1995;75:344-7.
37. Strumpf RK, Heuser RR, Eagan JT Jr. Angioscopy: a valuable tool in the deployment and evaluation of intracoronary stents. Am Heart J 1993;126:1204-10.
38. Resar JR, Brinker J. Early coronary artery stent restenosis: utility of percutaneous coronary angioscopy. Cathet Cardiovasc Diagn 1992;27:276-9.
39. Herrmann HC, Buchbinder M, Clemen MW, et al. Emergent use of balloon-expandable coronary artery stenting for failed percutaneous transluminal coronary angioplasty. Circulation 1992;86:812-9.
40. Schatz RA, Baim DS, Leon M, et al. Clinical experience with the Palmaz-Schatz coronary stent. Initial results of a multicenter study. Circulation 1991;83:148-61.
41. Den Heijer P, Van Dijk RB, Twisk SP, Lie KI. Early stent occlusion is not always caused by thrombosis. Cathet Cardiovasc Diagn 1993;29:136-40.
42. Den Heijer P, Foley D, Escaned J, et al. Angioscopic versus angiographic detection of intimal dissection and intracoronary thrombus. J Am Coll Cardiol 1994;24:649-54.
43. Uretsky BF, Denys BG, Counihan PC, Ragosta M. Angioscopic evaluation of incompletely obstructing coronary intraluminal filling defects: comparison to angiography. Cathet Cardiovasc Diagn 1994;33:323-9.

Chapter 3

RAMAN SPECTROSCOPY OF ATHEROSCLEROSIS: TOWARDS REAL-TIME *IN VIVO* HISTOCHEMISTRY AND PATHOLOGY

Tjeerd J. Römer, James F. Brennan III and Hendrik P.J. Buschman

Summary

The progression and regression of atherosclerotic plaques appear to be related to the amount and type of lipids that accumulate in the intima of arteries.[1-3] Although several therapies are available to treat atherosclerosis, diagnostic methods that reliably predict lesion progression do not exist. Currently, lesion composition rather than lesion area or volume is believed to determine whether a stable or slowly-growing plaque will rupture and cause an acceleration of clinical symptoms [4,5], but a method to study lesion composition in the living patient is not yet available. Clearly, an instrument is needed that can determine *in situ* the chemical composition of atherosclerotic lesions objectively and accurately. Raman spectroscopy has the potential to provide this information. It can quantify the biochemical composition of atherosclerotic plaque *in situ.*

This technique does not require tissue removal, or the use of dyes or labels. It is rapid, molecule specific, non-destructive, and optical fiber compatible, and thus provides a means to study artery disease at the chemical level in the living patient. A Raman spectroscopy instrument would be useful to clinicians and researchers in many applications, such as determining the risk of plaque rupture, providing information for determining the optimum

Van der Wall et al. (eds.),
Advanced Imaging in Coronary Artery Disease, 29-53.

form of medical intervention, and monitoring the effects of pharmacological and mechanical intervention techniques in the treatment of atherosclerotic vessel disease. In this chapter, a review is given of the basic principles and applications of Raman spectroscopy.

Introduction

Raman spectroscopy is a promising technique that can be used to characterize the chemical composition of biological tissue. A Raman spectrum of a given molecule is unique, which makes Raman spectroscopy ideal for detecting, identifying and diagnosing diseases that involve gross chemical changes in tissue, such as atherosclerosis.[6-9] Raman spectra of arterial tissue can be obtained by processing the collected light that is scattered from an artery as it is illuminated with a laser beam. With sensitive laboratory spectroscopic equipment, quality spectra can be collected in less than a second, and most spectral features are visible in spectra collected in only a few seconds via optical fiber catheters.[10-12] Since Raman spectroscopy is non-destructive, one can collect spectra of the tissue *in situ*, which can be processed to provide quantitative information about the chemical composition of an arterial wall.[13,14] This information has been used to identify pathological and morphological features of the atherosclerotic process.[15] Certainly, Raman spectroscopy has the potential of providing diagnostic capabilities that are not available with current medical techniques.

A Raman spectrum contains a wealth of information about the scattering material so it is not surprising that thousands of uses have been found for this spectroscopic technique. For instance, Raman spectroscopy can provide information about the structure of specific molecules and has been used to study various molecular configurations.[16,17] Processes can be remotely and actively monitored via optical fibers in biological and chemical samples.[18,19] Its ability to identify diseased tissue *in vitro* and *in vivo* is under study by several research groups. Raman spectra have been obtained from eye lenses,[20,21] viruses,[22] teeth and bone,[23,24] single living cells,[25,26] living salmon sperm,[27] DNA,[22,25,28] etc.

Although the Raman effect was discovered in the 1920s, it was difficult to apply, because one needed strong light sources and sensitive light detection equipment. Little sustained interest was aroused by the promising practical aspects of the Raman effect until the advent of lasers. Biological and clinical applications of Raman techniques wanted additional technology innovations, since instruments were needed that were convenient to use and capable to collect spectral information rapidly. In addition, Raman signal size was severely limited by the need to work at excitation intensities sufficiently low to avoid damage to biological samples.

Silicon-based CCD detectors have dramatically improved the instrumentation used to measure Raman spectra. The high sensitivity and negligible dark noise of these detectors have permitted spectra to be measured orders of magnitude faster than with earlier instrumentation. However, in materials such as biological tissue the Raman effect is often obscured by strong background fluorescence. In order to reduce this, recently investigators have used excitation wavelengths in the NIR range, 700 to 850 nm, where fluorescence is significantly reduced and silicon CCDs are still sensitive to the Raman scattered light (850 to 1000 nm).

Cardiovascular studies with Raman spectroscopy have been performed *in vitro* with arterial tissue, but successful *in vivo* measurements have long been impeded by the high background noise generated by scattering within the optical fibers used to construct intravascular Raman probes. Methods of reducing this background signal are under investigation by several research groups.[29] Recent developments indicate that adequate reduction of background signal is feasible,[30] and open the way for remote catheter based Raman spectral acquisition *in vivo*.

This review addresses some of our studies of arterial tissue with Raman spectroscopy. We will focus on our work with human coronary arteries. We provide a brief explanation of the Raman effect and direct the interested reader to the many illustrative papers on the subject. A short biography of Prof C.V. Raman is also given. We will briefly explain the Raman spectroscopy systems with which we performed these studies, and show spectra of arterial tissue in various stages of disease. We developed models to extract clinically useful information from the coronary artery spectra and will discuss two of these models: a quantitative chemical model and a semi-quantitative morphological model. We will show how this spectroscopic information can be used to provide *in situ* histopathology. We also investigated how deep Raman spectroscopy can detect cholesterol deposits in arterial wall to define the capacity of Raman spectroscopy to detect subsurface lesions.

The applications of Raman spectroscopy techniques in cardiology will be probably widespread. We will present some exploratory studies that illustrate some possible uses of this new diagnostic technique. This technique combined with intravascular ultrasound may be used to map the chemical composition of an arterial wall. We also show how Raman spectroscopy can provide a detailed chemical map of atherosclerotic lesions developed in transgenic mice, which may be used to monitor and evaluate the effects of lipid lowering agents on plaque progression and regression.

The Raman effect

The vibrations and rotations between atoms within a molecule can occur only at discrete frequencies, that are determined by factors such as the micro-environment of the molecule and the masses and attractive forces of the atoms.[31-33] These molecular motions store energy, like the flywheel on a gasoline engine stores energy. Since a molecule's internal motions are quantized, a molecule can absorb or emit energy in only discrete units as it changes from one vibrational state to another.

Light consists of discreet packets of energy called photons. The energy of a photon is inversely proportional to the wavelength of the light; an ultraviolet photon at a wavelength of 244 nm has more energy than an infrared photon at a wavelength of 900 nm. When a molecule radiatively changes state, the wavelength of the light that is emitted or absorbed during the transition changes by a discreet amount corresponding to the change in stored energy of the molecule. Since different molecules have distinct internal configurations, they have unique frequencies of internal motion and thus can be identified by their spectra.

The spectrum of light scattered from a molecule generally contains an elastic contribution, where the emitted frequency equals the incident frequency (Rayleigh scattering), together with several spectral components for which these frequencies differ (Stokes and anti-Stokes scattering), as illustrated in figure 1A. One source of this frequency-shifted light is a sequence of processes known as relaxed fluorescence, in which the frequency of the incident light falls within an electronic absorption band of the interacting molecule. The molecule is raised to an excited state as it absorbs an incident photon and, after losing some energy by making non-radiative molecular transitions, re-emits light at a different frequency.

Raman scattering is another source of frequency-shifted light. To Raman scatter, the incident light frequency need not be within the absorption band of the scattering molecule. The frequency difference between the incident and scattered light, which is commonly expressed in units of inverse wave length or wave numbers (cm^{-1}), corresponds to vibrational state transitions in the scattering molecule. During Raman scattering, a molecule changes state from one vibrational energy level to another. To conserve energy and momentum, the energies of the scattered photons are different from the incident photon energy by an amount equal but opposite to the molecular energy change.

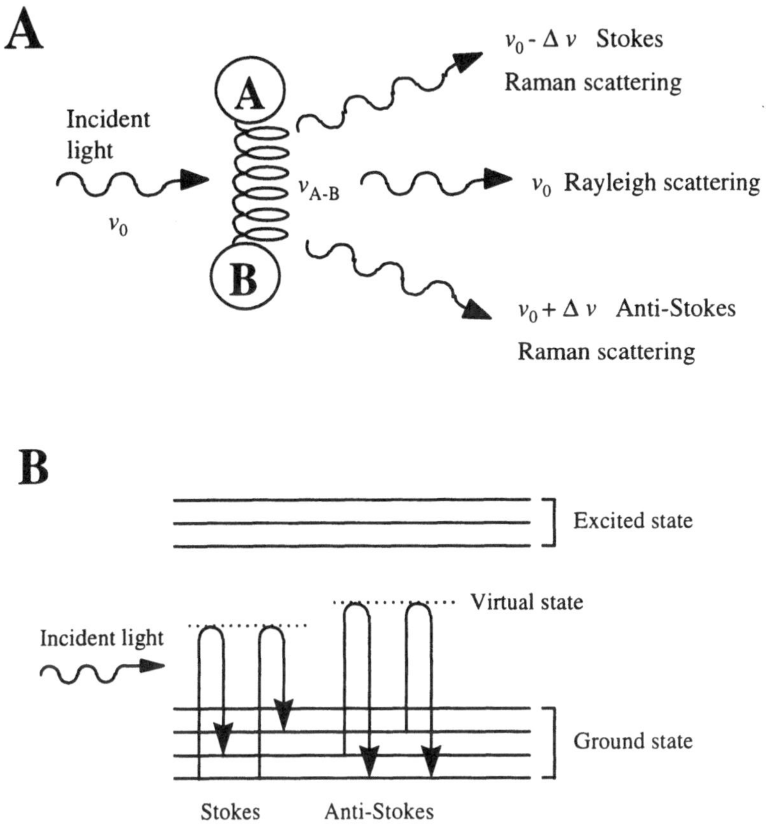

Figure 1. (A) *A schematic illustration of Raman and Rayleigh scattering. The scattered photon is like the incident photon in Rayleigh scattering, but in Raman scattering the scattered photon has a lower or higher frequency (v_0). The difference in energy between the incident and scattered photons is the same as the change in molecular vibrational energy.* ***(B)*** *A schematic illustration of the molecular energy levels and transitions during Raman scattering. The energy level of the virtual state is well below that of the excited electronic state. After a Raman event, the molecule has changed vibrational state, but remains in the electronic state.*

Rayleigh scattering can be looked on as an elastic collision between the incident photon and the molecule and is by far the strongest component of the scattered radiation. Since the rotational and vibrational energy of the molecule is unchanged in an elastic collision, the wavelength of the scattered photon is the same as that of the incident photon. When an incident photon interacts with a molecule in the lowest vibrational state of the molecule, the molecule absorbs the photon energy and is raised momentarily to some high level of energy which is not stable (a virtual state). The molecule immediately loses energy and returns to the lowest vibrational level, as it emits a photon at a wavelength which is the same as that of the incident photon.

The Raman effect can be viewed as an inelastic collision between the incident photon and the molecule, where, as a result of the collision, the vibrational or rotational energy of the molecule is changed. In some instances after a molecule absorbs a photon and enters an unstable state, it may fall to an excited vibrational state of the molecule and not to the lowest vibrational level (figure 1B). In this case, the scattered photon has less energy than the exciting photon and gives rise to a so-called Stokes line in the Raman spectrum, which is at a wavelength longer than that of the incident photon. If the molecule was initially in an excited vibrational state before it absorbed an incident photon and entered the virtual state, so-called anti-Stokes Raman scattering can occur where the emitted photon is at a wavelength shorter than that of the incident photon. This effect is usually much weaker than Stokes scattering and was not studied by us.

For illustration, we picture an imaginary compound with a single vibrational state. If this compound is illuminated with 850 nm light, a spectrum of the scattered light may contain a Rayleigh line at 11,765 cm^{-1} (850 nm) and a Stokes line at say 10,165 cm^{-1} (984 nm). The frequency difference between the incident and emitted photons (1600 cm^{-1}) would correspond to the vibrational energy change in the molecule. A Raman spectrum of a compound usually has several spectral peaks, and their positions and intensities can be used as a molecular fingerprint. For more information about the basic principles of Raman spectroscopy and its biological applications, the reader is referred to the book written by Anthony T. Tu.[17]

Prof. C.V. Raman

C.V. Raman was born in 1888 in Southern India, as one of seven children. He graduated in Physics at the University of Madras and went to Calcutta in 1907, where he became Professor and Head of the Department of

Physics of the Calcutta University of Science in 1917.[34] Before he detected the phenomenon that bears his name, he published more than 50 papers on light scattering and magnetism of liquid and solid media. With a quartz mercury lamp as light source, a simple set of lenses and filters, and a pocket spectroscope, he observed by eye that highly purified organic liquids, which were positioned in an incident light beam path, generated weak frequencies in the scattered light not present in the original incident light. He exposed photographic plates for hours, even days, to obtain his spectra. Prof. Raman first announced his discovery in an inaugural lecture entitled "A New Radiation" at a meeting of the South Indian Association in 1928.[35] In that same year he published two papers in Nature about the phenomenon, which made it known throughout the world.[36,37] He received the Nobel prize for his work in 1930.[38] At present, numerous publications on Raman spectroscopy have been published. Prof. Raman died in 1970, just before the wide exploration of biological applications of Raman spectroscopy started.[17]

Raman spectroscopy instrumentation

The methods used to collect Raman spectra are relatively easy to follow. Basically, light of a single wavelength is directed onto a sample, and then light scattered from the sample is collected and launched into a spectrometer. The spectrometer separates the light according to its wavelength, like a prism spreads sunlight into a rainbow. This rainbow of light is projected onto a detector which can record the intensities of each color of light. A plot of these intensities as a function of wavelength (or frequency) is called a spectrum.

Two types of instruments have been used for the below described studies; one system for laboratory studies and one for clinical use. The laboratory system was designed to collect the highest quality spectra possible. The clinical system was designed to collect *in vivo* Raman spectra in a clinical setting from peripheral and coronary arteries via optical fibers. Each system consists of three main components: a laser, a spectrometer-CCD detection system, and a personal computer for data storage and analysis. The laboratory system was extended with a confocal microscope[25], allowing spectroscopic studies of tissue samples at both macroscopic (~1mm^3), and microscopic (~1 µm^3) level. In our laboratory studies, we irradiated coronary artery tissue with near infrared laser light of ~830 nm or 850 nm (figure 2). The laser light was directed with mirrors to either the macroscopic set-up holding a piece of artery tissue, or launched into the microscope and focused onto a thin (6 µm) artery section. The Raman scattered light was collected with lenses. Special optical filters were used to remove the intense Rayleigh scattered light from the collected light before it was projected into a high-efficiency spectrometer. In the spectrometer, the light was collimated, separated spatially by wavelength with a diffraction grating, and imaged onto a charge coupled device (CCD) camera. This spectral information was stored and analyzed with a computer. In the microscope set-up the Raman scattered light was projected onto a pinhole (P) before being filtered and projected into the spectrometer. The aperture gives the microscope its confocal properties by rejecting Raman signal contributions from out-of-focus fields. With both systems Raman spectra with a high signal-to-noise ratio could be colleted in seconds (see below).

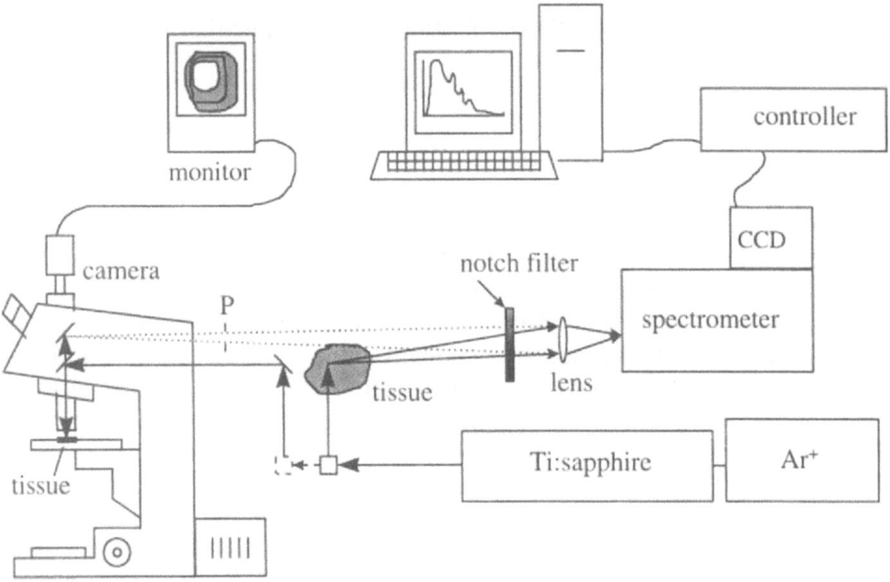

Figure 2. *Schematic diagram of the laboratory Raman instrumentation. Laser light of 850 nm or 830 nm from an Ar+ laser pumped Ti:sapphire laser system is passed through a holographic laser filter, and either directly focused onto an artery sample (macroscopic) or coupled into the microscope and focused onto a thin section of artery tissue with a 63x microscope objective. Light scattered by the tissue is collected by a lens, filtered and coupled into the spectrometer. Scattered light collected from the tissue under the microscope passes through a pinhole (P), which enables confocal detection, before it is filtered and projected into the spectrometer. A removable mirror in the microscope is used to either direct collected Raman light from the sample to the spectrometer, or white light images to the camera and monitor. Raman signals are collected with a personal computer and stored on hard disk for later analysis.*

The clinical system (not shown) was designed to be compact, mobile, and able to collect real-time Raman spectra via optical fiber probes in hospital settings. It consists of a system in which filters, lenses, spectrograph and CCD/controller are integrated, equipped with Raman optical fiber probes, a compact diode laser, and a note-book computer. In a number of *in vivo* pilot experiments infrared light (~830 nm) was delivered to and collected from tissue with an optical fiber probe consisting of six collection fibers surrounding a central delivery fiber.[10,11] The distal tip of the optical fiber probe was brought into contact with the tissue to be spectroscopically examined, collected with the surrounding fibers, coupled into the spectrometer, and analyzed.

The clinical system was able to detect the presence of hydroxy-apatite in calcified coronary artery in a 0.01 s signal collection time. Fiber background, however, severely limited the spectral quality.[10,39] Typically, the fiber background at ~1000 cm^{-1} is >30 times larger than the Raman spectral features of cholesterol. The tip of the probe that we currently use, is designed in such a way that the signal contribution of the fiber material itself is strongly suppressed.[30] The probe, a 7-around-1 design, has a central fiber of 400 μm core-diameter, guiding laser light to the tissue, and signal collection fibers of 300 μm core-diameter. The central fiber is coated with a dielectric narrow band pass filter, which transmits the laser light but blocks Raman signal from the fiber material. The signal collection fibers are coated with a dielectric high pass filter that blocks the laser wavelength and transmits the scattered tissue Raman light. An example of the effect of filtering is shown in figure 3.

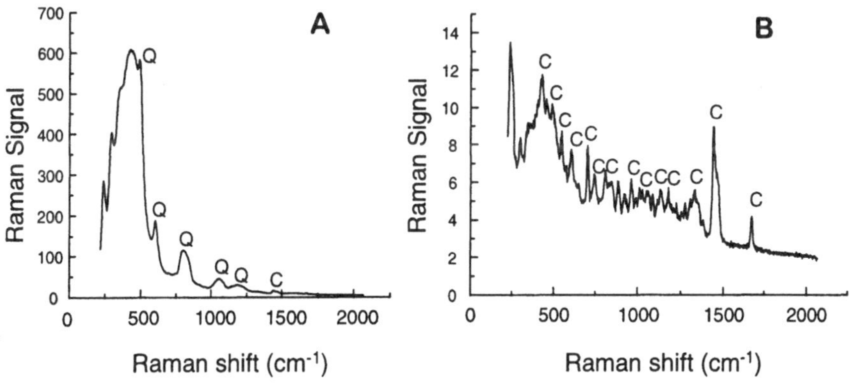

Figure 3. *Raman spectra obtained from pure cholesterol with **(A)** an unfiltered probe or **(B)** a filtered probe. Peaks from quartz and cholesterol are indicated by Q and C, respectively. Note the scale change.*

It clearly shows the dramatic reduction in Raman background as a result of the filtering, by which the spectral information of the sample that was examined was greatly enhanced.

Raman spectra of coronary artery

For most studies, we obtained coronary artery samples from explanted recipient hearts and stored these samples at -80 ^{0}C until spectroscopic examination. NIR Raman spectra, measured from three different types of human coronary artery, are shown in figure 4.

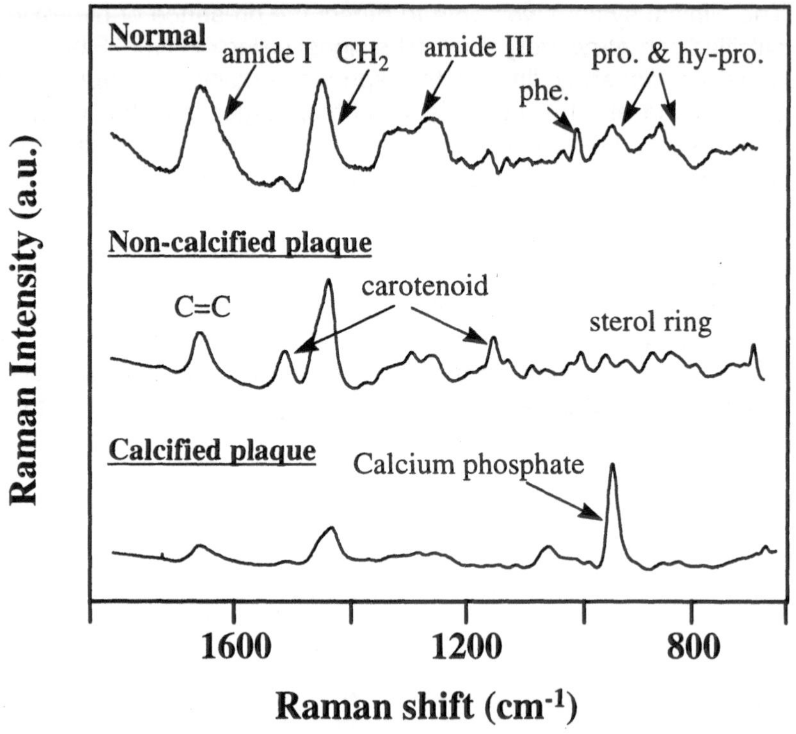

Figure 4. *Raman spectra of three different types of coronary artery. Spectral features can be assigned to specific molecular vibrations.*

The top spectrum was obtained from a sample of non-atherosclerotic coronary artery; the middle from a non-calcified atheromatous plaque; and the bottom from a calcified plaque. The spectra from these different artery types are distinct and provide clear features for determining the chemical composition and histological classification of the arterial wall. For example the normal coronary artery spectrum is dominated by protein features such as the amide I and III modes at ~1650 and 1250 cm^{-1}, respectively, and the CH_2 bending modes at ~1450 cm^{-1}. In non-calcified atheromatous plaques, spectral features of cholesterol and cholesterol esters constitute the major part of the spectrum. The symmetric stretch at 960 cm^{-1} of phosphate, which is a constituent of calcium hydroxy-apatite, dominates the spectrum of calcified plaques.

Raman spectral analysis

We macroscopically examined hundreds of coronary artery samples that represented various pathological states and obtained their spectra. To extract clinical useful information from these spectra, a number of models were developed each of which views an artery spectrum as a linear superposition of spectra of individual components or basis-spectra. These models differ in the set of basis-spectra. One model is based on the Raman spectra collected from chemical components that were isolated from artery wall. A second model uses basis-spectra from the different morphological structures that are present in artery wall.

Artery chemistry with Raman spectra

The chemical model uses individual chemical components from artery wall as basis-spectra. We found that spectra of seven arterial components were needed to model adequately all of the measured coronary artery spectra. These components were free cholesterol (FC), cholesterol esters (CE), calcium salts (CS), triglycerides and phospholipids (TG&PL), two delipidized artery segments (DA) and β-carotene.
The contribution of some components in a coronary artery spectrum, such as triglycerides or proteins, is difficult to model with spectra obtained from commercially available chemicals, because these components in the artery contain mixtures of related molecules in the class. Therefore, these components were extracted from the artery wall itself. The DA spectra were obtained from delipidized artery samples, one from non-atherosclerotic tissue (DA I) and another from non-calcified atherosclerotic tissue (DA II). Linear superpositions of the seven components modeled the measured coronary artery spectra well, judged by the residuals of the fit that are obtained by subtracting the model fit from the artery spectrum.

The spectra of the seven model compounds were then scaled appropriately with known weight mixtures of the seven compounds. The overall spectral model was validated by comparing chemical concentrations in coronary artery minces calculated from the Raman spectra to the actual concentrations measured with standard assay techniques. Excellent agreement was reached between the relative weights calculated with Raman spectroscopic techniques and those determined with standard assays conducted on the minces (figure 5). Details of the model and its validation with standard chemical assays have been described previously.[13,14,39]

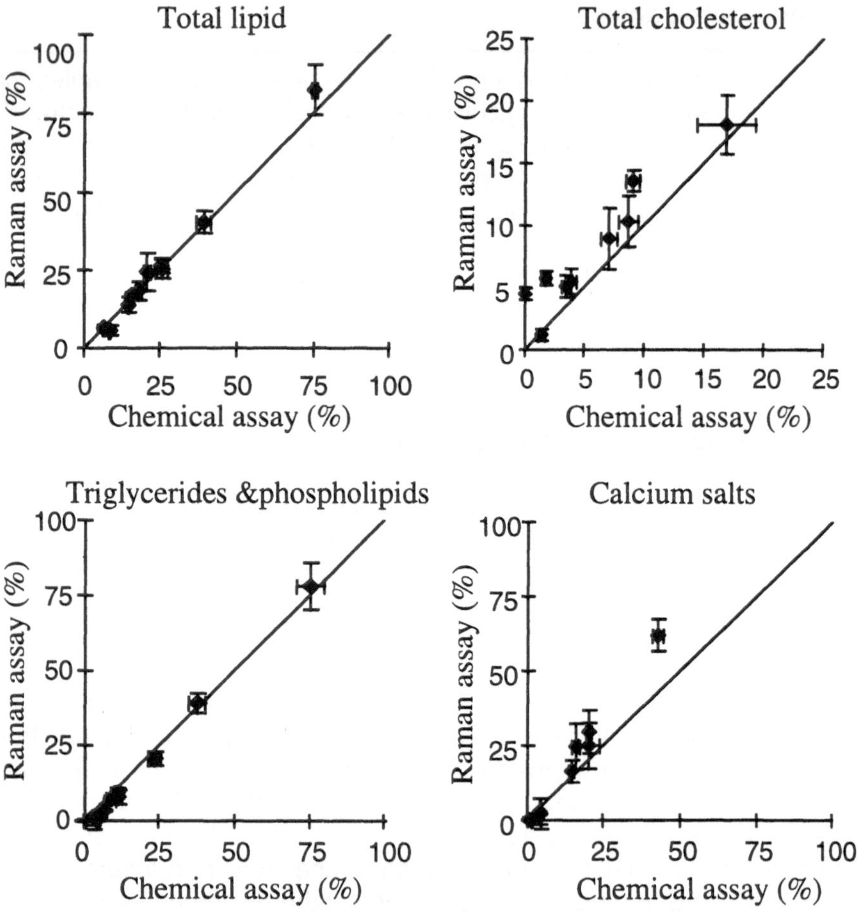

Figure 5. *Comparison of the percentage weights of lipids and calcium salts measured in coronary artery minces by Raman spectral analysis and standard chemical assay techniques.*

Histopathology with Raman spectra of coronary artery

In this study, we extracted quantitative chemical information from Raman spectra obtained from coronary artery in different stages of atherosclerosis and correlated this information with standard histological tissue diagnosis. To improve clinical utility, we developed an algorithm based on these chemical parameters that allows the classification of coronary artery atherosclerosis *in situ*, according to standard pathological classification schemes.

In figure 6, Raman spectra (dots) of intimal fibroplasia, non-calcified atheromatous plaque and calcified atheroscleromatous plaque are modeled with the above described model (line). The curve below each spectrum and model fit is the residual, obtained by subtracting the fit from the artery spectrum. Figure 6A shows a spectrum of intimal fibroplasia, that is dominated by protein and TG features visible at about 1650, 1250 and 1450 cm^{-1}. The TG's located in the adventitial layer are stronger Raman scatterers than the proteins in the intima and media, so the TG spectral features dominate the artery spectrum although the relative weight of TG is lower than that of proteins. In the spectrum of an atheromatous plaque shown in figure 6B, spectral features from the sterol rings of FC and CE are visible below 1000 cm^{-1}. The Raman spectral model calculated a 12% relative weight of FC and a 6% relative weight of CE. Raman spectra obtained from calcified plaque are distinguishable by the symmetric stretch vibration of phosphate (960 cm^{-1}) found in calcium salts, mainly calcium hydroxy-apatite. A large relative weight of CS was calculated from the spectrum of a highly calcified atheromatous plaque shown in figure 6C.

As shown, Raman spectra of coronary artery are fingerprints of the tissue's molecular composition. Figure 7 shows that the quantification of the chemical composition calculated from artery spectra correlates with standard histologic tissue classification. We found that an artery's cholesterol and calcium salts content is useful for classifying the artery as either non-atherosclerotic tissue, non-calcified plaque, or calcified lesion. Using these two chemical parameters, we made diagnostic algorithms that could calculate the probability that an area of interest in a coronary artery is in one of these three categories. These algorithms were successful in separating ~170 coronary artery samples into their proper diagnostic categories, as determined by the pathologist. This study suggests that the pathological state of a coronary artery site can be assessed successfully from its chemical composition determined with Raman spectra.[15]

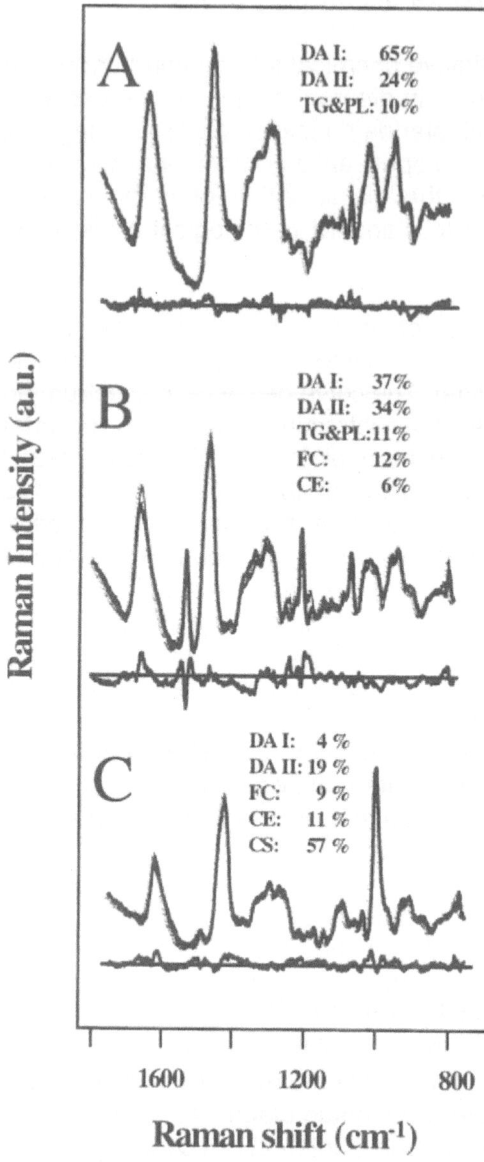

Raman spectroscopic analysis of tissue shows certain advantages over light microscopic examination.

A pathologist needs to observe lipid-bearing morphological structures, such as cholesterol crystals and foam cells, and calcification remnants in tissue sections to diagnose a given artery sample, but these telling structures may be missed on microscopic examination due to sampling error during tissue sectioning. Raman spectroscopy examines a large volume of tissue (~1 mm^3 in this study), so it is not subject to this type of sampling error. To examine the same volume of tissue, a pathologist would need to inspect hundreds of tissue sections.

Figure 6. *Raman spectra (dotted line) of intimal fibroplasia **(A)**, atheromatous plaque **(B)** and calcified plaque **(C)** modeled with the set of spectra from individual components (line) to quantify the chemical composition of the artery wall. The curve under each spectrum shows the difference of the spectrum and the model fit.*

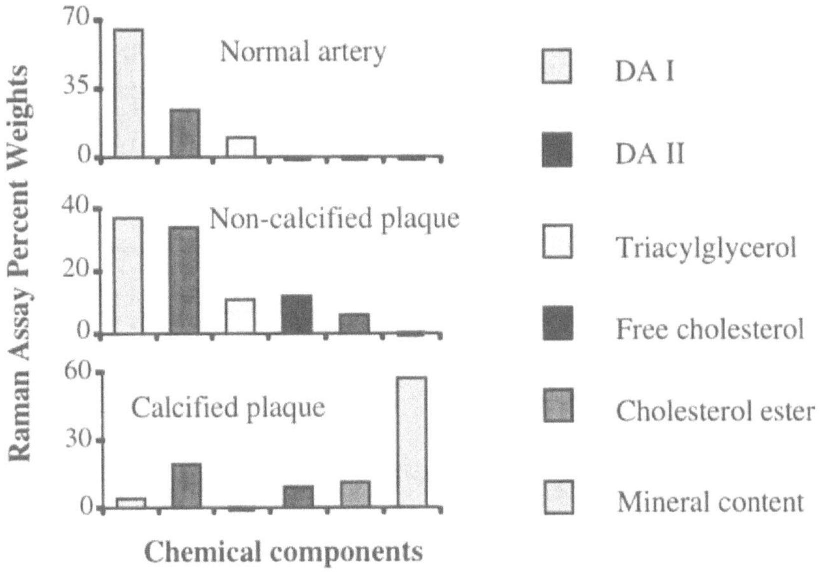

Figure 7. *Quantitative chemical information provided by Raman spectroscopy correlates to histopathology. DA indicates delipidized artery (see text)*

Artery morphology with Raman spectra

We are developing a new spectral method of analysis that exploits the capabilities of Raman spectroscopy to identify morphological structures instead of chemical components.[40] In this method a Raman spectrum is modeled as a linear superposition of the Raman line-shapes of the different morphological structures that were collected from artery tissue. The use of this morphological model may provide direct information about the fraction of morphological structures in the tissue, that can be used to give insight into the pathological condition of the artery. Raman spectra were obtained with the confocal microspectroscopic system described above. Thin (6 μm) unstained tissue sections were cut on a microtome, placed on a sample holder and covered with saline. Under the microscope a structure was selected for spectroscopic examination with white light illumination, and the laser spot was focused with a 63x refractive objective to a spot of about 1 μm, after which Raman spectra were obtained. Raman spectra were recorded from the internal elastic lamina (IEL), collagen fibers, foam cells, adventitial fat, necrotic core, cholesterol crystals, calcium mineralizations, and β-carotene mineralizations. Examples of Raman spectra from the IEL from different artery samples are shown in figure 8. The spectral features of the six spectra are very similar, indicating that the chemical composition of the IEL is very homogeneous in different artery tissue samples. Further spectral analysis assigns the combination of peaks to the chemical elastin.

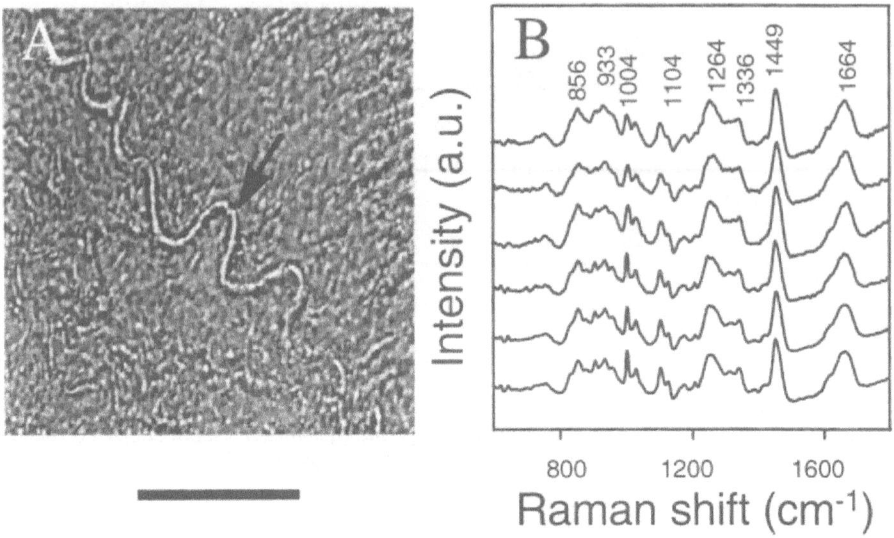

Figure 8. *Example of* ***(A)*** *a microphotograph of the internal elastic lamina (arrow) in an unstained coronary artery section of 6 μm, and* ***(B)*** *the Raman spectrum of this morphological structure from six different coronary artery samples. Scale bar: 20 μm.*

The Raman spectra from macroscopic artery samples expressing different stages of atherosclerosis (n=97) were modeled with a morphological model containing the lineshapes of the above structures, and showed excellent fits (not shown). With the fit-contribution of the morphological basis-spectra to each macroscopic Raman spectrum we constructed an algorithm to calculate the probability of these samples to belong to one of the three diagnostic categories described above. The accuracy of this algorithm was similar to that of the algorithm based on chemical components. These results suggest that Raman spectroscopy can provide morphological information from intact tissue that can be used to classify artery tissue to different pathological states.

Sampling depth

We also investigated how deep Raman spectroscopy can detect subsurface structures in an arterial wall. When we validated the above-discussed chemical model, we obtained spectra from homogeneous minces of coronary artery where the amount of a chemical compound was uniformly distributed throughout the sample.

Chemical amounts calculated by processing Raman spectra collected from intact, inhomogeneous plaques are more difficult to interpret, because the strength and shape of a spectrum measured at the surface of an artery wall is determined by a complex interaction between a number of physical factors (e.g. the compound's scattering cross-section, the depth of the scatterer, and the excitation/collection geometry). We studied how the relative weight of cholesterol calculated with Raman spectra is related to the depth of the cholesterol deposit into an arterial wall.[41]

The attenuation of a cholesterol deposit's contribution to a Raman spectrum seems to decrease roughly exponentially as a function of distance from the artery surface. We found that a 300 μm layer of non-atherosclerotic tissue attenuates the Raman signal of plaque cholesterol by ~50% at 850 nm excitation, which is in agreement with results found by other researchers.[9]

These results indicate that NIR Raman spectroscopy can detect subsurface structures that are ~1-1.5 mm beneath the artery surface and therefore should be capable of detecting atherosclerotic deposits under thick fibrous caps. Atherosclerotic plaques in coronary arteries vary in thickness and may reach a fibrous cap thickness of 200-300 μm and an underlying core thickness of ~400 μm.[42]

We compared cholesterol amounts calculated with Raman spectra of intact plaques to those calculated with quantitative absorption microscopy of tissue sections from these plaques that were specially stained to visualize cholesterol. If one properly accounts for the depth of a cholesterol deposit into an arterial wall, we showed that cholesterol amounts calculated with spectra correlate strongly to amounts determined with quantitative microscopy.

These results suggest that one may map *in vivo* chemical concentrations throughout the thickness of an arterial wall by combining Raman spectroscopic techniques with a non-destructive depth-sensing tool, such as intravascular ultrasound or optical coherence tomography.

Raman spectroscopy combined with intravascular ultrasound

Coronary intravascular ultrasound (IVUS) imaging provides tomographic information about vessel wall structure. Previous studies demonstrated that IVUS can detect intimal thickening, lipid deposits and calcific deposits.[43-46] For instance, the presence of a calcific deposit corresponds with a shadow behind an echodense area, and the presence of a deposit of lipids with an echolucent area. However, studies in which IVUS is compared with histologic examination under high-power magnification demonstrated that IVUS can detect these deposits only if they are at least 0.25 mm in diameter.[43] In addition, accurate determination of the size of calcific deposits was impossible with IVUS, since ultrasound waves are reflected mostly at the particle surface. The sensitivity in detecting lipid and calcific deposits was found to be low, 46% and 77% respectively.[43,47]

Future catheters could be designed to collect simultaneously Raman spectra via optical fibers and IVUS images. This powerful diagnostic tool would combine the quantitative chemical information provided by Raman spectroscopy and the morphologic information provided by IVUS.

We explored the feasibility of combining IVUS and Raman spectroscopy technologies. IVUS images were collected from intact coronary artery segments (a few cm long) in different stages of atherosclerosis. Before collecting the images, a steel needle was positioned in the adventitia as an angular bearing for future comparisons. The arteries were opened longitudinally, and Raman spectra were collected at 0.5 mm interval steps over the circumference of the locations marked with a needle, as shown in figure 9A. Figures 9B-D reveal the results of examining a calcified plaque with both IVUS and Raman spectroscopy. The IVUS image (figure 9B) shows a shadow, directly behind an echodense area, opposite the location of the needle, indicating the presence of a calcified deposit. The calcium salts amounts determined with Raman spectra indicate clearly the presence of calcified tissue in this region (figure 9C), and elevated cholesterol amounts (figure 9D) are present in the non-calcified regions that are not plainly visible in the IVUS image. Histologic sections, which were made through this circumferential cross-section and stained specifically for cholesterol, confirmed that an elevated level of cholesterol was present in these areas.

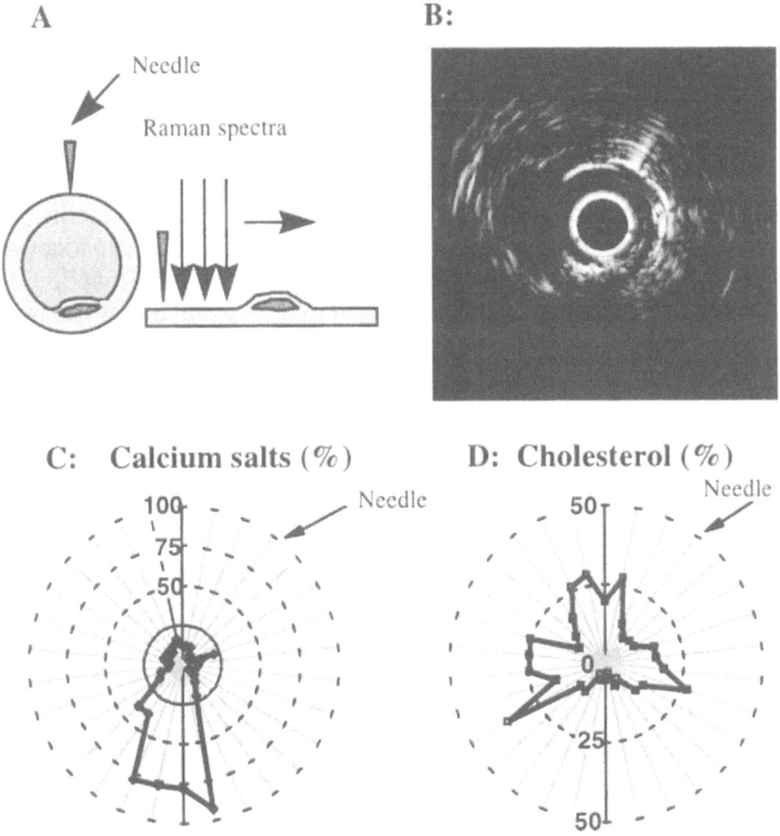

__Figure 9.__ IVUS images were obtained from an intact artery segment, which were marked by a needle. The artery was opened, and Raman spectra were collected from the artery's inner circumference __(A)__. The IVUS image shows a calcification __(B)__, in agreement with the CS detected with Raman spectroscopy __(C)__. In addition, cholesterol is detected with Raman spectroscopy but cannot be seen in the IVUS image __(D)__. (Note the difference in scale.)

Chemical mapping of transgenic mice aortas

Our chemical Raman spectral model that was developed on human coronary artery can be altered easily to quantify the chemical composition of aortas from APOE*3 Leiden transgenic mice. After they are fed with a high fat / cholesterol (HFC) diet, these mice are highly susceptible to diet-induced atherosclerosis and develop human-like atherosclerotic plaques within six months.[48] This animal model may be ideal to monitor and evaluate the effects of hypolipidemic, antithrombogenic and other drugs on plaque progression and regression.[49] The lipids in these plaques can be visualized with standard light microscopy after Oil Red O staining of ~10 μm thick sections. Raman spectroscopy adds an extra dimension to the assessment of atherosclerosis by quantifying the chemical composition of the plaque *in situ*. This information cannot be obtained with any other available technique. We fed groups of these mice with a HFC diet for 1 to 6 months. We followed the development of plaques in these mice with Raman spectroscopy, as illustrated in figure 10. To create this chemical map, a mouse that received the HFC diet for 6 months was sacrificed, and its aorta (~4 mm circumference) was flushed, prepared and cut open for spectroscopic examination. Raman spectra were obtained in 0.5 mm steps over the width and length of the aorta, starting from the aortic valve until ~8 mm distally. The Raman spectra were processed to quantify the relative amounts of cholesterol and calcium salts.[50]

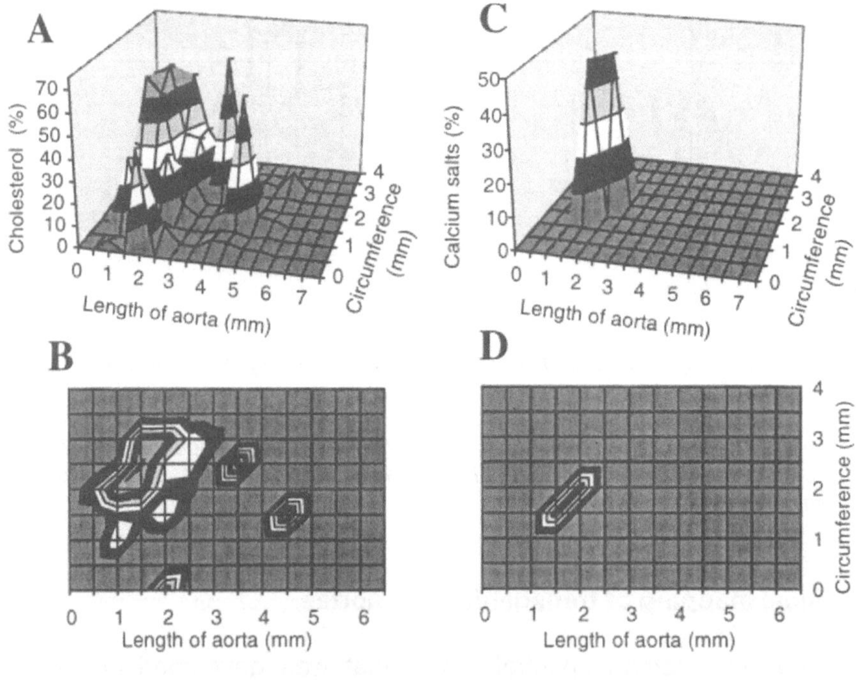

Figure 10. *Accumulation of cholesterol in the aorta of a APOE*3 Leiden transgenic mouse, just distally of the aortic valve, quantified with Raman spectroscopy* ***(A, and top view B)****. In the center of the plaque, a calcium salts deposit was found and quantified with Raman spectroscopy* ***(C and top view D)****.*

As shown in figure 10, a cholesterol-rich plaque with calcium salts deposits in its center developed just distally of the aortic valve at the inner circle of the arch. The relative weight of this calcified deposit amounted to >70% of the volume examined spectroscopically at that location. Aortas of mice that received normal chow did not exhibit elevated levels of cholesterol or calcium salts deposits (not shown).

As this study suggests, Raman spectroscopy can map the chemical composition of atherosclerotic plaques from transgenic mice, which could aid the study of atherogenesis and help assess hypolipidemic and anti-atherosclerotic therapies.

Conclusion

Since its discovery in the 1920's, Raman spectroscopy has been widely explored and utilized. Raman spectroscopy is reproducible, objective and thus independent of intra- and inter-observer variability. Over the last decade, technological advances have made Raman spectroscopy suitable for biomedical studies. Our group has performed a number of *in vitro* cardiovascular studies with Raman spectroscopy, and *in vivo* measurements with special Raman optical fiber probes are under way. In our studies, we modeled coronary artery spectra with spectra of arterial compounds and used the results of the model to quantify the chemical composition of arterial wall. The variation in fit-contribution of the basis-spectra was seen to vary with the type and extent of atherosclerotic disease in the arterial wall, which illustrated that Raman spectroscopy can provide *in situ* histopathology. Our results also indicated that NIR Raman spectroscopy can detect subsurface structures that are ~1-1.5 mm beneath the artery surface and therefore should be capable of detecting atherosclerotic deposits under thick fibrous caps.

The applications in cardiology of Raman spectroscopy techniques may be widespread, and we discussed some exploratory studies to illustrate its potential. Once *in vivo* closed vessel transluminal measurements become possible, Raman spectroscopy combined with intravascular ultrasound, may give the clinician unprecedented capabilities that could serve many purposes, such as chemical mapping of atherosclerotic plaques which may be used to monitor the effects of lipid lowering therapies, and identifying rupture-prone lesions, or lesions likely to restenose following angioplasty.

Acknowledgment

The authors wish to acknowledge the financial support by the Netherlands Heart Foundation (R93.310 and 95.134), the Interuniversity Cardiology Institute of the Netherlands (ICIN: D96.2158/MH), and the National Institutes of Health (NIH R01-HL51265 & NIH P41-RR02594). This work was carried out at the Cardiology department and Gaubius Laboratory/TNO-PG at the Leiden University Medical Center, Leiden, the Laboratory for Intensive Care Research and Optical Spectroscopy at the Dijkzicht Hospital, Rotterdam, and the G.R. Harrison Spectroscopy Laboratory, MIT, Cambridge, MA, U.S.A. Many collaborators were involved in this work, but we wish to thank Michael Feld, John Kramer, Gerwin Puppels, Arnoud van der Laarse and Albert Bruschke in particular.

References

1. Small DM. George Lyman Duff memorial lecture. Progression and regression of atherosclerotic lesions. Insights from lipid physical biochemistry. Arteriosclerosis 1988;8:103-29.
2. Steinberg D, Witztum JL. Lipoproteins and atherogenesis. Current concepts. JAMA 1990;264:3047-52.
3. Stary HC. Composition and classification of human atherosclerotic lesions. Virchows Arch A Pathol Anat Histopathol 1992;421:277-90.
4. Loree HM, Tobias BJ, Gibson LJ, Kamm RD, Small DM, Lee RT. Mechanical properties of model atherosclerotic lesion lipid pools. Arterioscler Thromb 1994;14:230-4.
5. Libby P. Molecular bases of the acute coronary syndromes. Circulation 1995;91:2844-50.
6. Manoharan R, Baraga JJ, Rava RP, Dasari RR, Fitzmaurice M, Feld MS. Biochemical analysis and mapping of atherosclerotic human artery using FT-IR microspectroscopy. Atherosclerosis 1993;103:181-93.
7. Manoharan R, Baraga JJ, Feld MS, Rava RP. Quantitative histochemical analysis of human artery using Raman spectroscopy. J Photochem Photobiol B 1992;16:211-33.
8. Baraga JJ, Feld MS, Rava RP. Rapid near-infrared Raman-spectroscopy of human tissue with a spectrograph and a CCD detector. Appl Spectrosc 1992;46:187-90.
9. Baraga JJ, Feld MS, Rava RP. In situ optical histochemistry of human artery using near infrared Fourier transform Raman spectroscopy. Proc Natl Acad Sci USA 1992;89:3473-7.
10. Brennan JF 3rd, Wang Y, Dasari RR, Feld MS. Near-infrared Raman spectrometer systems for human tissue studies. Appl Spectrose 1997;51:201-8.
11. Kramer JR, Brennan JF 3rd, Römer TJ, Wang Y, Dasari RR, Feld MS. Spectral diagnosis of human coronary artery: a clinical system for real-time analysis. Proc SPIE 1995;2395:376-82.
12. Puppels GJ, van Aken T, Wolthuis R, et al. In vivo tissue characterization by Raman spectroscopy. Proc SPIE. In press, 1998.
13. Brennan JF 3rd, Römer TJ, Tercyak AM, et al. In situ histochemical analysis of human coronary artery by Raman spectroscopy compared with biochemical assay. Proc SPIE 1995;2388:105-9.
14. Brennan JF 3rd, Römer TJ, Lees RS, Tercyak AM, Kramer JR Jr, Feld MS. Determination of human coronary artery composition by Raman spectroscopy. Circulation 1997;96:99-105.
15. Römer TJ, Brennan JF 3rd, Fitzmaurice M, et al. Histopathology of human coronary atherosclerosis by quantifying its chemical composition with Raman spectroscopy. Circulation. In press 1998.
16. Carey PR. Biochemical applications of Raman and resonance Raman spectroscopies. New York: Academic Press; 1982.
17. Tu AT. Raman spectroscopy in biology. New York: J Wiley; 1982.
18. Fehrmann A, Franz M, Hoffmann A, Rudzik L, Wust E. Dairy product analysis: identification of microorganisms by mid-infrared spectroscopy and determination of constituents by Raman spectroscopy. J AOAC Int 1995;78:1537-42.

19. Nave SE, O'Rourke PE, Toole WR. Sampling probes enhance remote chemical analysis. Laser Focus World 1995;12:83-8.
20. Yaroslavsky IV, Yaroslavsky AN, Otto C, et al. Combined elastic and Raman light scattering of human eye lenses. Exp Eye Res 1994;59:393-9.
21. Duindam HJ, Vrensen GF, Otto C, Puppels GJ, Greve J. New approach to assess the cholesterol distribution in the eye lens: confocal Raman microspectroscopy and filipin cytochemistry. J Lipid Res 1995;36:1139-46.
22. Thomas GJ Jr, Agard DA. Quantitative analysis of nucleic acids, proteins, and viruses by Raman band deconvolution. Biophys J 1984;46:763-8.
23. Van der Veen MH, ten Bosch JJ. The influence of mineral loss on the autofluorescent behaviour of in vitro demineralised dentine. Caries Res 1996;30:93-9.
24. Tsuda H, Ruben J, Arends J. Raman spectra of human dentin mineral. Eur J Oral Sci 1996;104:123-31.
25. Puppels GJ, de Mul FF, Otto C, et al. Studying single living cells and chromosomes by confocal Raman microspectroscopy. Nature 1990;347:301-3.
26. Bakker Schut TC, Puppels GJ, Kraan YM, Greve J, van der Maas LL, Figdor CG. Intracellular carotenoid levels measured by Raman microspectroscopy: comparison of lymphocytes from lung cancer patients and healthy individuals. Int J Cancer 1997;74:20-5.
27. Egeberg KD, Springer BA, Martinis SA, Sligar SG, Morikis D, Champion PM. Alteration of sperm whale myoglobin heme axial ligation by site-directed mutagenesis. Biochemistry 1990;29:9783-91.
28. Peticolas WL. Raman spectroscopy of DNA and proteins. Methods Enzymol 1995;246:389-416.
29. Lewis IR, Griffiths PR. Raman spectrometry with fiber-optic sampling. Appl Spectrosc 1996;50:A12-A30.
30. Wach ML, Marple ET; inventors. Visionex Enviva biomedical Raman probe. US Patent Application WO 97/34175.
31. Loudon R. The quantum theory of light. 2nd ed. Oxford: Oxford University Press;1983.
32. Marcuse D. Principles of quantum electronics. New York: Academic Press, 1980.
33. Yariv A. Quantum electronics. 3rd ed.) New York: Wiley; 1989.
34. Chakravarti RN. Fifty years of Raman effect: 1928-1978. J Inst Chem (India) 1978.
35. Raman CV. A new radiation. Indian J Phys 1928;2:387-98.
36. Raman CV, Krishnan KS. A new type of secondary radiation. Nature 1928;121:501-2.
37. Raman CV. A change of wave-length in light scattering. Nature 1928;121:618.
38. Raman CV. The molecular scattering of light. Nobel Lecture. Stockholm: Imprimerie Royale, P.A. Norstedt; 1930.
39. Brennan JF 3rd. Near infrared Raman spectroscopy for human artery histochemistry and histopathology. Cambridge, USA: Massachusetts Institute of Technology, 1995.
40. Buschman HPJ, Deinum G, van der Laarse A, Bruschke AVG, Dasari RR, Feld MS. Chemical modelling of Raman spectra of morphological structures in human coronary artery. Cardiologie 1997;10:482.
41. Römer TJ, Brennan JF 3rd, Bakker Schut TC, et al. Raman spectroscopy for quantifying cholesterol in intact coronary artery wall. Submitted.

42. Tracy RE, Kissling GE. Age and fibroplasia as preconditions for atheronecrosis in human coronary arteries. Arch Pathol Lab Med 1987;111:957-63.
43. Peters RJ, Kok WE, Havenith MG, Rijsterborgh H, van der Wal AC, Visser CA. Histopathologic validation of intracoronary ultrasound imaging. J Am Soc Echocardiogr 1994;7:230-41.
44. Mintz GS, Popma JJ, Pichard AD, et al. Patterns of calcification in coronary artery disease. A statistical analysis of intravascular ultrasound and coronary angiography in 1155 lesions. Circulation 1995;91:1959-65.
45. Nissen SE, Gurley JC, Booth DC, De Maria AN. Intravascular ultrasound of the coronary arteries: current applications and future directions. Am J Cardiol 1992;69:18H-29H.
46. Nissen SE, De Franco AC, Tuzco EM, Moliterno DJ. Coronary intravascular ultrasound: diagnostic and interventional applications. Coron Artery Dis 1995;6:355-67.
47. Benkeser PJ, Churchwell AL, Lee C, Abouelnasr D. Resolution limitations in intravascular ultrasound imaging. J Am Soc Echocardiogr 1993;6:158-65.
48. Groot PH, van Vlijmen BJ, Benson GM, Hofker MH, et al. Quantitative assessment of aortic atherosclerosis in APOE*3 Leiden transgenic mice and its relationship to serum cholesterol exposure. Arterioscler Thromb Vasc Biol 1996;16:926-33.
49. Jukema JW, Zwinderman AH, van Boven AJ, et al. Evidence for a synergistic effect of calcium channel blockers with lipid-lowering therapy in retarding progression of coronary atherosclerosis in symptomatic patients with normal to moderately raised cholesterol levels. The REGRESS Study Group. Arterioscler Thromb Vasc Biol 1996;16:425-30.
50. Römer Tj, Buschman HP, Puppels GJ, et al. Raman spectroscopy provides chemical mappings of atherosclerotic plaques in APOE*3 Leiden transgenic mice [Abstract]. Circulation. In press 1998.

Chapter 4

Coronary Vascular Function in Stable and Unstable Angina

Stefan H.J. Monnink, Hendrik Buikema, Ad J. van Boven and Wiek H. van Gilst

Introduction

Angina pectoris and acute myocardial infarction are the main cardiac manifestations of atherosclerosis. Atherosclerosis is a pathological condition that underlies several important disorders including coronary artery disease, cerebrovascular disease, and diseases of the aorta and peripheral arterial circulation. Since Edward Jenner first attributed angina pectoris to coronary artery disease in 1786, there is a growing understanding about the pathophysiology of coronary artery disease and its complications. The first coronary artery disease manifestation in women is more likely to be angina, whereas in men it more often presents as a myocardial infarction. Even after surviving the acute stage of myocardial infarction, the incidence of re-infarction, sudden death, angina pectoris and cardiac failure are all substantial. Further innovations in diagnosis and treatment of coronary disease will undoubtedly improve the outlook of patients surviving the initial attack.

Pathogenesis of atherosclerosis

Atherosclerosis begins as intimal lipid deposits (fatty streaks of mainly cholesterol and its esters) in childhood and adolescence. In middle age, fatty streaks in some arterial sites are converted into fibrous plaques by continued accumulation of lipids and proliferation of smooth muscle cells

Van der Wall et al. (eds.),
Advanced Imaging in Coronary Artery Disease, 55-66.

and connective tissue, some of which produce the terminal occlusive episode as a consequence of plaque rupture and thrombosis [1] on its intimal surface. The knowledge that atherosclerosis begins early in life stimulated interest in risk factors (serum lipoproteins, smoking and blood pressure) management with two fundamental objectives. First, reduction of ischemic symptoms due to a fixed flow-limiting coronary stenosis, abnormal epicardial vessel tone, intermittent arterial vasospasm, microvascular dysfunction or incomplete collateral development. Second, prevention of clinical events such as cardiac death, myocardial infarction or worsening angina pectoris towards unstable angina due to plaque rupture. The primary locus of the atherosclerotic disease process is the tunica intima covered by a monolayer of cells lining the inside of all blood vessels - the vascular endothelium.

The endothelium

Originally viewed simply as a passive barrier, the endothelium is now considered to be a multifunctional organ whose function is essential to normal vascular physiology. Changes in endothelial structure and function provoked by pathophysiological stimuli can result in localized, acute and chronic alterations in the interaction with blood components and the vessel wall. These alterations include increased permeability to plasma lipoproteins, hyperadhesiveness for leukocytes and a functional imbalance in local pro- and antithrombotic factors, growth stimulators and inhibitors, and vasoactive (dilator, constrictor) substances. These manifestations, collectively termed endothelial dysfunction, play an important role in the initiation and progression of vascular disease.

Role of the endothelium in vasomotor tone

In 1980, Furchgott and Zawadzki described that the presence of endothelial cells was required to elicit relaxation in an isolated artery in response to acetylcholine (figure 1). This discovery triggered a major inquiry into the role of endothelial cells in the local control of vasomotor tone. Endothelium-dependent relaxation was shown to be due to the release of one or more vasodilator substances termed endothelium-derived relaxing factors (EDRF). In recent years it has become evident that not only acetylcholine but also a host of other neurohumoral mediators can trigger the release of these substances. The principle of endothelium-mediated vasodilatation is now established not only in vitro but also in the whole organism, and in particular in human subjects.

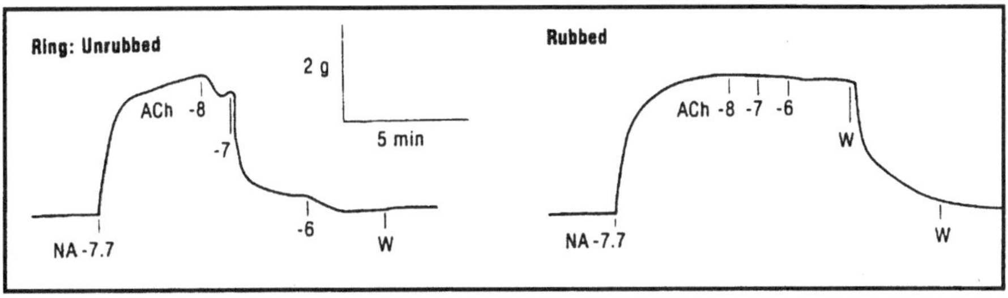

Figure 1. The classic demonstration of Furchgott and colleagues showing that rings of rabbit aorta require endothelial cells (unrubbed) to relax to acetylcholine [35]*.*
Ach = acetylcholine; NA = norepinephrine; W = washout

Nitric oxide (NO) was found to have major similarities to EDRF: NO is responsible for the vasodilator effects of nitrates; it activates the same enzyme as EDRF; like EDRF it is destroyed by certain free radicals; endothelial cells can provide NO and inhibitors of the synthesis of NO prevent most endothelium-dependent relaxations. For these reasons, the EDRF described by Furchgott and Zawadzki has been identified as NO. The release of NO in response to acetylcholine has been demonstrated in many arteries. NO has a very short half-life (5 - 15 seconds) and is destroyed by superoxide anions. It is formed enzymatically in the endothelial cell from a semi-essential amino acid: L-arginine. The enzyme involved has been called NO synthase, and is constitutive in normal endothelial cells. This enzymatic transformation can be inhibited competitively by the L-arginine analogs, such as L-NMMA and NLA. NO acts on the smooth muscle by stimulating a cytosolic enzyme, a soluble guanylate cyclase. Activation of this enzyme accelerates the formation of a cyclic neuropeptide, cyclic 3,5 guanosine monophosphate (cyclic GMP) which causes inhibition of the contractile apparatus. NO can not only be destroyed by superoxide anions, but also scavenged by oxyhemoglobin (figure 2).

Role of NO in vasomotor tone

The described pharmacological observation has major functional repercussions. The endothelial cell secretes NO not only towards the underlying vascular smooth muscle but also into the blood vessel lumen. Under physiological conditions, the presence of oxyhemoglobin in the erythrocytes neutralizes the NO which only has a physiological role at the interface between the endothelial cells and the blood content. In particular

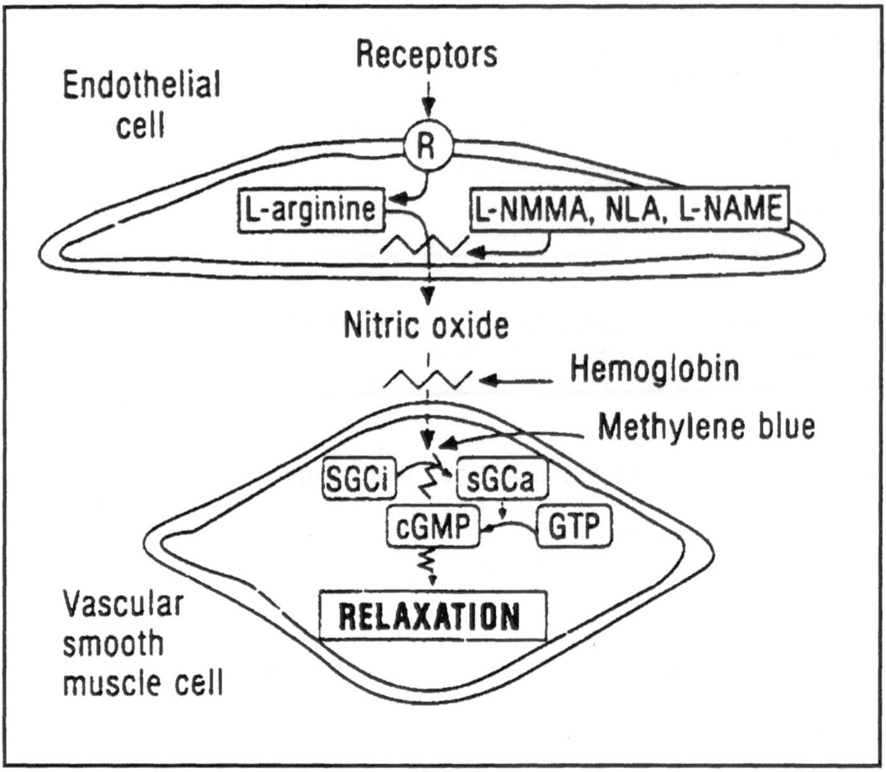

Figure 2. *Production of nitric oxide by endothelial cells and its action on smooth muscle cells [36]. Endothelial receptor, (R); competative analogous of L-arginine (L-NMMA, NLA, L-NAME); inactive (i) or active (a) soluble guanylate cyclase (sGC).*

NO inhibits the adhesion of platelets and leukocytes to the endothelium. It also acts synergistically with prostacyclin to strongly inhibit platelet aggregation. The contribution of NO to vasodilatation in vivo has been demonstrated, when using inhibitors of NO synthesis [2]. Although the discovery of the role of endothelium in local vasomotor control was based on the in vitro response to acetylcholine, it is unlikely, in the intact organism, that acetylcholine ever reaches the endothelial cells. Cholinergic nerve endings are found only in the adventitia of blood vessels and acetylcholine is destroyed by cholinesterase before it can activate the endothelial muscarine receptors. Nevertheless, there are a number of other factors, which can release NO. In the metabolic control of coronary blood flow, shear stress of blood on the arterial wall is one of the main factors in the release of NO [3]. The conclusion was reached that an increased flow rate through an isolated artery substantially increases NO release. A similar result is obtained if a stable flow rate is replaced by a pulsatile one [4,5] (figure 3).

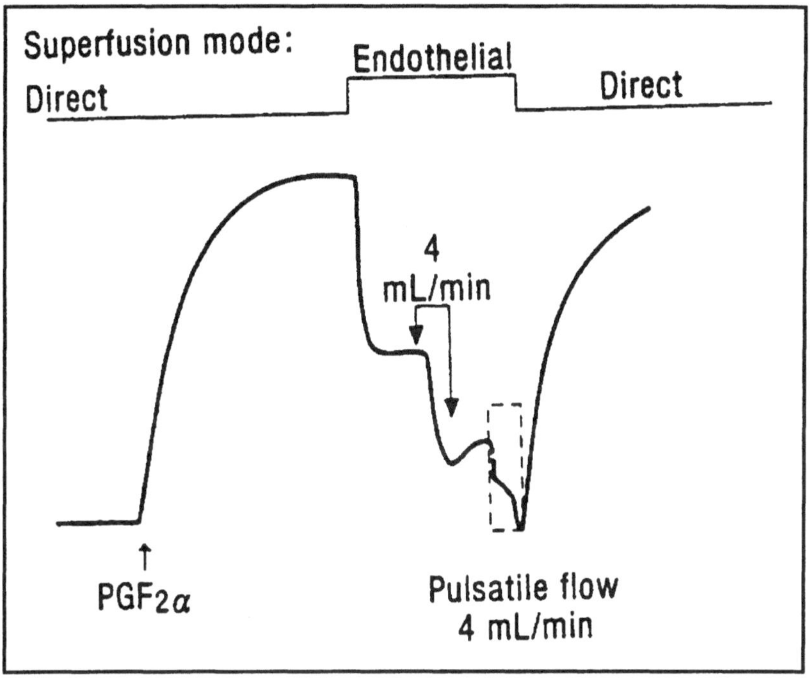

Figure 3. *Relaxation of an endothelium-denuded* $PGF_{2\alpha}$*-precontracted coronary artery ring through stimulation with the perfusate of a endothelium-intact femoral artery segment during increased (2 and 4 ml/min) and pulsatile flow* [5].

NO release by shear stress explains why flow-induced vasodilatation is endothelium-dependent in the intact organism. Thus the resistance vessels in a peripheral organ suddenly dilate, and the resulting source of blood causes dilation of the large arteries leading to that organ. This dilatation is not observed in arteries without endothelium.

Another factor in the release of NO is due to activation of endothelial receptors. The endothelial cell membrane contains many receptors acting to a variety of endogenous substances such as hormones, autacoids or platelet products. The receptors are connected to NO synthesis by various kinds of coupling proteins. Some responses mediated by the endothelium can be inhibited by pertussis toxin, a well-known inhibitor of a subgroup of these coupling proteins. The hormones that contribute to endothelium-dependent regulation at increased oxygen demand are the catecholamines (epinephrine and norepinephrine) [6-8] and vasopressin. The autacoids histamine and bradykinin, responsible for local vasodilatation, are also potent stimulators of the release of NO. In the prevention of unwanted intravascular thrombosis, thrombin and the release products of activated platelets (serotonin and ADP) trigger NO release. NO exerts a negative feedback on platelet aggregation and vasodilatation helps to flush the microaggregates away (figure 4).

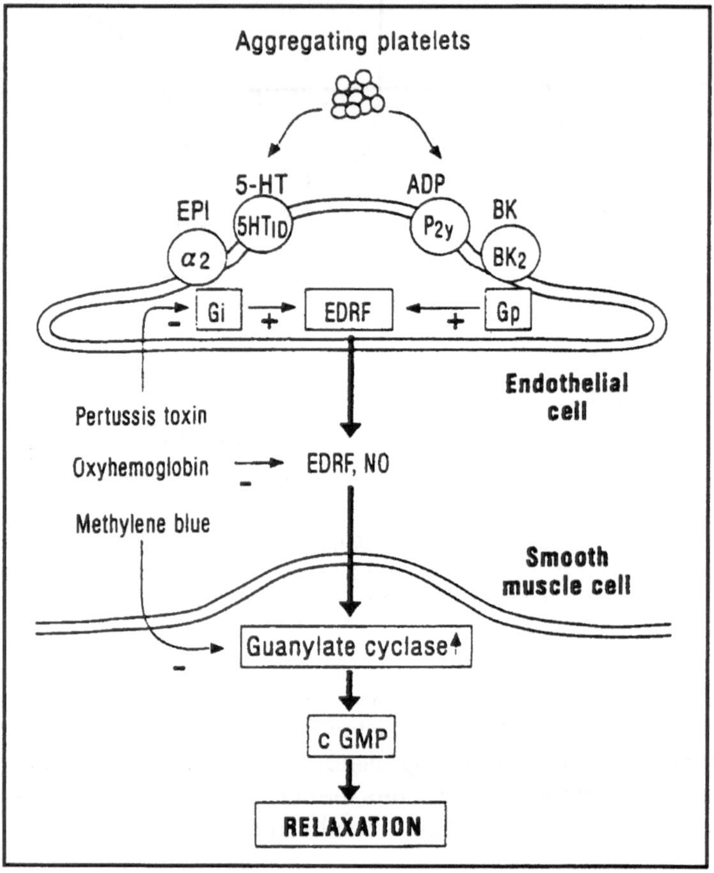

Figure 4. *Illustration showing the paracrine function of the endothelium and some of the processes involved* [37]*. Epinephrine (EPI); α_2 adrenergic receptor (α_2); serotonin (5-HT); serotonin receptor (5-HT_{1D}); adenosine diphosphate (ADP); purinergic receptor (P_{2y}); bradykinin (BK); kinin receptor (BK_2); transducer proteins Gi and Gp; endothelium derived relaxing factor (EDRF); nitric oxide (NO); cyclic GMP (cGMP).*

Abnormal endothelium-dependent responses have been reported in many models of vascular disease studied to date

During the aging process, endothelial cells tend to disappear and are replaced by the growth of surrounding cells. Following the removal of coronary artery endothelium, endothelial regrowth was satisfactory and the number of endothelial cells in the formerly denuded area is approximately double that of the control area. Unfortunately, these regenerated cells have lost some of their ability to release NO, in particular using the pertussis toxin-sensitive response via thrombin and platelet aggregation. There are clinical consequences to this inability of regenerated endothelium in response to platelet aggregation. The area of the regenerated endothelium becomes a site of predilection for triggering exaggerated vasoconstriction in response to platelet aggregation. It is interesting to note that one of the early characteristics of human coronary artery disease is a tendency to hyperconstriction in response to serotonin or acetylcholine [9]. Endothelial dysfunction, as demonstrated by the abnormal response to ergonovine [10], is believed to be the fundamental step in the progression of atherosclerosis. Aging, coupled with risk factors such as hypertension, smoking and stress, accelerate endothelial aging and hence the process of endothelial regeneration, endothelial dysfunction and atherosclerosis [11-13]. The development of atherosclerosis and especially coronary artery disease, which continues to be a leading cause of morbidity and mortality, is one presentation in a continuum of events that can lead to end-stage heart disease [14-17]. Therefore it is of clinical importance to improve or restore endothelial function in the prevention of end-stage heart disease.

Reversal of endothelial dysfunction

Endothelial dysfunction is associated with cholesterol levels in humans [18,19] and endothelium-dependent dilatation in hypercholesterolemic patients can be restored by short-term administration of the EDRF substrate L-arginine[20]. In symptomatic men with significant coronary atherosclerosis and normal to moderately elevated serum cholesterol, Jukema et al. observed less progression of coronary atherosclerosis and fewer new cardiovascular events in the group of patients treated with lipid lowering drugs [21]. Treasure et al. demonstrated that cholesterol lowering significantly improved endothelium-mediated responses in the coronary arteries of patients with atherosclerosis. Such improvement in the local regulation of coronary arterial tone could potentially relieve ischemic symptoms and signal the stabilization of the atherosclerotic plaque [22], which was demonstrated by

Van Boven et al. They showed a reduced transient myocardial ischemia in men with documented coronary artery disease and optimal lipid lowering therapy[23].

Also medical intervention by angiotensin-converting enzyme (ACE) inhibition may improve endothelial function. This was not only demonstrated in the TREND study in normotensive patients who did not have severe hyperlipidemia or evidence of heart failure [24,25] but also in patients who had evidence of heart failure [26]. The benefits of ACE inhibition are likely to be due to attenuation of the contractile effects and superoxide-generating effects of angiotensin II and to enhancement of endothelial cell release of NO secondary to diminished breakdown of bradykinin.

Future directions

Despite all efforts of risk factor management, improvement or restoration of endothelial function, and (aggressive) treatment by anti-ischemic medication, coronary balloon angioplasty even with stent implantation or coronary bypass surgery, coronary artery disease is still of major importance in total morbidity and mortality. In a recently published trial it was demonstrated that, 5 years after successful coronary angioplasty, a substantial number of patients developed recurrent ischemia [27]. However, recurrent ischemia may occur in the absence of restenosis, probably due to coronary endothelial dysfunction at the dilated coronary segment. Nowadays, intracoronary stents are implanted in 50-60% of all coronary angioplasty procedures, and substantially reduce angiographically detected restenosis [28-30]. After successful balloon angioplasty, a drug-induced coronary artery spasm at the dilated segment is frequently associated with restenosis [31]. This suggests that initial endothelial dysfunction is associated with subsequent restenosis of the lesion. Balloon angioplasty in experimental studies causes denudation of endothelial cells in the acute phase [32], but re-endothelialization occurs in weeks with a reversal to normal function within 4 - 6 weeks [33]. Also after stent implantation endothelial cells regenerate, but their function will be impaired shortly after implantation [34]. The long-term effect of stents on the human coronary endothelial function at the site of the implantation and on the segments adjacent to the stent was never studied before. It was hypothesized that a long time after re-endothelialization of the stent surface, the endothelial function of the adjacent segments is restored. However, two recent studies by Caramori et al. [38], and Monnink et al. (1998 submitted) showed a marked coronary endothelial dysfunction six months after stent implantation without a loss of vasodilative capacity. This endothelial dysfunction might be caused by a downstream release of mediators from the site of the stent implantation that chronically affect the distal endothelial function. These findings may be of clinical importance since stents are implanted more frequently during angioplasty procedures without a proven benefit on cardiac mortality, when compared to conventional balloon angioplasty. Furthermore, endothelial dysfunction might be associated with restenosis, post-angioplasty angina pectoris and ischemia. Therefore additional therapy directed towards normalization of endothelial function may reduce cardiac morbidity and mortality in the future.

General literature

V. Fuster, R. Ross and E.J. Topol. Atherosclerosis and Coronary Artery Disease. Pennsylvania, USA: Lippincott-Raven Publishers, 1996.

C.M. Boulanger and P.M. Vanhoutte. The endothelium: a pivotal role in health and cardiovascular disease. Courbevoie Cedex, France: Servier International, 1994.

References

1. Weitz JI. Activation of blood coagulation by plaque rupture: mechanisms and prevention. Am J Cardiol 1995; 75:18B-22B.
2. Quyyumi AA, Dakak N, Andrews NP, Gilligan DM, Panza JA, Cannon RO 3rd. Contribution of nitric oxide to metabolic coronary vasodilation in the human heart. Circulation 1995; 92:320-6.
3. Olsson RA, Bunger R. Metabolic control of coronary blood flow. Prog Cardiovasc Dis 1987; 29:369-87.
4. Canty JM Jr, Schwartz JS. Nitric oxide mediates flow-dependent epicardial coronary vasodilation to changes in pulse frequency but not mean flow in conscious dogs. Circulation 1994; 89:375-84.
5. Rubanyi GM, Romero JC, Vanhoutte PM. Flow-induced release of endothelium-derived relaxing factor. Am J Physiol 1986; 250:H1145-9.
6. Vita JA, Treasure CB, Yeung AC, et al. Patients with evidence of coronary endothelial dysfunction as assessed by acetylcholine infusion demonstrate marked increase in sensitivity to constrictor effects of catecholamines. Circulation 1992; 85:1390-7.
7. Vatner SF. Regulation of coronary resistance vessels and large coronary arteries. Am J Cardiol 1985; 56:16E-22E.
8. Cocks TM, Angus JA. Endothelium-dependent relaxation of coronary arteries by noradrenaline and serotonin. Nature 1983; 305:627-30.
9. Yasue H, Matsuyama K, Matsuyama K, Okumura K, Morikami Y, Ogawa H. Responses of angiographically normal human coronary arteries to intracoronary injection of acetylcholine by age and segment. Possible role of early coronary atherosclerosis. Circulation 1990; 81:482-90.
10. Nobuyoshi M, Tanaka M, Nosaka H, et al. Progression of coronary atherosclerosis: is coronary spasm related to progression? J.Am.Coll.Cardiol. 1991; 18:904-10.
11. Vita JA, Treasure CB, Nabel EG, et al. Coronary vasomotor response to acetylcholine relates to risk factors for coronary artery disease. Circulation 1990; 81:491-7.
12. Quyyumi AA, Dakak N, Andrews NP, et al. Nitric oxide activity in the human coronary circulation. Impact of risk factors for coronary atherosclerosis. J Clin Invest 1995; 95:1747-55.
13. Zeiher AM, Drexler H, Saurbier B, Just H. Endothelium-mediated coronary blood flow modulation in humans. Effects of age, atherosclerosis, hypercholesterolemia, and hypertension. J Clin Invest 1993; 92:652-62.
14. Ontkean M, Gay R, Greenberg B. Diminished endothelium-derived relaxing factor activity in an experimental model of chronic heart failure. Circ Res 1991; 69:1088-96.

15. Drexler H, Hayoz D, Munzel T, et al. Endothelial function in chronic congestive heart failure. Am J Cardiol 1992; 69:1596-601.
16. Treasure CB, Alexander RW. The dysfunctional endothelium in heart failure. J Am Coll Cardiol 1993; 22 (4 Suppl A):129A-134A.
17. Drexler H, Hornig B. Importance of endothelial function in chronic heart failure. J Cardiovasc Pharmacol 1996; 27 Suppl 2:S9-12.
18. Steinberg HO, Bayazeed B, Hook G, Johnson A, Cronin J, Baron AD. Endothelial dysfunction is associated with cholesterol levels in the high normal range in humans. Circulation 1997; 96:3287-93.
19. Voors AA, Oosterga M, Buikema H, et al. Dyslipidemia and endothelium-dependent relaxation in internal mammary arteries used for coronary bypass surgery. Cardiovasc Res 1997; 34:568-74.
20. Drexler H, Zeiher AM, Meinzer K, Just H. Correction of endothelial dysfunction in coronary microcirculation of hypercholesterolaemic patients by L-arginine. Lancet 1991; 338:1546-50.
21. Jukema JW, Bruschke AV, van Boven AJ, et al. Effects of lipid lowering by pravastatin on progression and regression of coronary artery disease in symptomatic men with normal to moderately elevated serum cholesterol levels. The Regression Growth Evaluation Statin Study (REGRESS). Circulation 1995; 91:2528-40.
22. Treasure CB, Klein JL, Weintraub WS, et al. Beneficial effects of cholesterol-lowering therapy on the coronary endothelium in patients with coronary artery disease. N Engl J Med 1995; 332:481-7.
23. Van Boven AJ, Jukema JW, Zwinderman AH, Crijns HJ, Lie KI, Bruschke AV. Reduction of transient myocardial ischemia with pravastatin in addition to the conventional treatment in patients with angina pectoris. REGRESS Study Group. Circulation 1996; 94:1503-5.
24. Rajagopalan S, Harrison DG. Reversing endothelial dysfunction with ACE inhibitors. A new trend. Circulation 1996; 94:240-3.
25. Mancini GB, Henry GC, Macaya C, et al. Angiotensin-converting enzyme inhibition with quinapril improves endothelial vasomotor dysfunction in patients with coronary artery disease. The TREND (Trial on Reversing ENdothelial Dysfunction) Study [published erratum appears in: Circulation 1996;94:1490]. Circulation 1996; 94:258-65.
26. Mulder P, Elfertak L, Richard V, et al. Peripheral artery structure and endothelial function in heart failure: effect of ACE inhibition. Am J Physiol 1996; 271:H469-77.
27. Five-year clinical and functional outcome comparing bypass surgery and angioplasty in patients with multivessel coronary disease. A multicenter randomized trial. Writing Group for the Bypass Angioplasty Revascularization Investigation (BARI) Investigators. JAMA 1997; 277:715-21.
28. Fischman DL, Leon MB, Baim DS, et al. A randomized comparison of coronary-stent placement and balloon angioplasty in the treatment of coronary artery disease. Stent Restenosis Study Investigators. N Engl J Med. 1994; 331:496-501.
29. Serruys PW, de Jaegere P, Kiemeneij F, et al. A comparison of balloon-expandable-stent implantation with balloon angioplasty in patients with coronary artery disease. Benestent Study Group. N Engl J Med 1994; 331:489-95.

30. Serruys PW, Emanuelsson HU, van der Giessen W, et al. Heparin-coated Palmaz-Schatz stents in human coronary arteries. Early outcome of the Benestent-II Pilot Study. Circulation 1996; 93:412-22.
31. Bertrand ME, Lablanche JM, Fourrier JL, Gommeaux A, Ruel M. Relation to restenosis after percutaneous transluminal coronary angioplasty to vasomotion of the dilated coronary arterial segment. Am J Cardiol 1989; 63:277-81.
31. El Tamimi H, Davies GJ, Crea F, Maseri A. Response of human coronary arteries to acetylcholine after injury by coronary angioplasty. J Am Coll Cardiol 1993; 21:1152-7.
33. Weidinger FF, McLenachan JM, Cybulsky MI, et al. Persistent dysfunction of regenerated endothelium after balloon angioplasty of rabbit iliac artery. Circulation 1990; 81:1667-79.
34. Jenkins JS, Webel R, Laughlin MH, et al. The effects of intravascular stents on vasomotion in porcine coronary arteries. J Invasive Cardiol 1995; 7:200-6.
35. Furchgott RF, Zawadzki JV. The obligatory role of endothelial cells in the relaxation of arterial smooth muscle by acetylcholine. Nature 1980; 288:373-6.
36. Vanhoutte PM, Eber B. Endothelium-derived relaxing and contracting factors. Wien Klin Wochenschr 1991; 103:405-11.
37. Vanhoutte PM. Serotonin, hypertension and vascular disease. Neth Med 1991; 38:35-42.
38. Caramori PR, Lima VC, Seidelin PH, Newton GE, Adelman AG. Endothelial dysfunction distal to stents implanted for more than six months [abstract]. Circulation 1997;96 (8 Suppl):I756.

Chapter 5

THE ROLE OF IMAGING TECHNIQUES IN THE DIAGNOSIS OF ATHEROSCLEROSIS

Han J.G.H. Mulder, Albert V.G. Bruschke, Martin J. Schalij
and Ernst E. van der Wall

Introduction

Atherosclerosis is the leading cause of morbidity and mortality in the Western world. The disease is a syndrome with a variety of clinical expressions dependent on the stage and activity of the pathological process. These expressions may vary from asymptomatic, minor plaque formation to acute myocardial infarction. An important challenge for the contemporary imaging technique is the creation of an image of the atherosclerotic lesions which are "hot". That is the identification of lesions that are prone to rupture, thereby implying an increased risk for the individual patient for an acute cardiovascular event.

The pathophysiological basis of the wide range of clinical expressions can be found, among others, in the combination of arterial wall anatomy and functionality. In the past, emphasis was placed on techniques that identified encroachment of vessel lumen. However, while lumen patency is considered to be a surrogate indicator of atherosclerosis, it is not always coherent with the current and future clinical expression of the disease. Techniques, providing functional information of the supposed culprit lesions, yield a different kind of information about the present state of the atherosclerosis and complement the "luminographic" information. Knowledge of both anatomy and function will lead to a better prediction of the disease process, so that it can be better monitored and interventions can be undertaken which are neither premature or delayed.

Van der Wall et al. (eds.),
Advanced Imaging in Coronary Artery Disease, 67-99.

Coronary atherosclerosis is part of the generalized syndrome of atherosclerosis. The imaging of this subterritory of atherosclerosis presents a special challenge. Not only to establish enough accuracy because of the very critical importance of this subset of vessels, but also because of the complicating imaging aspects of coronary vessels themselves, i.e. small caliber and continuous motion. This chapter will focus on the coronary arteries themselves.

Atherosclerosis

Arteriosclerosis, a generic term for the thickening and hardening of the arterial wall, is responsible for the majority of deaths in most Westernized societies. One type of arteriosclerosis is atherosclerosis, the disorder of the larger arteries that primarily forms the basis of the coronary artery disease.

Ever since Virchow's initial statement about the disease in the mid-eighteenth century, the etiology of the syndrome atherosclerosis has remained a controversial topic. Atherosclerosis today is seen as an advancing, chronic inflammatory condition of the vascular wall. This generally, stable, quiescent condition can abruptly be converted into an acute clinical event by plaque "instability". Instability, with or without plaque rupture, leads to micro-aggregate formation or even complete obstruction of the epicardial conductance vessels as a result of massive local thrombosis.[1,2] At present, the basic mechanisms initiating the sequence of atherogenesis are thought to involve low-density lipoproteins and oxidative processes.[3]

Atherogenesis

The process of atherogenesis starts with oxidation of low-density lipoprotein particles after these have become entrapped in the subendothelial space. During the process of oxidation the low-density lipoprotein particle loses its innate specific properties (apo-B oxidation), which results in it being "absorbed" by recruited macrophages and smooth muscle cells without any feedback. This unrestricted process results in "foam cell" formation, the pathological hallmark of atherosclerosis.[3]

Altogether these foam cells form fatty streaks, and these initially small "plaques", which expand through the imbedding of new, mononuclear cells, lead to the proliferation of already existing macrophages and smooth muscle cells and the formation of a necrotic core. Finally, thrombosis may occur, initiated by "activated", unstable plaques which is often accompanied by plaque rupture.[1,2]

The role of the vascular endothelial cells and their dysfunction seems to become more and more important in relation to the rate of events of the clinical sequelae in coronary artery disease. This inner lining of the cardiovascular system seems to participate actively in both normal and disrupted vascular physiology as well in the pathogenesis of vascular diseases such as atherosclerosis.[4]

Clinical sequelae of atherosclerosis

When the pathophysiological processes of atherogenesis are categorized according to resulting clinical sequelae, three primary processes evolve. First, there is slow encroachment of the coronary artery lumen by plaque expansion. Secondly there is progressive dysfunction of the coronary artery wall, and thirdly there is acute local thrombosis caused by plaque rupture and severe dysfunctional endothelium.

Stable angina pectoris is probably the result of the first and second category processes. Slow encroachment causes ever more myocardial ischemia and a lesser tolerance for increased oxygen demand. Attributing to this intolerance is the dysfunctional vessel wall, which may react inadequately to, for example, circulating stress hormones causing vasoconstriction instead of vasodilation.[5] This vessel wall dysfunction might just surpass the critical level of lumen narrowing, causing a decrease in the oxygen supply to a critical level.[6]

The pathological substrate of *unstable angina* is plaque rupture and/or plaque activation with subsequent platelet activation and thrombus formation.[7] This local thrombosis can result in transient lumen obstruction or, if all endogenous thrombolytic measures fail, in a more permanent obstruction. Unstable angina pectoris is related to the above-mentioned second and third category processes. The role of the dysfunctional endothelium (second category) has to be seen in the perspective of modulation of the thrombotic/thrombolytic process. Platelet aggregation, for example, triggers nitric oxide release in the healthy endothelium.[8]

This effect is due to the release of substances by aggregating platelets. Normally these substances cause, through interaction with healthy endothelium, vasodilation, inhibition of platelet aggregation, and inhibition of platelet adhesion to the vessel wall. This results in elimination of the micro-aggregate and, thereby, the prevention of progressive vascular occlusion. The opposite is true in case of endothelial dysfunction where the synthesis of counteracting substances is compromised.

Diagnosis of coronary atherosclerosis
Despite the availability of a variety of tests, detection of atherosclerosis usually awaits one of the clinical events that occur after a critical decrease of blood flow in an involved vessel. This has resulted in improved knowledge of the prevalence and incidence of arteriosclerosis and most of the inferences concerning its causes derived from tabulations of the appearance of its sequelae.

The other way around is also true. Generally all patients with myocardial infarction, as defined by electrocardiographic and enzymatic changes, have coronary atherosclerosis. Therefore, the presence of myocardial infarction is a strong marker for the presence of coronary atherosclerosis. Most other events, like chest pain attributed to coronary artery disease, are less strong indicators of the presence of coronary atherosclerosis. They might also be of other pathophysiological origin.

Consequently, atherosclerosis is most often determined by "surrogate" markers. For example, myocardial infarction or radiopaque calcium particles observed at coronary angiograms are very strong markers for the presence of atherosclerosis, whereas high blood pressure or a dilated ventricle are weak ones. Not only being markers for the presence of atherosclerosis, they are also indicators of the risk of a cardiovascular event. However, an increased presence of a marker is not always consistent with increased risk. The relation between risk and marker is very variable among the markers.

Markers derived from "scans" obtained from imaging modalities also have implications for the detection and quantification of atherosclerosis and the prediction of the clinical prognosis. The best known marker is probably the presence of coronary artery stenosis at angiograms obtained with coronary angiography. This marker is a strong indicator of the presence of atherosclerosis. The traditional view that the clinical course of coronary artery disease is closely linked to the severity of coronary artery occlusion, however, has been recently partially abandoned.[9] In addition, mild stenosis can lead to acute events. For the individual patient this has implications with respect to the diagnostic techniques which assess the presence and activity of atherosclerosis. Apparently, additional markers are needed, next to percentage stenosis, in order to achieve better insight into the possible future occurrence of adverse events.

The present imaging modalities range from traditional "luminography" (angiography) to positron emission tomography (PET) imaging of arterial wall metabolism. They all measure aspects of the ongoing atherosclerotic process, from a different perspective. In this article, we will focus on the imaging techniques of atherosclerosis in coronary arteries, especially on imaging of the coronary anatomy and local vascular function.

Atherosclerosis and imaging

Currently visualized aspects of coronary atherosclerosis (table 1,graph 1)

	Coronary vessel morphology / structure		Vessel inner surface	Molecular exploration of the vessel wall			Patho-physio-logy
	Longitudinal	Cross sectional		Calcium pockets	Chemical Composition	Meta-bolism	
Cine-angiography	Yes	No	No	Yes[+]	No	No	No
Cine-angiography +endothelial function analysis	No Yes	No No	No No	No Yes[+]	No No	No No	No Yes
Angioscopy	Yes	No	Yes	No	No	No	No
Intra-coronary ultrasound	Yes	Yes	No	Yes	No	No	Yes
Electron beam computed tomography	Yes	No	No	Yes	No	No	No
Magnetic resonance imaging	Yes[*]	Yes[*]	No	Yes[*]	Yes[*]	No	No
Raman Imaging	No	No	No	Yes[#]	Yes[#]	No	No
Nuclear Imaging	No	No	No	No	No	Yes[*]	No
Optical coherence tomography	Yes[*]	Yes[*]	No	No	No	No	No

+ Only major pockets

* Possible future developments

Feasibility in vivo unknown yet

***Table 1.** Visualized aspects of coronary atherosclerosis and imaging modalities*

Visualized aspects of coronary atherosclerosis

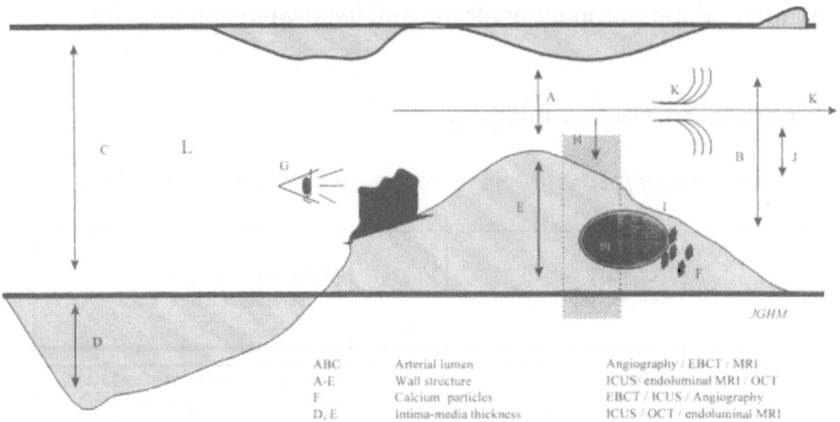

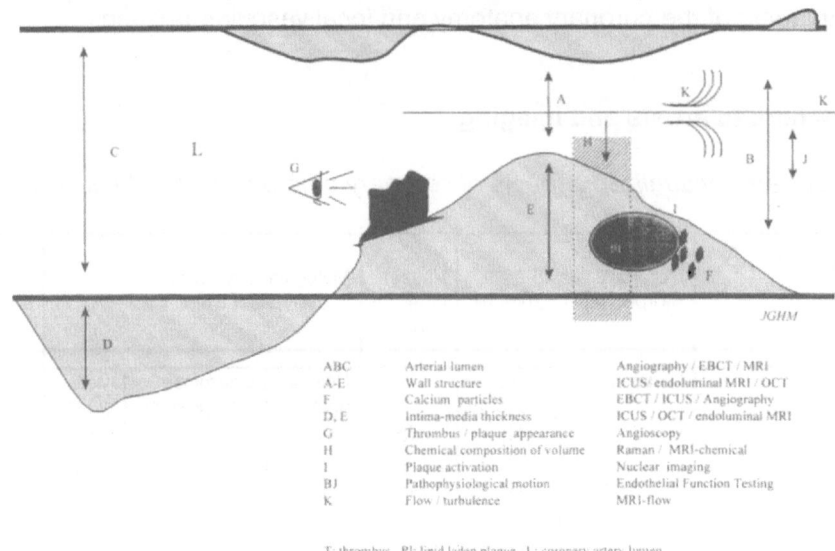

ABC	Arterial lumen	Angiography / EBCT / MRI
A-E	Wall structure	ICUS/ endoluminal MRI / OCT
F	Calcium particles	EBCT / ICUS / Angiography
D, E	Intima-media thickness	ICUS / OCT / endoluminal MRI
G	Thrombus / plaque appearance	Angioscopy
H	Chemical composition of volume	Raman / MRI-chemical
I	Plaque activation	Nuclear imaging
BJ	Pathophysiological motion	Endothelial Function Testing
K	Flow / turbulence	MRI-flow

T: thrombus. Pl: lipid laden plaque, L: coronary artery lumen
CD : Compensatory enlargement
EBCT: electron beam computed tomography, MRI: Magnetic resonance imaging,
ICUS: intra-coronary ultrasound, OCT: Optical coherence tomography

Graphic 1

It is difficult to make direct and exact assessments of the presence of atherosclerosis in the coronary artery. Almost all present techniques determine “surrogate” markers for this disease. This is no major problem given the pragmatic purpose of atherosclerotic imaging, which is the assessment of present risk and functional importance of the disease process. In daily practice, all markers derived from imaging techniques are judged valuable in relation to their ability to predict the risk and functional importance of the disease process. This is the reason why many markers have evolved and vanished in the course of time, even though some of them, with respect to pure patho-anatomical atherosclerosis diagnosis, might have been very useful.

Deformity of the arterial lumen

Imaging the coronary artery lumen is probably the oldest and still most utilized method of assessing coronary atherosclerosis. The imaging of coronary vessel lumen has proven to be an accurate method for assessing coronary stenosis, with high validity and reproducibility. This resulted in the frequent use as a parameter in trials to monitor progression/regression of coronary atherosclerosis.

However, despite impressive developments in lumen imaging (e.g. quantitative coronary angiography, electron beam computed tomography), the validity for identification of early (noninvasive) disease with "luminography" is poor. Also, advanced disease of the wall of the coronary artery that does not "invade" the lumen is overlooked.[10] The recognition of the process known as remodeling, or compensatory enlargement, made it clear that "luminography" overlooks a significant part of developing atherosclerosis. It was demonstrated that coronary vessels can remodel and accommodate plaque without compromising luminal patency of "stenoses" up to 40%.[11] (graphic 1, CD) Therefore, it is not relevant how high the temporal or spatial resolution is with a certain "luminographic" imaging technique or to which high level of accuracy the images are being analyzed. The inability to measure the "underground" development is inherent to the measured parameter, which entirely depends on the encroachment of the lumen.

Structural composition of the arterial walls

Another approach to assess coronary atherosclerosis is the visualization of the coronary artery wall anatomy/structure. When atherosclerosis develops, changes occur in the macro/micro structure of the wall, which can be assessed by various imaging techniques. The parameters derived from these images can be both qualitative and quantitative.

A qualitative parameter is the appearance of the coronary plaque on these *"images"*. For example the, lipid-laden, *"soft"* lesions, which do not necessarily have to compromise arterial lumen to a great extent, are an important finding of present atherosclerosis. They are related to the occurrence of coronary thrombosis.[2]

A simultaneous qualitative and quantitative parameter is the presence of *calcium* pockets/layers in the coronary artery wall. The presence of calcium in the coronary artery wall is the result of reorganization of local small thrombi, appearing every time a plaque rupture happens. The occurrence of these, mainly clinically silent, plaque ruptures can be frequent [12] and the reorganization process results in deposition of fibrous matrix and calcium deposits. In addition, the process of atherogenesis itself is accompanied by the creation of calcium deposits in time. Therefore, calcium is seen as a marker of advancing atherosclerosis. Nevertheless, demonstration of calcification does not always indicate the presence of atherosclerosis, and complete luminal obstruction may occur in the absence of any calcification.[13]

Detection of calcification is most valuable in persons less than 40 years old in whom modification of risk factors may be important and the absence of calcification in coronary arteries may diminish the need for further testing.[14] In addition, the progression and possible regression of calcification can be used as an indicator of the progress/regress of the atherosclerotic process. At this moment, no fully validated method for determining the quantity of coronary calcium is available and we do not know whether the amount of calcium is a consistently accurate reflection of the extent of the local atherosclerosis. Furthermore, the prognostic significance of coronary calcium in any given atherosclerotic lesion remains to be established.

A quantitative parameter, derived from coronary artery wall scanning is the *arterial intima-media thickness (IMT).* There is increasing evidence that an increment in arterial intima-media thickness represents early atherosclerotic involvement of the vessel wall. The clinical importance of this measurement is, however, still being debated.[15] The IMT seems, at least in peripheral vessels like the carotid arteries, to represent a valuable parameter within the framework of future coronary heart disease[16, 17] and has already proven its use for monitoring purposes. With the development of high-resolution imaging techniques, it has become possible to assess this parameter accurately in coronary arteries.[18] Future trials will prove its significance.

Optical aspects of the vascular wall

The earliest optically detectable lesions of coronary atherosclerosis are the fatty streaks. In due time, the typical crescent-shaped plaques also become visible. The qualitative aspects derived from optical, intracoronary observation can be separated into plaque appearance and the possible presence of thrombus.

Normal coronary arteries appear smooth and white with angioscopy. The *atherosclerotic plaque* however, is more yellowish.[19] Gray-white lesions represented fibrous plaque with a small amount of plaque degeneration. The yellow color is closely related to degenerated plaque or atheroma and is associated with unstable coronary syndromes.[20] In the case of unstable angina the plaque underlying intracoronary thrombus is usually yellow and/or disrupted, which supports in vitro observations that lipid-rich plaques are highly thrombogenic and that disruption of these plaques is associated with in situ thrombosis.[21]

Local *thrombus* is a next finding in angioscopy. The red thrombus, in particular is important because this is a sign of atherosclerotic plaque instability, and has clear clinical implications. For example, angioscopically-protruding thrombus at the angioplasty site is significantly associated with greater "late loss" in coronary artery lumen diameter.[22] Furthermore, it has been shown that the presence of yellow color and thrombus at site of the culprit lesions are associated with an eight-fold increase in risk of adverse outcome of the angioplasty.[23]

Molecular components of the vascular wall
The improvement of present techniques and the development of new ones will enable researchers to directly assess the chemical composition of the vessel wall. The chemical composition can inform us about the presence and quantity of cholesterol, etc. This results in a direct "chemical picture" of the vessel wall. These pictures seem to be strongly correlated with the grade of atherosclerosis and, certain composition profiles are correlated with plaques compositions which have proven to be at risk. Monitoring of substances involved in the biochemical process of atherogenesis and plaque activation is another application. The scintigraphic monitoring of radioisotope-labeled low-density lipoprotein is such an example.

Coronary flow disturbances
Marked luminal narrowing can cause predictable decreases in coronary flow. This is intimately related with other hemodynamic parameters like pressure drop over the stenosis, coronary flow reserve and flow profile disturbances in the post stenotic area. Therefore, assessment of one of these parameters gives information on present stenosis. Unfortunately the degree of stenosis does not reflect the thrombogenic potential, which may lead to acute myocardial ischemic syndromes.[2] However, because some new techniques can assess disturbances noninvasively, it could potentially add to the monitoring of major changes of coronary vessel morphology.

Pathophysiology of the vascular wall
Atherosclerosis induced, pathophysiological changes can be visualized by means of provocation or monitoring.
The vessel can be *provoked* to respond to impulses. One such as impulse can be the intracoronary infusion of acetylcholine. This "double agent" provokes the coronary arteries to display different reactions, depending on

the degree of disease of the coronary artery wall. Especially assessment of "functional" significance of an atherosclerotic coronary artery lesion seems to be a promising parameter.[24]

Monitoring of the pathophysiology can be established by the registration of infrared (heat) emitted locally from the coronary wall. Because atherosclerosis is a chronic inflammatory condition, the metabolism at active lesions is relatively higher than elsewhere. Hence, it offers the possibility of identifying activated lesions through imaging of slight temperature differences.

Imaging derived information

The most extensively recognized form of coronary atherosclerosis is the development of plaques. This is one of the reason why coronary angiography has developed into the "gold standard" for detecting atherosclerotic lesions in coronary arteries. As discussed earlier, this imaging modality can only provide information on vessel morphology, which is not necessary consistent with the true extent of the atherosclerotic plaque or the functional integrity of the coronary vessel wall. Many other imaging techniques have been developed and, by providing different kinds of information on the ongoing atherosclerotic process, some of them have complemented the shortcomings of angiography.

The categorizing of different kinds of information, provided by the different imaging techniques, can be done on basis of the "object" studied, like vessel lumen, molecular composition, or vasomotion. In a more generalized point of view the information can be divided into primarily anatomic (lumen, wall structure, molecular composition) information or primarily functional (vasomotion, increased metabolism) information. In addition, this information can be derived at a local site of the coronary artery or from a generalized area related to a coronary artery system or even the whole heart.

Performing this categorization results in four groups of imaging derived information, related to atherosclerosis:

A. Anatomic generalized information

General vessel morphology (e.g. classic angiography/electron beam computed tomography)

B. Anatomic local information

Local vessel morphology (e.g. Intravascular ultrasound/Raman spectroscopy)

C. Functional generalized information
Segment/global heart (dys)function (e.g. exercise electrocardiography/ scintigraphy)
D. Functional local information
Local vessel (dys)function (e.g. endothelial function assessment)

The imaging modalities described between the brackets are examples. Some of these modalities also yield information of other categories, but in general, they primarily provide information belonging to the category to which they are assigned.

Methodological aspects of imaging coronary atherosclerosis
Imaging modalities "scan" the entity of interest and produce an image of the process, with information depicted for which the "technique" of the modality is sensitive. In this respect, the term imaging can be viewed broadly. A method producing temperature reading at a certain point of the coronary vessel is as much an image as a picture of the lumen of a coronary artery.

Coronary artery imaging has certain complicating challenges compared with imaging of peripheral vessels. Primarily, there is the generally smaller caliber of the coronary arteries (4-5 mm). Furthermore, there is the frequent tortuosity. However, most disturbing is the almost continuous, complex movement of the vessels in the three-dimensional space. Spatial displacement during the heart cycle is in the range of 1-2 cm. The displacement happens with peak velocities of more than 20 cm/s during certain phases such as the rapid cardiac contraction.[25] This is the reason why some modalities for imaging atherosclerosis are only applicable to peripheral vessels at the present state of the technique.

The three-dimensional motion of the coronary vessels is the result of two major contributing factors; respiration and heart muscle contraction. Both can be regular and predictable. The opposite can also happen. To capture the image with sufficient detail, the techniques have to have enough spatial and temporary resolution. Coronary angiography is a technique with sufficient capabilities of both. The image is acquired within milliseconds, which is short enough to "freeze" the movement of the coronary artery. The resolution also is well below clinical necessity.

Other techniques like magnetic resonance imaging need more time to acquire an image. The problem of movement during acquisition is circumvented through application of electrocardiography and respiration gated techniques, which makes it possible to divide acquisition time into acceptable individual parts of the cycle. Only upon the cyclic return to the same spatial position of the artery, information is acquired. This moment of acquisition should be short enough to "freeze" the artery movement. Adding the captured information over a period of time, assuming the spatial position of the artery to be the same at every moment of acquisition, results in a good and clear "image". In reality the "gated" techniques are more difficult than might be expected. The problems have different origins. For example, in appropriate timing of the acquisition period may occur as a result of incorrect prediction of the next moment of identical spatial position of the coronary tree. This might be due to irregular breathing, misregistration between breath holds and beat-to-beat heart variability. The technique of the imaging modalities often develops stepwise with respect to temporal and spatial resolution. Probably, most of the techniques will arrive some time (in the near or far future) at a point where they will be capable of adequately acquiring an image, in a period short enough to prevent the need for gating.

Three-dimensional reconstruction is another interesting development in current imaging techniques, coming within the reach of the clinician since the development of ever-faster computers. However, the techniques that depend on gated acquisitions of two-dimensional slices for three-dimensional reconstruction, face the same problems as the previously mentioned gated acquisition techniques.

Imaging modalities for imaging coronary atherosclerosis

Before 1970, fluoroscopy and invasive angiography were the only widely used imaging modalities for assessment of coronary atherosclerosis. Since then techniques have advanced rapidly resulting in several modalities of imaging atherosclerosis in the coronary artery. One of the interesting developments was the appearance of noninvasive techniques to assess the disease process. Current noninvasive modalities can, reasonably successfully, screen for serious obstructive coronary artery disease by detecting stress-provoked ischemic changes in electrical repolarization, wall motion, or myocardial radiolabeled tracer uptake. Unfortunately, it appears that morbid events such as unstable angina pectoris and myocardial infarction are poorly related to these phenomena. However, the invasive modalities, which might produce a better assessment of event risk, have potential inherent risks for the patient because of their invasive nature. New, noninvasive modalities, assessing other qualities of the disease process, might fill this diagnostic gap (e.g. nuclear imaging of "active" coronary plaques) (table 2).

	Ionizing radiation required	Contrast media needed	Acquisition time per scan	Invasive
Angiography	Yes	Yes	Seconds	Yes
Angioscopy	No	No	Real-time	Yes
Electron beam CT	Yes	Yes	Seconds	No
Intracoronary ultrasound	No	No	Real time	Yes
Magnetic resonance imaging	No	No*	Minutes	No

Table 2. *Technical aspects of currently used clinical imaging modalities. *For myocardial perfusion imaging contrast agents are needed.*

Anatomical/structural imaging modalities for coronary atherosclerosis

Angiography

Angiographic visualization of lumen deformities in the coronary vessels still remains the "golden standard" for describing coronary atherosclerosis. The generally applied method is the contrast-enhanced, x-ray cine-angiography. This involves the injection of a radio-opaque contrast agent directly into a specific coronary artery using a catheter. The contrast agent is injected during recording of the radiographic image and each coronary artery is usually viewed in several projections to permit assessment of the severity of asymmetric stenosis and to minimize overlap of adjacent vessels. The acquisition time of a single picture (frame) of the film is short enough to "freeze" the vessel motion with more than sufficient spatial resolution. Still improving techniques now permits the visualization and assessment of arteries as small as 0.5 mm in diameter.

The main information displayed with coronary angiography is vessel lumen, but major calcifications can also be identified. Quantitative coronary angiography (QCA), the computer-assisted stenosis analysis technique, is presently a common feature in many coronary angiography systems. It allows automatic detection of the boundaries of the stenosis, interpolation of the expected dimensions of the coronary vessel at the point of obstructions, and angiographically derived estimation of the size of the atheromatous plaque (figure 1). However, in comparative analyses with ICUS (intracoronary ultrasound) it appears that, at the site of maximal obstruction, QCA underestimates plaque size. Furthermore, it appears that atherosclerotic disease is consistently present at the angiographic start of the stenosis. Thus, the site identified by automated stenosis analysis as the start of the stenosis does not represent a disease-free site but rather the place where compensatory vessel enlargement fails to preserve luminal dimensions.[26,27] Another drawback is its inability of angiography to detect activated lesions.

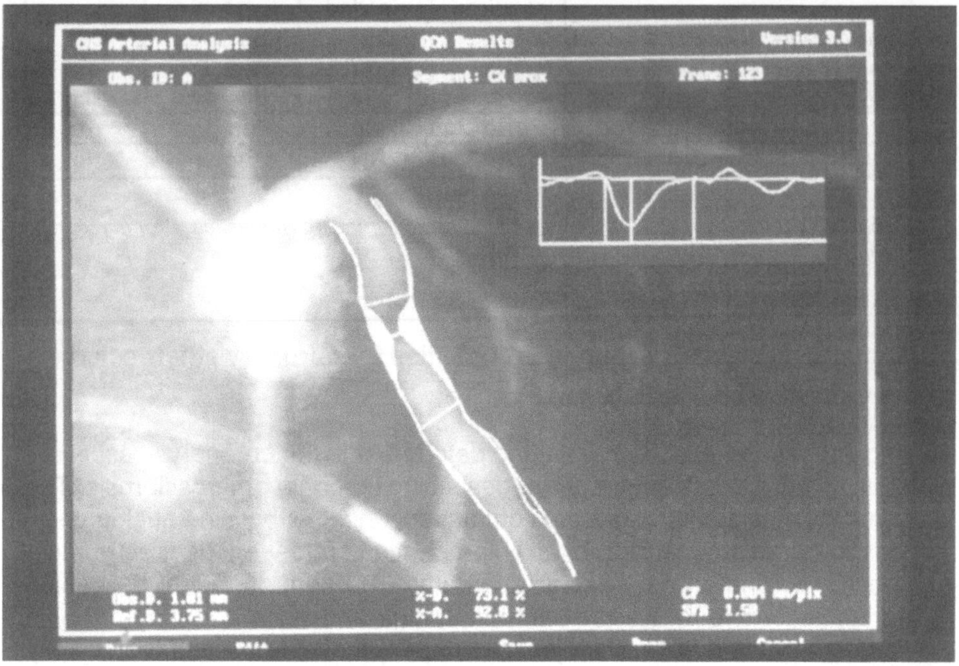

Figure 1. *Quantitative Coronary Angiography (QCA). With courtesy of The Laboratory for Clinical and Experimental Image Processing, Leiden, The Netherlands*
(See also Colour Plates, p. 338)

Despite these drawbacks, coronary angiography adequately describes severe stenosis and has proven to be relevant in the assessment of the relation between arterial disease and the clinical outcome. In addition, the method has proven to be sufficiently reliable and reproducible to support clinical trials in the past and present.

Angioscopy

Coronary angioscopy evaluates the composition of the atherosclerotic plaque by direct examination of the arterial wall. With the aid of a percutaneous transluminal fiber optic system, a view of the mid and distal segments of the coronary arteries is provided. One major limitation associated with the technique of angioscopy is the need for vessel occlusion during the imaging procedure, which may produce myocardial ischemia. Furthermore, there is presently no reliable method for quantifying angioscopic findings.

The optical visualized aspects of coronary atherosclerosis are plaque color, plaque disruption, plaque protrusion, and the presence of thrombus. The importance of the technique at this moment is mainly in the area of interventional cardiology. For example, in the prediction of angioplasty outcome, angioscopic features like plaque rupture and thrombus appeared to be superior to parameters derived from angiography.[23,28] The appearance of a thrombus at site of intervention is associated with an unfavorable early angiographic outcome in patients who undergo coronary angioplasty. [29] This can be detected with more accuracy than using angiography or ultrasound.[30]

Ultrasound

Among the physical entities for scanning tissue are acoustical waves (ultrasound). Differences in the acoustic impedance of various tissues localize the signal reflection and reflect the tissue boundaries. Ultrasound images are created from a series of acoustic beams emitted circumferentially from a catheter positioned in the coronary vessel. The ultrasound beams are emitted perpendicular to the axis of the catheter from a transducer mounted on the tip of the catheter. Both mechanical and annular array techniques are used to manipulate the direction of the emitted beam.

The transducer at the tip of the catheter contains a piezo-electric crystal that interconverts electrical and mechanical (i.e. sound) energy, functioning both as the transmitter of sound and as the receiver of reflected waves. Recent advances in microelectronics and piezo-electric technology have resulted in the development of a miniature ultrasound device capable of real-time tomographic intracoronary imaging.

With the technique called ICUS (intracoronary ultrasound), a high-frequency (20-30 MHz) ultrasound transducer placed on the tip of a flexible catheter is advanced down the coronary artery during cardiac catheterization. Axial resolution, that is the ability to distinguish two neighboring objects in line with the beam, can be approximately 150 μ, establishing detailed cross-sectional (tomographic) images of the coronary artery wall. Like QCA the same kind of image quantifying software is now being developed for echocardiographic images. (VDA = Videodensitometric analysis) (figure 2).

The technique of ICUS visualizes acoustic properties, but no specific tissues, so care has to be taken with interpretation. For example, atheroma and thrombus may appear echogenically the same. Thus ultrasound can delineate the thickness and echogenicity of vessel wall structure but does not provide actual histology.[31]

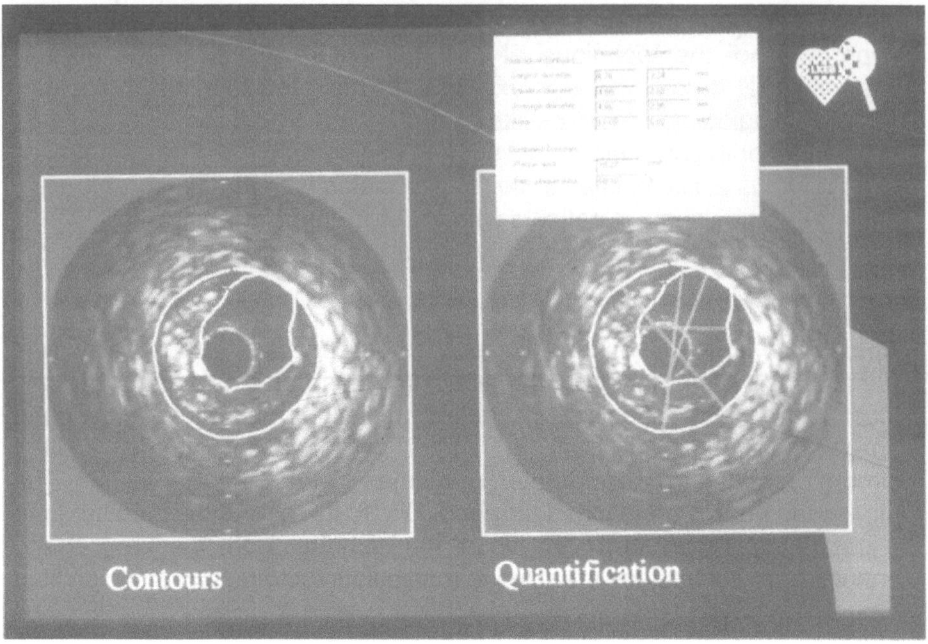

Figure 2. *Intracoronary ultrasound. Quantification of plaque with ICUS. With courtesy of The Laboratory for Clinical and Experimental Image Processing, Leiden, The Netherlands*

(See also Colour Plates, p. 339)

An ultrasound image of a normal coronary artery shows a trilaminar or a monolayered vessel wall. The innermost vessel band on the echo-image represents reflections from the internal elastic lamina, while the middle sonolucent layer is principally composed of the vessel media. The deepest layer of the arterial wall represents the (peri)adventitia with its characteristic "onion skin" appearance.

One of the qualitative parameters, derived from echocardiographic images is the classification of different coronary atheromata into three categories; soft, fibrous and calcified plaques. These are recognizable in ultrasound images as, respectively, less echogenic, equal and more echogenic than the echogenicity of the peripheral adventitia (figure 3). The soft, lipid-laden, sonolucent plaque is especially associated with a high incidence of acute ischemic syndromes.[32] However, its appearance is mimicked by technical factors and other tissue types, and the appearance is very dependent on gain, transmission power, and the intervening tissue. The same holds for the visualization of thrombus. It can be difficult to differentiate thrombus from the plaque itself in the two-dimensional tomographic image.[33] Despite its limitations, the qualitative aspects of ultrasound imaging have given much insight into the mechanisms underlying the effects of interventional techniques. For example, ICUS has indicated that vessels with a remnant arc of disease-free wall are dilated mainly by wall stretching compared with other types of vessels and in this manner are associated with a smaller lumen gain.[34] From the point of view of atherosclerosis, it should be mentioned that the currently available ultrasound technology can not discriminate stable plaques from unstable ones.[35]

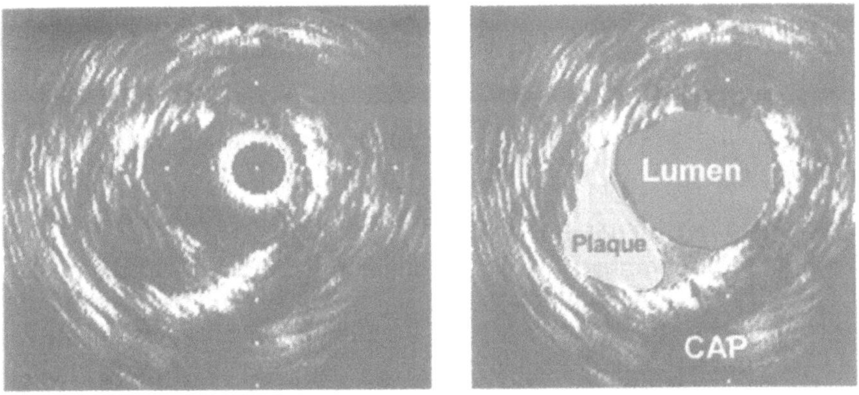

Figure 3. *Intracoronary ultrasound. Ruptured lipid cap of the left main coronary artery. Reprinted by permission from Gorge et al.*[74]
(See also Colour Plates, p. 339)

Calcification, another qualitative imaging aspect, is easily identified by ultrasound because of its high echogenicity. The total attenuation of the ultrasound image distal to the calcium is referred to as "shadowing". Because of its ease of recognition, this is the most studied aspect with ICUS. The delineation and radial location of coronary calcification can not be made by any other imaging technique at this moment. However, ICUS is only good at detecting dense calcifications. In the case of micro-calcification, a pattern of small flecks of plaque calcium often present in developing atherosclerosis, the sensitivity is much lower.[36] Quantification of the total calcium burden is also a problem because deeper structures that may or may not be calcified are hidden in the shadow of more superficially calcified regions. Therefore, quantification of calcification by ICUS can only be done by the semi-quantitative expression "arc length".[37] The arc-length is the angle, expressed in degrees, from the point of view of the transducer, in which the tissue is calcified. This is of course a very rough indication.

One quantitative marker derived from ICUS images is coronary wall thickness. The thickness of the inner echogenic plus sonolucent layers on the ICUS image, represent the intimal plus medial thickness as observed by histology. So the use of this value may be appropriate in the assessment of coronary wall thickening associated with atherosclerosis[18] The first trials on the use of coronary IMT are underway.[38]

In summary, it is possible to assess both the nature of an atherosclerotic lesion (endothelial cells, lipid content, fibrous tissue, and calcifications) and the extent of the disease. Delineation of plaque area and calcification are easily acquired, whereas the destruction between thrombus, soft plaque and hard plaque can be problematic.

X-ray computed tomography

Computed tomography (CT), is a technique in which a two dimensional picture is reconstructed mathematically from many, one-dimensional data assessments. In the case of x-ray CT, the reconstruction is assembled from data of x-ray attenuation, acquired after the beams have pierced the body. The great advantage over conventional x-ray techniques is the avoidance of superimposing structures.

A relative new development in CT techniques is electron beam computed tomography (EBCT) or ultrafast x-ray transmission CT. In contrast to conventional computed tomography, EBCT scanners do not have a rotating x-ray tube to acquire the attenuation data from several angles. It is this mechanical movement which limits the imaging speed of conventional CT. In EBCT a powerful electron beam is generated by an electron gun which is then magnetically focused, angled and steered to sweep a series of metal (tungsten) targets which are arranged around the patient. The energy of the electron beam striking the targets creates x-rays that are collimated to pass through the heart of the patient and then measured by an array of detectors opposite to the metal elements. The electron beam can sweep the metal targets in a very short time interval. Without the nuisance of mechanical movement of conventional CT, the acquisition time of an image can be reduced to 50-100 ms, witch is fast enough to eliminate the motion artifact related to cardiac contraction.[39] The tomograms currently have a high spatial resolution and the density resolution permits separation of about 2000 gray levels. Also, the temporal resolution of 17 frames per second is impressive. The imaging procedure itself includes one to three 30-second breath-holds in which 20-40, 3-mm thick electrocardiography gated images are acquired.

Electron-beam computerized tomographic imaging provides a sensitive means of detecting coronary calcifications, (figure 4) not only for dense calcifications but also for the micro-calcifications in the coronary artery wall.[40] Efforts are being made to quantify the measured calcium, which is expressed in parameters such as Hounsfield Units or Agatston calcium scores. Calcium presence as assessed with EBCT has a highly negative predictive power for the presence of coronary artery disease, but it does have a limited ability to predict disease severity.[41]

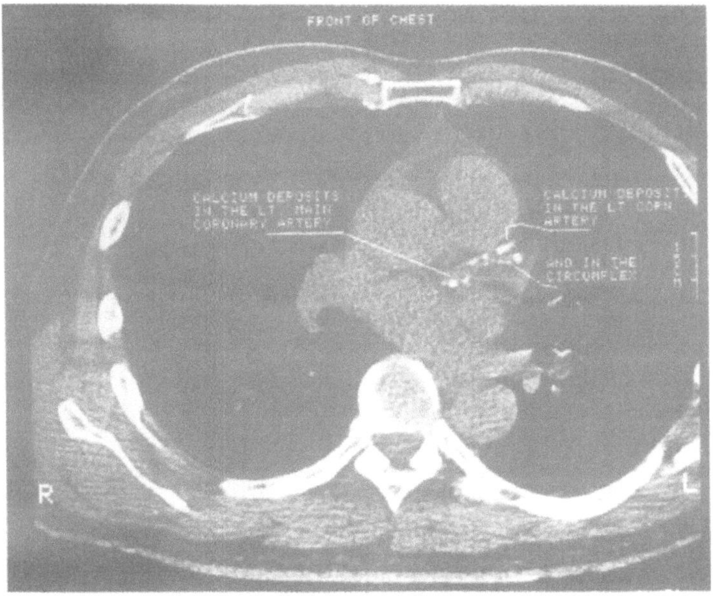

Figure 4. *Electron beam computed tomography: Calcium. Unenhanced EBCT-image which demonstrates calcium deposits. Reprinted by permission from Brundage et al.*[75]

The EBCT technique can also produce three-dimensional pictures of the coronary vessel lumen. The reconstruction is made from many two-dimensional tomographic slices, acquired through the gated assessment technique. High quality three-dimensional images can be constructed with EBCT. To enhance contrast between the coronary lumen and the surrounding tissue even more, intravenous contrast is given, administered by infusion at the site of the cubital vein. Although gated techniques have the disadvantage of blurring (loss of resolution) this technique delivers results that are in reasonable close correlation to those of the gold standard, quantitative coronary analysis of coronary angiograms (figure 5, 6 and 7).[42,43] This is valid at least for the left main coronary artery and the left anterior descending coronary artery. The other coronary vessels are less well correlated to angiography, probably because they have a smaller caliber, a faster and bigger spatial motion and are more superimposed on veins (contrast in cubital vein!). In comparative studies it has been demonstrated that the diameters of these other small vessel are underestimated, using the EBCT technique, which prohibits exact quantification of high-grade stenoses. In view of noninvasively detecting, high-grade stenoses however, EBCT is an accurate, new and promising technique.[44]

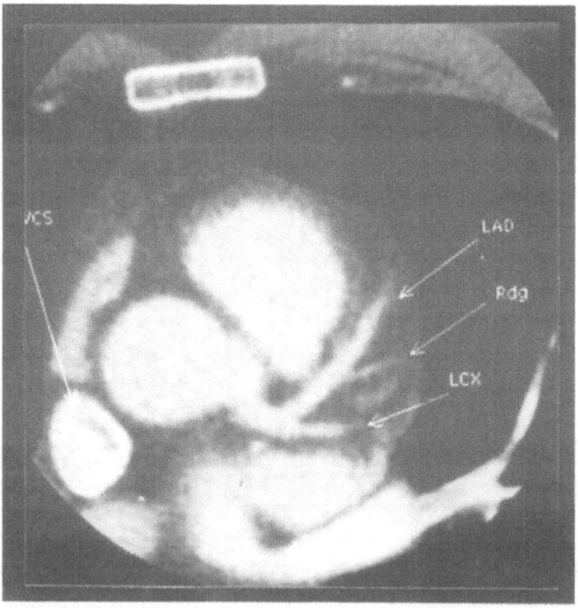

Figure 5. *Electron beam computed tomography: morphology. Axial two-dimensional cross-section obtained after intravenous contrast injection. Reprinted by permission from Achenbach et al.*[42]

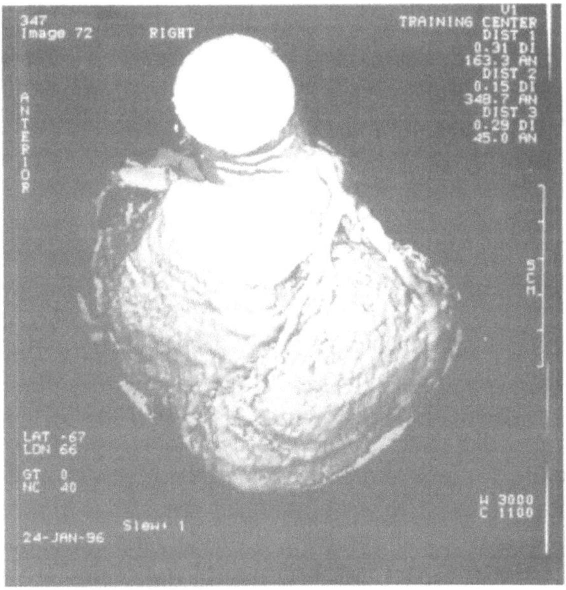

Figure 6. *Electron beam computed tomography: morphology. Three dimensional reconstruction of the same patient as in figure 5. Reprinted by permission from Achenbach et al.*[42]

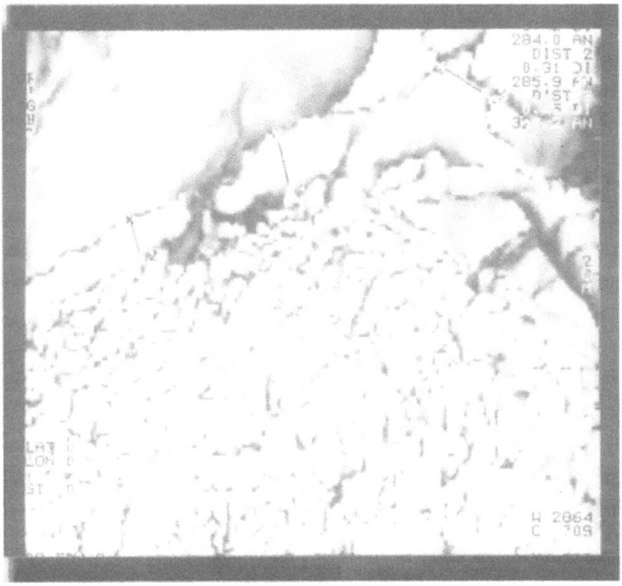

Figure 7. *Electron beam computed tomography: morphology. Luminal measurements. Reprinted by permission from Achenbach et al.* [42]

For a technique to be utilized in the monitoring of the atherosclerotic process, it has to prove itself with respect to reproducibility, reliability and accuracy. One of the first studies using EBCT to monitor atherosclerosis is the FAPS study. In this Felodipine Atherosclerosis Prevention Study, the progression of coronary atherosclerosis is monitored by changes in calcium presence, and assessed by EBCT.[45]

Future developments in anatomy

Three-dimensional reconstructions of intravascular ultrasound (3D-ICUS) images have recently been introduced. These reconstructions provide spatial visualization of the longitudinal and volumetric measurement of lumen and plaque dimensions (figure 8). The images can be acquired during continuous or electrocardiography-gated withdrawals of the ICUS imaging catheter, and a discrimination between the blood pool and structures of the vascular wall can be achieved by the application of different quantifying techniques. Currently there are still major problems with the 3D-imaging technique but new approaches, like combining data obtained from 3D-ICUS and biplane angiography seem to be very promising for the future.[46 47]

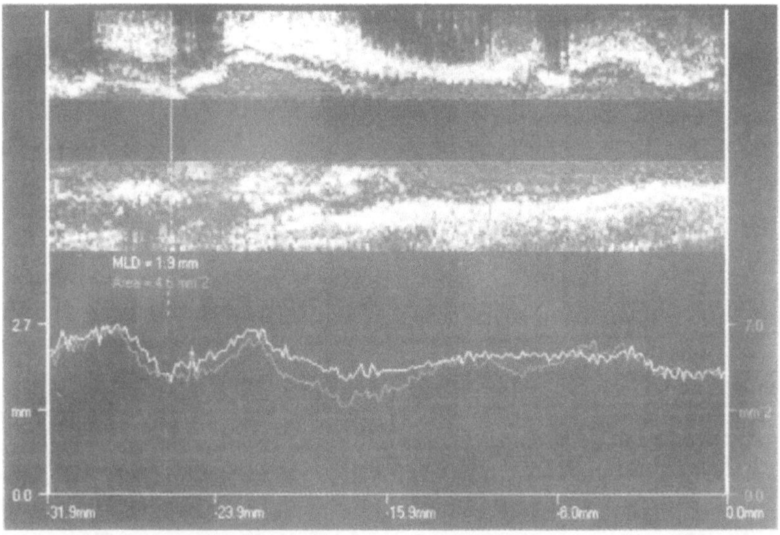

Figure 8. *Intracoronary ultrasound: three-dimensional reconstruction. Longitudinal view of the proximal left descending coronary artery. The image was obtained during a motorized pull-back. Visible are large calcified plaques and a stenosis at 5 cm from the coronary ostium. Blood pool: red, lumen diameter: yellow line, area measurement: green line. Reprinted by permission from Di Mario et al.*[76]

(See also Colour Plates, p. 340)

Optical coherence tomography (OCT) is a new form of ultrasound imaging technique. The difference is the wavelength, used to image the object of interest. Instead of acoustic waves, like with ICUS, infrared light is used. The primary advantage of infrared waves over acoustic waves is the achievable axial spatial resolution of only 20 μ. This resolution allows small vascular structural details such as the width of intimal caps and the presence of fissures to be determined. The extent of lipid collections is also well visualized and like normal ICUS it does not require direct vessel wall contact (figure 9). Although still in the research phase, the properties of EBCT as by providing a high contrast among tissue constituents, a high resolution, and a high ability of penetrating heavily calcified tissue are promising.[48 49 50]

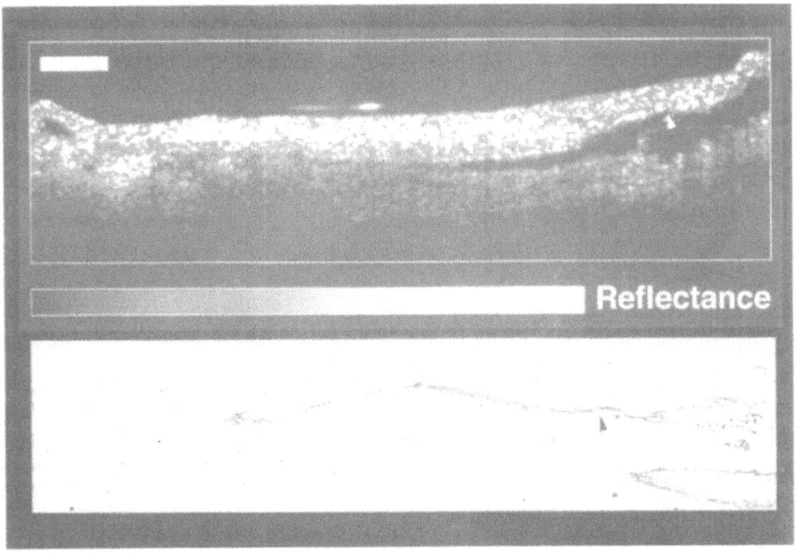

Figure 9. *Optical coherence tomography. Image of a human coronary artery and corresponding histology. The reflectance pattern shows good difference between tissue transitions zones (arrow) and tissue type. Reprinted by permission from Di Mario et al.*[76]
(See also Colour Plates, p. 340)

Magnetic resonance imaging (MRI) is based upon the radiofrequency (RF) signal emitted by hydrogen nuclei of tissues after they have been disturbed by exogenous RF pulses in the presence of a strong magnetic field. The emitted RF signal has certain characteristics called relaxation times (T1,T2), and these are variable among the different tissues. The signal intensity of one tissue compared to another (contrast) can be manipulated by varying the elapsed time between the application of the exogenous RF pulses (repetition time). And varying the time between an RF pulse and the sampling of the emitted signal (echo delay time). MR imaging is a form of computed tomography. By analyzing emitted radiosignals from nuclei, it mathematically constructs a cross-sectional (tomographic) picture of the body.

Magnetic resonance angiography (MRA) is the collectively known name for magnetic resonance imaging techniques which evaluate the anatomy and flow of vessels. Many attempts have been made to use MRA for visualizing coronary arteries, but it is technically still cumbersome to achieve good results[51] (figure 10). Despite the high expectations at the beginning of the 1990s, an MRI technique has not yet emerged which can provide a sensitivity and specificity for coronary lesions that compares with traditional contrast angiography.[52,53]. MRA has been successful in the detection of congenital coronary artery variants and the imaging of coronary stents and bypass grafts.[54] Even three-dimensional reconstructions have been explored in this field.

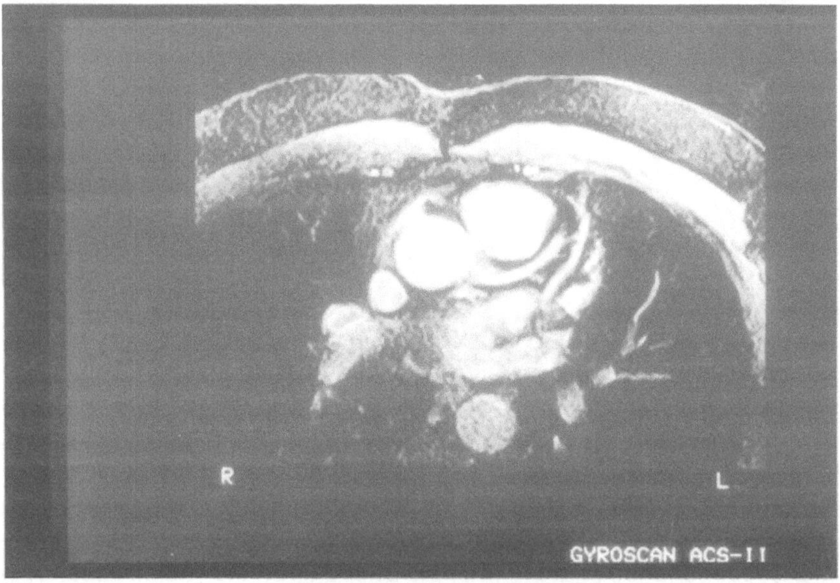

***Figure 10.** Magnetic resonance imaging: coronary angiography*

Magnetic resonance imaging of the lumen is called intravascular MRI. An ex vivo analysis of human femoral arteries, with receiver coils mounted to an inflatable balloon is able to differentiate the coronary wall layers and plaque components.[55] [56] [57] Its feasibility in coronary arteries in humans still is unknown due to predictable problems caused by the motion of intracoronary placed, endoluminal receiver coil.

Functional/molecular imaging modalities for coronary atherosclerosis
Current clinical diagnostic imaging modalities, such as MRI, CT and ICUS, provide predominantly anatomical information: CT images produce primarily x-ray attenuation distribution in the body, whereas ultrasound localizes echo reflections. As discussed in the section Introduction there is a need for functional imaging techniques that provide information that complements the acquired anatomical information. However, what the imaging techniques of local, coronary artery dysfunction have in common is the fact that they are not yet utilized clinically to a great extent. They are predominantly in the research phase. This is in contradiction to the imaging procedures like myocardial perfusion scintigraphy, which is already widely accepted as a tool to evaluate the functional consequences of coronary atherosclerosis.

Functional imaging of coronary atherosclerosis

Endothelial function as assessed with vasomotion
Endothelium-dependent vasomotion may be regarded as one of the "thermometers" of endothelial health. For this parameter to be used effectively and comparably, it is necessary to quantify the "degree" of endothelium-dependent vasorelaxation. This is established by giving endothelium-dependent provocation impulses [chemical (acetylcholine) or physical (flow increase)] to the endothelium and subsequently comparing the response to a reference. The physiologically maximal achievable vasodilation is used as a reference, which is comparable to the situation in which the endothelial cells would produce an abundance of endothelium derived nitric oxide. This situation can be simulated by endothelium-independent vasodilators like nitroglycerin.[24]

Invasive assessment of endothelial function of epicardial conductance vessels.
In the case of the invasive assessment of the coronary artery function as developed by Ludmer et al. [58] acetylcholine is used as a provocative agent. The changing of vessel dimensions are observed by means of coronary angiography. After the baseline angiograms are established, graded concentrations of acetylcholine are infused. After each infusion, an angiogram is taken, which is analyzed with QCA. The quantified endothelium-dependent vascular response to acetylcholine can then be compared to the quantified endothelium-independent vascular response to nitroglycerin (figure 11).

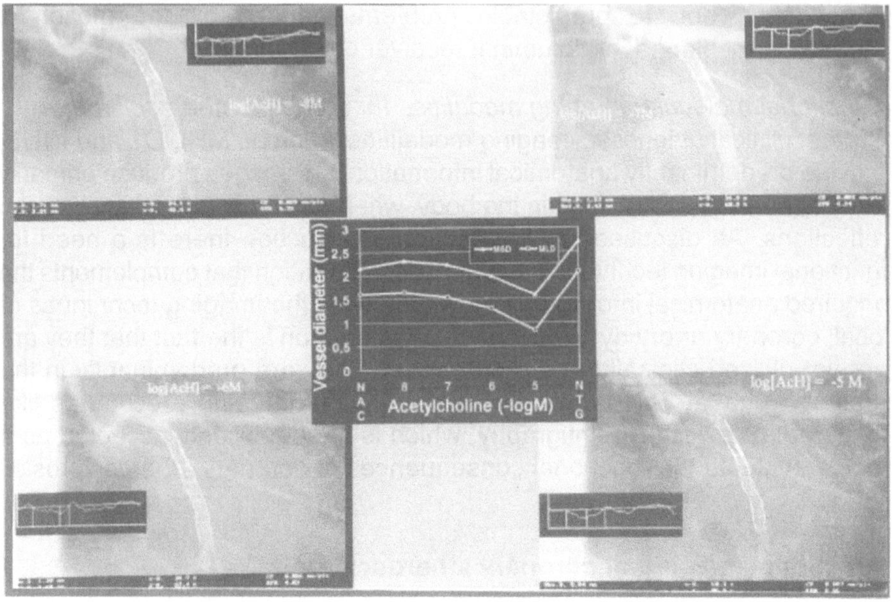

Figure 11. Endothelial function assessment with angiography. Compilation of the infusions sequence angiograms made of one patient and the quantitative coronary angiography results. MSD, mean segment diameter; MLD, minimum lumen diameter; NAC, saline; NTG, nitroglycerin. PREFACE study, preliminary results. Reprinted by permission from Mulder et al.[24]

Another method is to study at the coronary vasodilation after an increase in coronary blood flow. Flow dependent dilation is an endothelial cell dependent form of vasodilation that is mediated through shear stress-sensitive receptors located at the surface of the endothelial cells. Flow dependent dilation is caused through increased "shear stress" or viscous drag. This longitudinal force exerted by the blood flow upon the endothelial cell layer can be achieved by increasing the coronary blood flow.[59] This can be done by distal infusion of for example *adenosine,* which causes a strong peripheral vasodilation.[60] The method of endothelial function assessment has already been used to monitor atherosclerosis in several trials.[61-64]

Magnetic resonance flow imaging

Emerging techniques in magnetic resonance imaging [phase-contrast magnetic resonance imaging (PC-MRI)] have made it possible to noninvasively measure the absolute flow in the vessels of the thoracic cavity. In rather stationary vessels like coronary bypasses, phase velocity mapping is already a promising clinical tool in the noninvasive assessment of graft patency and function.[65] The patency is indirectly derived from the existence/non-existence of flow at certain parts of the vessel. Calculations of this "flow" profile could ultimately result in the prediction of degree of stenosis of a certain vessel. The challenging coronaries have also been within reach of this technique. At this moment, it is possible to distinguish open from occluded infarct-related coronary arteries, or even to measure absolute coronary arterial flow and flow reserve in the proximal left anterior descending artery. The sensitivity of the technique is high enough to display pharmacologically induced changes in coronary artery flow.[54,66,67]

Molecular imaging of coronary atherosclerosis

Magnetic resonance imaging: chemical imaging

When the resolution of MRI improves drastically, this modality might be very promising for identifying and imaging specific biochemical components of the atherosclerotic plaque because the components have certain atoms with nuclei with only one specific resonance frequency (chemical-shift imaging). In vitro experiments have demonstrated that the capability of this technique to discriminate different plaque components like triglycerides, unesterified/esterified cholesterol and phospholipids is very high.[68 69] In vivo, promising progress is also being made with MRI being capable of distinguishing lipid cores, fibrous caps, calcifications, normal media and adventitia in human atheromatous in carotid plaques.[70]

Nuclear imaging: radiopharmaceutical imaging

Nuclear imaging is the monitoring of radiolabeled substances (tracers) involved in various processes like atherosclerosis. In the future two major nuclear imaging modalities will be involved in the imaging of these tracers. The SPECT (single photon emission computed tomography) technique, which depends on gamma-emitting radionuclides attached to the tracer molecules, and the positron emission tomography (PET) technique, which depends on positron emitters attached to the tracer molecules. The PET technique has proven to have a higher sensitivity and spatial resolution than the SPECT modality.

The scintigraphic identification and monitoring of atherosclerosis is still in an early stage. Though labeling of low-density lipoprotein-particles and platelets is technically possible, clinical imaging of coronary hot spots in vivo is still in the phase of pre-clinical research. One complicating factor is the limited response time of the atherosclerosis-involved cellular blood constituents (platelets, monocytes) with the vascular surface at the injury site. In recent years, a large number of techniques and radiolabeled tracers has been tested. Except for platelet labeling, no technique has evolved to any clinical significance, although preliminary results indicate that radionuclide techniques may be of great benefit in the future in elucidating functional aspects of the disease.

Raman spectroscopy

Raman spectroscopy is a technique that is able to qualify and quantify the chemical composition of plaques, through the analysis of spectra emitted by a plaque compounds after being radiated with a laser beam. Still under research, this technique, based on the imaging of differences of emitted electromagnetic waves frequencies (Raman effect), holds great promise for the future. The clinician will have an instant (real time) picture of the chemical composition of the plaque with high accuracy.

Infrared catheter

In vivo, atherosclerotic plaques show thermal heterogeneity, according to local metabolic activity. The higher the local metabolic activity, the more activated macrophages either on the plaque surface or under a thin cap. The activation of macrophages is related to the possible risk of an acute local thrombotic event. The imaging of surface temperature heterogeneity can be performed with infrared sensitive catheters. Initial experiments have already been done.[71]

Conclusion

It is estimated that a large portion of the people with coronary artery disease dies suddenly and unexpectedly.[72] Atherosclerosis, the most important condition underlying coronary artery disease, is therefore a dangerous and unpredictable condition, with a relatively early onset in live.[73] In order to improve treatment and prognosis, adequate and timely assessment of the present "activity" and extent of the atherosclerotic process is necessary. This has been a challenging endeavor for imaging modalities for many years and the answer has yet not been found in one single assessment method. The assessment of both functional and anatomical aspects of atherosclerosis could result in an insight in the ongoing disease process, allowing the individualization of risk and the decision to treat.

References

1. Fuster V, Badimon L, Badimon JJ, Chesebro JH. The pathogenesis of coronary artery disease and the acute coronary syndromes (2). N Engl J Med 1992;326:310-8.
2. Fuster V, Badimon L, Badimon JJ, Chesebro JH. The pathogenesis of coronary artery disease and the acute coronary syndromes (1). N Engl J Med. 1992;326:242-50.
3. Berliner JA, Navab M, Fogelman AM, et al. Atherosclerosis: basic mechanisms. Oxidation, inflammation, and genetics. Circulation 1995;91:2488-96.
4. Schiffrin EL. The endothelium and control of blood vessel function in health and disease. *Clin Invest Med* 1994;17:602-20.
5. Vita JA, Treasure CB, Yeung AC, et al. Patients with evidence of coronary endothelial dysfunction as assessed by acetylcholine infusion demonstrate marked increase in sensitivity to constrictor effects of catecholamines. Circulation. 1992;85:1390-7.
6. Gould KL. Quantification of coronary artery stenosis in vivo. *Circ Res.* 1985;57:341-53.
7. Fuster V, Badimon L, Badimon JJ, Chesebro JH. The pathogenesis of coronary artery disease and the acute coronary syndromes. N Engl J Med 1992;326:242-250, 310-318
8. Cohen RA, Shepherd JT, Vanhoutte PM. Vasodilatation mediated by the coronary endothelium in response to aggregating platelets. Bibl Cardiol 1984;38:35-42.
9. Levine GN, Keaney JF Jr, Vita JA. Cholesterol reduction in cardiovascular disease. Clinical benefits and possible mechanisms. N Engl J Med 1995;332:512-21.
10. Crouse JR 3rd, Thompson CJ. An evaluation of methods for imaging and quantifying coronary and carotid lumen stenosis and atherosclerosis. Circulation. 1993;87: (3 Suppl):II17-33.
11. Glagov S, Weisenberg E, Zarins CK, Stankunavicius R, Kolettis GJ. Compensatory enlargement of human atherosclerotic coronary arteries. N Engl J Med. 1987;316:1371-75.
12. Fuster V, Stein B, Ambrose JA, Badimon L, Badimon JJ, Chesebro JH. Atherosclerosis plaque rupture and thrombosis. Evolving concepts. Circulation 1990;82:(3 Suppl):II47-59.
13. Frink RJ, Achor RW, Brown AL Jr, Kincaid OW, Brandenburg RO. Significance of calcification of the coronary arteries. Am J Cardiol 1970;26:241-7.
14. Stanford W, Thompson BH, Weiss RM: Coronary artery calcification: clinical significance and current methods of detection. AJR Am J Roentgenol 1993;161:1139-46.
15. Gnasso A, Irace C, Mattioli PL, Pujia A. Carotid intima-media thickness and coronary heart disease risk factors. Atherosclerosis 1996;119:7-15.
16. Chambless LE, Heiss G, Folsom AR, et al. Association of coronary heart disease incidence with carotid arterial wall thickness and major risk factors: the Atherosclerosis Risk in Communities (ARIC) Study, 1987-1993. Am J Epidemiol 1997;146:483-94.
17. Visona A, Pesavento R, Lusiani L, et al. Intimal medial thickening of common carotid artery as indicator of coronary artery disease. Angiology 1996;47:61-6.

18. Kawano S, Yamagishi M, Hao H, Yutani C, Miyatake K. Wall composition in intravascular ultrasound layered appearance of human coronary artery. Heart Vessels. 1996;11:152-9.
19. Lablanche JM, Van Belle E, McFadden E, et al. Angioscopie coronaire. Arch Mal Coeur Vaiss 1997;90 Spec No 2:29-33.
20. Thieme T, Wernecke KD, Meyer R, et al. Angioscopic evaluation of atherosclerotic plaques: validation by histomorphologic analysis and association with stable and unstable coronary syndromes. J Am Coll Cardiol 1996;28:1-6.
21. Waxman S, Mittleman MA, Zarich SW, et al. Angioscopic assessment of coronary lesions underlying thrombus. Am J Cardiol 1997;79:1106-9.
22. Bauters C, Lablanche JM, McFadden EP, Hamon M, Bertrand ME. Relation of coronary angioscopic findings at coronary angioplasty to angiographic restenosis. Circulation 1995;92:2473-79.
23. Waxman S, Sassower MA, Mittleman MA, et al. Angioscopic predictors of early adverse outcome after coronary angioplasty in patients with unstable angina and non-Q-wave myocardial infarction. Circulation. 1996;93:2106-13.
24. Mulder HJ, Schalij MJ. Endothelial (dys)function, lipid reduction and balloon angioplasty. In: Van der Wall EE, Manger Cats V, Baan J, editor: Vascular Medicine - From endothelium to myocardium. Dordrecht, Kluwer Academic Publishers; 1997, p 55-82.
25. Paulin S, von Schulthess GK, Fossel E, Krayenbuehl HP. MR imaging of the aortic root and proximal coronary arteries. AJR Am J Roentgenol 1987;148:665-70.
26. Escaned J, Baptista J, Di Mario C, et al. Significance of automated stenosis detection during quantitative angiography. Insights gained from intracoronary ultrasound imaging. Circulation 1996;94:966-72.
27. Mintz GS, Popma JJ, Pichard AD, et al. Limitations of angiography in the assessment of plaque distribution in coronary artery disease: a systematic study of target lesion eccentricity in 1446 lesions. Circulation 1996;93:924-31.
28. Feld S, Ganim M, Carell ES, et al. Comparison of angioscopy, intravascular ultrasound imaging and quantitative coronary angiography in predicting clinical outcome after coronary intervention in high risk patients. J Am Coll Cardiol 1996;28:97-105.
29. Larrazet FS, Dupouy PJ, Dubois-Rande JL, Ducot B, Kvasnicka J, Geschwind HJ. Angioscopy variables predictive of early angiographic outcome after excimer laser-assisted coronary angioplasty. Am J Cardiol 1997;79:1343-49.
30. Emanuelsson H. Future challenges to coronary angioplasty: perspectives on intracoronary imaging and physiology. J Intern Med. 1995;238:111-9.
31. Nissen SE, Tuzcu EM, DeFranco AC. Detection and quantification of atherosclerosis: the emerging role for intravascular ultrasound. In: Fuster V, editor. Syndromes of atherosclerosis. Armonk: Futura; 1996.
32. Hodgson JM, Reddy KG, Suneja R, Nair RN, Lesnefsky EJ, Sheehan HM. Intracoronary ultrasound imaging: correlation of plaque morphology with angiography, clinical syndrome and procedural results in patients undergoing coronary angioplasty. J Am Coll Cardiol 1993;21:35-44.
33. Kimura BJ, Bhargava V, DeMaria AN. Value and limitations of intravascular ultrasound imaging in characterizing coronary atherosclerotic plaque. Am Heart J 1995;130:386-96.

34. Baptista J, Di Mario C, Ozaki Y, et al. Impact of plaque morphology and composition on the mechanisms of lumen enlargement using intracoronary ultrasound and quantitative angiography after balloon angioplasty. Am J Cardiol 1996;77:115-21.
35. De Feyter PJ, Ozaki Y, Baptista J, et al. Ischemia-related lesion characteristics in patients with stable or unstable angina. A study with intracoronary angioscopy and ultrasound. Circulation 1995;92:1408-13.
36. Friedrich GJ, Moes NY, Muhlberger VA, et al. Detection of intralesional calcium by intracoronary ultrasound depends on the histologic pattern. Am Heart J 1994;128:435-41.
37. Metz JA, Yock PG, Fitzgerald PJ: Intravascular ultrasound: basic interpretation. Cardiol Clin 1997;15:1-15.
38. Takagi T, Yoshida K, Akasaka T, Hozumi T, Morioka S, Yoshikawa J. Intravascular ultrasound analysis of reduction in progression of coronary narrowing by treatment with pravastatin. Am J Cardiol 1997;79:1673-6.
39. Thompson GR, Forbat S, Underwood R. Electron-beam CT scanning for detection of coronary calcification and prediction of coronary heart disease. QJM. 1996;89:565-70.
40. Baumgart D, Schmermund A, Goerge G, et al. Comparison of electron beam computed tomography with intracoronary ultrasound and coronary angiography for detection of coronary atherosclerosis. J Am Coll Cardiol 1997;30:57-64.
41. Simon A, Levenson J: Early detection of subclinical atherosclerosis in asymptomatic subjects at high risk for cardiovascular disease. Clin Exp Hypertens 1993;15:1069-76.
42. Achenbach S, Moshage W, Ropers D, Bachmann K: Comparison of vessel diameters in electron beam tomography and quantitative coronary angiography. Int J Card Imaging 1998;14:1-7.
43. Chernoff DM, Ritchie CJ, Higgins CB. Evaluation of electron beam CT coronary angiography in healthy subjects. AJR Am J Roentgenol 1997;169:93-9.
44. Achenbach S, Moshage W, Bachmann K. Detection of high-grade restenosis after PTCA using contrast-enhanced electron beam CT. Circulation 1997;96:2785-88.
45. Wong ND, Teng W, Abrahamson D, et al. Noninvasive tracking of coronary atherosclerosis by electron beam computed tomography: rationale and design of the Felodipine Atherosclerosis Prevention Study (FAPS). Am J Cardiol 1995;76:1239-42.
46. Von-Birgelen C, Erbel R, Di Mario C, et al. Three-dimensional reconstruction of coronary arteries with intravascular ultrasound. Herz 1995;20:277-89.
47. Prause GP, DeJong SC, McKay CR, Sonka M. Towards a geometrically correct 3-D reconstruction of tortuous coronary arteries based on biplane angiography and intravscular ultrasound. Int J Card Imaging 1997;13:451-62.
48. Brezinski ME, Tearney GJ, Weissman NJ, et al. Assessing atherosclerotic plaque morphology: comparison of optical coherence tomography and high frequency intravascular ultrasound. Heart 1997;77:397-403.
49. Brezinski ME, Tearney GJ, Bouma BE, et al. Optical coherence tomography for optical biopsy. Properties and demonstration of vascular pathology. Circulation 1996;93:1206-13.
50. Fujimoto JG, Brezinski ME, Tearney GJ, et al. Optical biopsy and imaging using optical coherence tomography. Nat Med 1995;1:970-2.
51. van-der-Wall EE, Vliegen HW, de Roos A, Bruschke AV. Magnetic resonance imaging in coronary artery disease. Circulation 1995;92:2723-39.

52. Dinsmore RE: Noninvasive coronary arteriography--here at last? Circulation 1995;91:1607-08.
53. Doyle M, Pohost GM. Magnetic resonance coronary artery imaging. In: Fuster V, editor. Syndromes of atherosclerosis. Armonk: Futura; 1996.
54. Duerinckx AJ. MRI of coronary arteries. Int J Card Imaging 1997;13:191-7.
55. Zimmermann GG, Erhart P, Schneider J, von Schulthess GK, Schmidt M, Debatin JF. Intravascular MR imaging of atherosclerotic plaque: ex vivo analysis of human femoral arteries with histologic correlation. Radiology 1997;204:769-74.
56. Atalar E, Bottomley PA, Ocali O, et al. High resolution intravascular MRI and MRS by using a catheter receiver coil. Magn Reson Med 1996;36:596-605.
57. Ocali O, Atalar E. Intravascular magnetic resonance imaging using a loopless catheter antenna. Magn Reson Med 1997;37:112-8.
58. Ludmer PL, Selwyn AP, Shook TL, et al. Paradoxical vasoconstriction induced by acetylcholine in atherosclerotic coronary arteries. N Engl J Med 1986;315:1046-51.
59. Drexler H, Zeiher AM, Wollschlager H, Meinertz T, Just H, Bonzel T. Flow-dependent coronary artery dilatation in humans. Circulation 1989;80:466-74.
60. Wilson RF, Wyche K, Christensen BV, Zimmer S, Laxson DD. Effects of adenosine on human coronary arterial circulation. Circulation 1990;82:1595-06.
61. Mancini GB, Henry GC, Macaya C, et al. Angiotensin-converting enzyme inhibition with quinapril improves endothelial vasomotor dysfunction in patients with coronary artery disease. The TREND (Trial on Reversing ENdothelial Dysfunction) Study [published erratum appears in: Circulation 1996;94:1490].. Circulation 1996;94:258-65.
62. Mulder JG, Schalij MJ, Visser RF, et al. Endothelium-dependent vasomotion, 3 months after PTCA in humans. A randomized, double blinded study of the effects of pravastatin on the restoration of the endothelial function. The PREFACE study [abstract]. Eur Heart J 1997;18 (abstract Suppl):16.
63. Anderson TJ, Meredith IT, Yeung AC, Frei B, Selwyn AP, Ganz P. The effect of cholesterol-lowering and antioxidant therapy on endothelium-dependent coronary vasomotion. N Engl J Med 1995;332:488-93.
64. Leung WH, Lau CP, Wong CK. Beneficial effect of cholesterol-lowering therapy on coronary endothelium-dependent relaxation in hypercholesterolaemic patients. Lancet 1993;341:1496-500.
65. Galjee MA, van Rossum AC, Doesburg T, Van Eenige MJ, Visser CA. Value of magnetic resonance imaging in assessing patency and function of coronary artery bypass grafts. An angiographically controlled study. Circulation 1996;93:660-6.
66. Hundley WG, Lange RA, Clarke GD, et al. Assessment of coronary arterial flow and flow reserve in humans with magnetic resonance imaging. Circulation 1996;93:1502-8.
67. Dendale P, Franken PR, Meusel M, van der Geest R, de Roos A. Distinction between open and occluded infarct-related arteries using contrast-enhanced magnetic resonance imaging. Am J Cardiol 1997;80:334-6.
68. Trouard TP, Altbach MI, Hunter GC, Eskelson CD, Gmitro AF. MRI and NMR spectroscopy of the lipids of atherosclerotic plaque in rabbits and humans. Magn Reson Med 1997;38:19-26.

69. Yuan C, Petty C, O'Brien KD, Hatsukami TS, Eary JF, Brown BG. In vitro and in situ magnetic resonance imaging signal features of atherosclerotic plaque-associated lipids. Arterioscler Thromb Vasc Biol 1997;17:1496-503.
70. Toussaint JF, LaMuraglia GM, Southern JF, Fuster V, Kantor HL. Magnetic resonance images lipid, fibrous, calcified, hemorrhagic, and thrombotic components of human atherosclerosis in vivo. Circulation 1996;94:932-38.
71. Casscells W, Hathorn B, David M, et al. Thermal detection of cellular infiltrates in living atherosclerotic plaques: possible implications for plaque rupture and thrombosis. Lancet 1996;347:1447-51.
72. Castelli W, Leaf A. Identification and assessment of cardiac risk: an overview. Cardiol Clin 1985;3:178.
73. McNamara JJ, Molot MA, Stimple JF. Coronary artery disease in combat casualties in Vietnam. JAMA 1971;216:1185-7.
74. Gorge G, Ge J, Haude M, et al. Intravascular ultrasound for evaluation of coronary arteries. In: Reiber JH, Van der Wall EE, editors. Cardiovascular imaging. Dordrecht: Kluwer Academic Publishers; 1996, p. 283-300.
75. Brundage BH. What is the current role of ultrafast CT in coronary imaging? In: Reiber JH, Van der Wall EE, editors. Cardiovascular imaging. Dordrecht: Kluwer Academic Publishers; 1996, p. 531-44.
76. Di Mario C, Fitzgerald PJ, Colombo A. New developments in intracoronary ultrasound, in Reiber JH, Van der Wall EE, editors. Cardiovascular imaging. Dordrecht; Kluwer Academic Publishers; 1996, p. 257-75.

Chapter 6

The Coronary Microcirculation and Myocardial Ischemia

Paolo G. Camici and Ornella Rimoldi

Introduction

In normal human beings baseline myocardial energy expenditure in the anterior wall of the left ventricle, calculated from arterial and great cardiac vein substrate concentration and blood flow, amounts to 34±5 cal/min, which means roughly 2-3 times as much for the whole left ventricle. In the post-absorptive state energy is derived almost entirely from free fatty acids and 301±53 μmol/min of oxygen are required for their oxidation. If heart rate is doubled by atrial pacing from 80 to 160 beats per minute, energy expenditure increases to 64±7 cal/min and oxygen consumption to 593±71 μmol/min. These changes occur despite a fall in transmyocardial oxygen extraction from 71+3 to 64+3% from baseline to pacing tachycardia. The additional oxygen required can therefore be delivered only through an increase in myocardial blood flow which, in this particular case, is more than doubled[1].

Coronary vasodilator reserve

Generally, the heart is well protected by its coronary vasodilator reserve (a measure of the maximal ability of the coronary circulation to dilate in response to a vasodilator drug). After the administration of a vasodilator, assuming that vasodilation is maximal and perfusion pressure and cardiac

Van der Wall et al. (eds.),
Advanced Imaging in Coronary Artery Disease, 101-107.

workload are constant, the ratio of hyperemic to resting blood flow can be calculated and is defined as the coronary vasodilator reserve. These changes in myocardial blood flow occur through changes in resistance of the coronary microcirculation [2].

Under normal circumstances, the small coronary arterioles below 450 μm in diameter are the principal determinants of coronary vascular resistance whereas resistance is practically negligible in large epicardial arteries which are also known as "conductance vessels" [3, 4]. A 50% drop in perfusion pressure, relative to aortic, may be observed in vessels between 70 and 440 μm in diameter, which is consistent with 40-50% of total coronary vascular resistance being located in prearterioles greater than 100 μm in diameter [5]. Nearly all of the remaining resistance lies in vessels less than 100 μm in diameter which are also those responsible for autoregulation of myocardial blood flow[4] (figure 1).

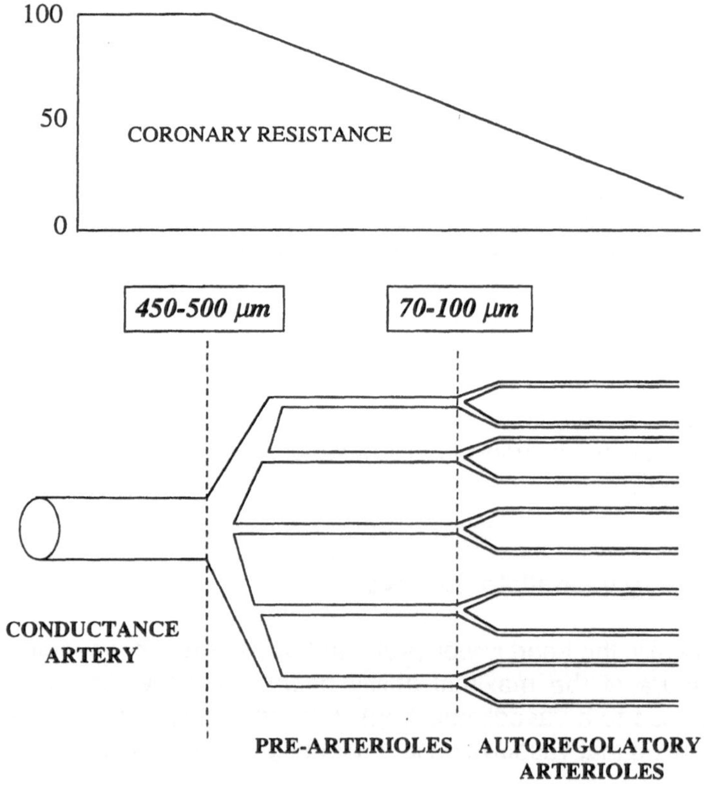

Figure 1. *Microcirculation*

In addition to intravascular resistance, myocardial perfusion is also influenced by extravascular forces, particularly due to the intramyocardial pressure which is generated throughout the contractile cycle[6]. Intramyocardial pressure is maximal in systole and in the subendocardial layers where it exceeds ventricular pressure [2] (figure 2).

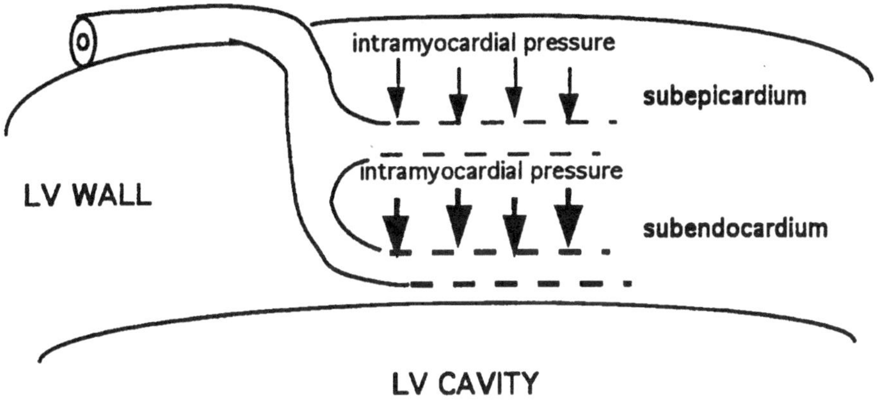

Figure 2. *Intramyocardial pressure and extravascular coronary resistance*

Mechanisms of myocardial ischemia

Myocardial ischemia occurs when the workload of the heart is not matched by an adequate oxygen delivery through myocardial blood flow. The best known mechanism of myocardial ischemia is that associated with atherosclerotic coronary disease. Studies in animals and patients with coronary artery disease have demonstrated that there is an inverse relation between the severity of a coronary stenosis and coronary vasodilator reserve [7-9]. The pressure drop across the stenosis is initially compensated for by a drop in coronary resistance through vasodilation of autoregulatory vessels. However, at stenosis equal or greater than 80% of the luminal diameter, the coronary vasodilator reserve becomes exhausted [9]. Under these circumstances an increase in cardiac workload cannot be met by an adequate increase in blood flow leading to myocardial ischemia.

The coronary microcirculation and myocardial ischemia

Recent clinical studies have suggested that constriction of small coronary arterioles may play a role in the genesis of myocardial ischemia in patients with coronary artery disease. In addition, symptoms and signs typical of myocardial ischemia can be demonstrated in patients without angiographic evidence of coronary disease (e.g. hypertensives) [2, 10].

Mechanisms of microvascular dysfunction

Reduction in the caliber of the small coronary arterioles can be due to a series of different mechanism including: 1- Active vasoconstriction or loss of vasodilator capacity; 2- Remodeling of the vessel wall (e.g. medial hypertrophy with lumen/wall ratio reduction); 3- Abnormal intramyocardial pressure (extravascular resistance).

1- Active vasoconstriction or loss of vasodilator capacity

It has been proposed that constriction of the small vessels can be induced by: a) drop in perfusion pressure distal to the epicardial stenosis; b) endothelial dysfunction [11, 12]; and c) neurohumoral factors (e.g. endothelin[13] neuropeptide Y [14], serotonin [15]). In addition, the small coronary arterioles receive autonomic inervation and their diameter may be altered by stimulation of these nerves [16-24].

2- Remodeling of the vessel wall

The structural remodeling of the coronary microcirculation, as that observed in hypertensive heart disease, includes changes in the arteriolar wall and a relative reduction in the total number of vessels, probably as a consequence of the disproportionate growth of myocytes without a corresponding increase in the available blood supply. Medial thickening of intramural coronary arteries in myocardial biopsy specimens from humans with hypertension has recently been confirmed, with an increase in the wall/lumen ratio which correlates with the increase in the resistance to coronary blood flow, and the reduction in coronary flow reserve. This clinical data confirms previous reports in post-mortem specimens where marked thickening of arterioles of 50-200 μm has been reported in patients with chest pain and hypertensive heart disease [25-27].

3- Abnormal intramyocardial pressure (extravascular resistance)

Both in the presence of coronary autoregulation and during maximal coronary vasodilation the subendocardial to subepicardial flow ratio is close to unity and ranges from 0.8 to 1.2 [28-31]. This occurs despite the higher extravascular intramyocardial pressure which is present in the subendocardial myocardium and is probably due to a greater vascularity in this layer [32]. During maximal vasodilation, however, if coronary perfusion pressure falls below the "subendocardial opening pressure" (i.e. the perfusion pressure required to open the subendocardial vessels which is higher than the pressure required to open the subepicardial vessels) selective subendocardial hypoperfusion occurs [32]. This will produce a drop in the subendocardial to subepicardial ratio to levels below 0.8 (transmural steal). A greater fall of perfusion pressure below the "subepicardial opening pressure" will cause transmural hypoperfusion [32].

References

1. Camici P, Marraccini P, Marzilli M, et al. Coronary hemodynamics and myocardial metabolism during and after pacing stress in normal humans. Am J Physiol 1989;257:E309-17.
2. De Silva R, Camici PG. Role of positron emission tomography in the investigation of human coronary circulatory function. Cardiovasc Res 1994;28:1595-612.
3. Chilian WM, Eastham CL, Layne SM, Marcus ML. Small vessel phenomena in the coronary microcirculation: phasic intramyocardial perfusion and microvascular dynamics. Prog Cardiovasc Dis 1988;31:17-38.
4. Marcus ML, Chilian WM, Kanatsuka H, Dellsperger KC, Eastham CL, Lamping KG. Understanding the coronary circulation through studies at the microvascular level. Circulation 1990;82:1-7.
5. Chilian WM, Eastham CL, Marcus ML. Microvascular distribution of coronary vascular resistance in beating left ventricle. Am J Physiol 1986;251:H779-88.
6. Hoffmann JI. Transmural myocardial perfusion. Prog Cardiovasc Dis 1987;29:429-64.
7. Lipscomb K, Gould KL. Mechanism of the effect of coronary artery stenosis on coronary flow in the dog. Am Heart J 1975;89:60-7.
8. Gould KL, Lipscomb K, Hamilton GW. Physiologic basis for assessing critical coronary stenosis. Instantaneous flow response and regional distribution during coronary hyperemia as measures of coronary flow reserve. Am J Cardiol 1974;33:87-94.
9. Uren NG, Melin JA, De Bruyne B, Wijns W, Baudhuin T, Camici PG. Relation between myocardial blood flow and the severity of coronary artery stenosis. N Engl J Med 1994;330:1782-8.
10. Camici PG. Microcirculation: what is the role of calcium antagonists? Eur Heart J 1997;18 Suppl A:A51-5.
11. Kuo L, Davis MJ, Cannon MS, Chilian WM. Pathophysiological consequences of atherosclerosis extend into the coronary microcirculation. Restoration of endothelium dependent responses by L-arginine. Circ Res 1992;70:465-76.
12. Zeiher AM, Drexler H, Wollschlager H, Just H. Endothelial dysfunction of the coronary microvasculature is associated with impaired coronary blood flow regulation in patients with early atherosclerosis. Circulation 1991;84:1984-92.
13. Larkin SW, Clarke JG, Keogh BG, et al. Intracoronary endothelin induces myocardial ischemia by small vessel constriction in the dog. Am J Cardiol 1989;64:956-8.
14. Clarke JG, Davies GJ, Kerwin R, et al. Coronary artery infusion of neuropeptide Y in patients with angina pectoris. Lancet 1987;1:1057-9.
15. McFadden EP, Clarke JG, Davies GJ, Kaski JC, Haider AW, Maseri A. Effect of intracoronary serotonin on coronary vessels in patients with stable angina and patients with variant angina. N Engl J Med 1991;324:648-54.
16. Chilian WM, Layne SM, Eastham CL, Marcus ML. Heterogeneous microvascular coronary alpha-adrenergic vasoconstriction. Circ Res 1989;64:376-88.
17. Nabel EG, Ganz P, Gordon JB, Alexander RW, Selwyn AP. Dilation of normal and constriction of atherosclerotic coronary arteries caused by cold presser test. Circulation 1988;77:43-52.

18. Zeiher AM, Drexler H, Wollschlager H, Saurbier B, Just H. Coronary vasomotion in response to sympathetic stimulation in humans: importance of the functional integrity of the endothelium. J Am Coll Cardiol 1989;14:1181-90.
19. Vita JA, Treasure CB, Yeung AC, et al. Patients with evidence of coronary endothelial dysfunction as assessed by acetylcholine infusion demonstrate marked increase in sensitivity to constrictor effects of catecholamines. Circulation 1992;85:1390-7.
20. Murray PA, Vatner SF. Alpha-adrenoreceptor attenuation of the coronary vascular response to severe exercise in the conscious dog. Circ Res 1979;45:654-60.
21. Heyndrickx GR, Muylaert P, Pannier JL. Alpha-advenergic control of oxygen delivery to myocardium during exercise in conscious dogs. Am J Physiol 1982;242:H805-9.
21. Gwirtz PA, Overn SP, Mass HJ, Jones CE. Alpha 1-adrenergic constriction limits coronary flow and cardiac function in running dogs. Am J Physiol 1986;250:H1117-26.
22. Dai XZ, Sublett E, Lindstrom P, Schwartz JS, Homans DC, Bache RJ. Coronary flow during exercise after selective alpha1- and alpha2-adrenergic blockade. Am J Physiol 1989;256:H1148-55.
23. Duncker DJ, Van Zon NS, Crampton M, Herrlinger S, Homans DC, Bache RJ. Coronary pressure-flow relationship and exercise: contribution of heart rate, contractility and alpha 1-adrenergic tone. Am J Physiol 1994;266:H795-810.
25. Strauer BE, Schwartzkopff B, Motz W, Vogt M. Coronary vascular changes in the progression and regression of hypertensive heart disease. J Cardiovasc Pharmacol 1991;18 Suppl 3:S20-7.
26. Schwartzkopff B, Motz W, Frenzel H, Vogt M, Knauer S, Strauer BE. Structural and functional alterations of the intramyocardial coronary arterioles in patients with arterial hypertension. Circulation 1993;88:993-1003.
27. Folkow B. 'Structural factor' in primary and secondary hypertension. Hypertension 1990; 16:89-101.
28. Domenech RJ, Hoffman JI, Noble MI, Saunders KB, Henson JR, Subijanto S. Total and regional coronary blood flow measured by radioactive microspheres in conscious and anesthetized dogs. Circ Res 1969;25:581-96.
29. Bache RJ, Cobb FR, Greenfield JC Jr. Myocardial blood flow distribution during ischemia-induced coronary vasodilation in the unanesthetized dog. J Clin Invest 1974;54:1462-72.
30. Cobb FR, Bache RJ, Greenfield JC Jr. Regional myocardial blood flow in awake dogs. J Clin Invest 1974;53:1618-25.
31. Buckberg GD, Fixler DE, Archie JP, Hoffman JI. Experimental subendocardial ischemia in dogs with normal coronary arteries. Circ Res 1972;30:67-81.
32. L'Abbate A, Marzilli M, Ballestra AM, et al. Opposite transmural gradients of coronary resistance and extravascular pressure in the working dog's heart. Cardiovasc Res 1980; 14:21-9.

Chapter 7

Myocardial Ischemia and Cholesterol Lowering Therapy

Hans-Marc J. Siebelink and Ad J. van Boven

Introduction

Only recently a causal relation between cholesterol and ischemic heart disease has been accepted [1,2]. Large intervention trials have shown that cholesterol lowering therapy in patients with elevated and with moderately elevated plasma cholesterol levels decreases cardiovascular morbidity and mortality [3-5]. Together with smoking, hypertension, dietary factors, sedentary life style and family history of vascular disease, elevated cholesterol is one of the major risk factors for atherosclerosis. High serum lipid levels facilitate atherosclerotic plaque formation and are associated with endothelial dysfunction, inflammation and thrombosis.
With new therapeutic strategies to lower cholesterol levels, the process of atherosclerosis and thrombosis can be modified, reducing the incidence of ischemic heart disease. This chapter will focus on different mechanistic aspects of cholesterol and its relation to ischemic heart disease.

Cholesterol and coronary circulation

The atherosclerotic process affects macro- and microcirculation. The hallmark of atherosclerosis in macrocirculation is the atherosclerotic plaque. The pathophysiological process of atherosclerosis is characterized by inflammation that causes damage to the vessel wall. Plaque formation occurs at the site of injury which is greatly influenced by low density

Van der Wall et al. (eds.),
Advanced Imaging in Coronary Artery Disease, 109-120.

lipoprotein (LDL) cholesterol, in particular by its oxidized modification [6]. When modified LDL passes the damaged endothelial barrier it is taken up by macrophages creating the metabolic active foam cell inside the plaque. Macrophages release cytokines which enhance the chronic inflammatory process and are chemotactic to other leucocytes [7]. Activated macrophages cause smooth muscle cell proliferation and neovascularization of the plaque[8]. As a result the plaque size increases. However obstructive atherosclerotic lesions (> 70%) seldom lead to acute coronary events. Plaque stability seems one of the most important factors since lesions less than 50% contribute for two-thirds of all acute myocardial infarction [9,10]. Plaque rupture is determined by several factors [11,12,13]. The plaques prone to rupture are eccentric, contain greater content of lipids, contain more macrophages and have a thinner fibrous cap covering the plaque. High esterified lipid concentrations at the edge of the plaque are associated with macrophage activity [13]. Macrophages are able to synthesize metalloproteinases which increase breakdown of the extracellular matrix so that the plaque weakens and ruptures [14]. The underlying mechanism of acute coronary events such as myocardial infarction is a ruptured plaque with subsequent thrombosis leading to occlusion of the coronary vessel. Although atherosclerosis and thrombosis in the macrocirculation are thought to be responsible for the majority of cardiovascular events, microcirculatory dysfunction might also be a factor for cardiac morbidity. Without overt macrocirculatory abnormalities, the process of atherosclerosis in the coronary microcirculation becomes more important.

In the microcirculation no atherosclerotic plaque is found. Hypercholesterolemia and other risk factors cause impaired endothelial function. Endothelial dysfunction is generally accepted as an early atherosclerotic manifestation and is present in macro- and microcirculation[15]. Endothelium derived nitric oxide (NO) has important vasodilator functions but also protects the artery from injury by inhibiting chemokines, adhesion of molecules, platelet adhesion and aggregation, and vascular smooth muscle proliferation. In unaffected coronary arteries the endothelium is able to dilate the coronary artery by releasing NO under physiological conditions. In dysfunctional endothelium the NO production is decreased and vasodilatation is impaired or even reversed to vasoconstriction. This phenomenon was first demonstrated by Furchgott and Zawadzki by damaging the endothelium and infusion of acetylcholine, a specific endothelium mediated vasomotor substance [16]. Vita et al.[17] and Steinberg et al. [18] showed that degree of endothelial dysfunction in coronary arteries correlated with cholestesterol levels. Oxidized LDL cholesterol was found to impair endothelium mediated vasodilatation in coronary arterioles of pigs [19]. Moreover Zeiher et al. showed that endothelial dysfunction was also present in patients with minimal coronary artery disease with normal cholesterol levels [20]. Results from our own institution demonstrated that coronary flow reserve with dipyridamole is impaired in hypercholesterolemic non coronary artery disease (CAD) patients compared to normals measured with positron emission tomography (PET). This suggests an impaired microcirculatory response possibly due to endothelial dysfunction.

Cholesterol and thrombosis

Hypercholesterolemia is associated with hypercoagulability and enhanced platelet aggregation. Hypercoagulability can be explained by increased humoral thrombogenic and hypofibrinolytic factors found in hypercholesterolemic patients [21]. Higher resting levels of thromboxane B2 and beta-thrombomodulin suggest that high blood cholesterol levels induce platelet activation [22]. In vitro experiments showed that baseline thrombus formation was significantly higher in hypercholesterolemic patients compared to controls [23]. The mechanism for this increased thrombosis is not yet completely known, but it is suggested that impaired endothelial function also plays a significant role.

Effect of cholesterol lowering therapy

Lipid lowering therapy with fibrates and HMG-CoA reductase inhibitors greatly affects plasma lipid levels. By lowering LDL cholesterol levels the amount of LDL cholesterol available for atherosclerotic plaque formation will be reduced. In a plaque containing less cholesterol, less oxidized LDL cholesterol and less foam cells will be formed. On cholesterol lowering therapy high density lipoprotein (HDL) cholesterol levels generally increase. Since HDL cholesterol transports cholesterol from tissue back to the liver, the amount of cholesterol in plaques can be reduced. Cholesterol lowering therapy is also associated with other beneficial effects such as immune modulation affecting plaque stability, reduction of growth factor production, enhancement of endothelial function and reduction of thrombosis.

Experimental studies
Convincing evidence that atherosclerosis can be reduced with lipid lowering therapy is derived from experimental studies with animals. Atherosclerosis can be induced by cholesterol-rich diet in a group of animals. As plasma lipid levels rise, the composition of the coronary artery changes and

contains more collagen, elastin and cholesterol. When animals are fed on a cholesterol low diet plasma lipid levels drop to normal values and changes in coronary arteries partly regress over 20-40 months [24,25]. In hypercholesterolemic rabbits progressive atherosclerosis and impairment of endothelial function was found.
By feeding these rabbits with NO precursor L-arginine regression of lesions, improvement of endothelium dependent relaxation and reduction of superanion generation was observed. This indicates that NO therapy can modify endothelial function and the process of atherosclerosis [26]. Consequently, if in animal studies progression of atherosclerosis can be reduced or even reversed and endothelial function can be restored, this could have great impact on incidence of ischemic heart disease in humans.

Cholesterol lowering trials
Major effects on the incidence of coronary heart disease were first demonstrated in the Helsinki Heart Study with gemfibrozil in asymptomatic men with dyslipidemia. In this study a reduction of 34% in coronary heart disease was shown [3]. It is well known that fibrates lower trigycerides and that HMG-CoA reductase inhibitors lower LDL cholesterol levels. HDL cholesterol levels are increased by fibrates and to a lesser extend by HMG-CoA reductase inhibitors. Results form the 4S [4], WOSCOP [5], CARE [27] and LIPID [28] studies show that cholesterol lowering therapy with HMG-CoA reductase inhibitors results in reduction of reintervention rates, myocardial infarction, and cardiac death.

These results are applicable to symptomatic and asymptomatic CAD patients, patients with elevated and average cholesterol levels and non-CAD patients. The 4S-study even reports a decrease in total death in the treated group and in this group of patients cholesterol lowering reduces the risk independently of age and smoking.

Angiographical and Holter studies
Several studies evaluating cholesterol lowering therapy angiographically report that treatment with lovastatin and pravastatin results in less progression of lesions and a reduction of new lesions compared to placebo[29-31]. In addition to angiographical changes the REGRESS investigators also found a reduction in cardiovascular events in the statin treated group [30]. In angiographical studies a minimal but significant reduction of atherosclerosis, combined with substantial reduction of events, suggests that not only angiographical changes but also other factors are influenced positively by cholesterol lowering therapy [32].

From the REGRESS study it was also reported that in patients treated with pravastatine, Holter monitoring demonstrated less ischemic episodes and that duration of ischemia was significantly reduced compared to placebo (figure 1) [33]. These findings were supported by Andrews et al [34].

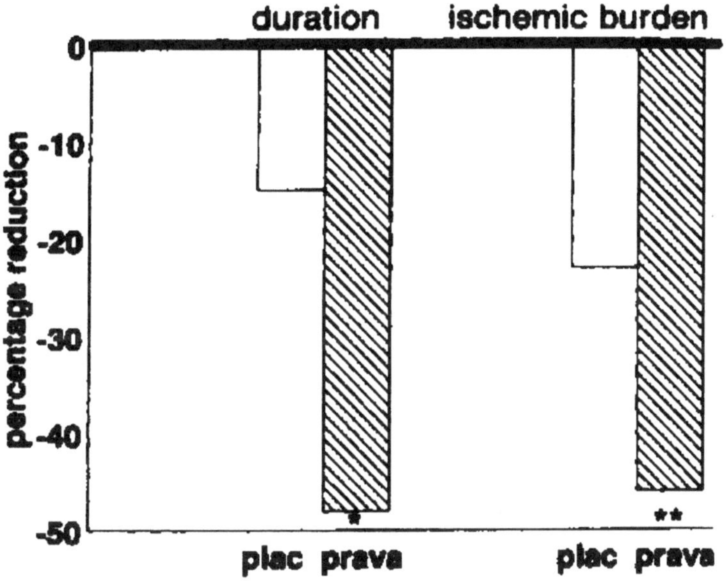

Figure 1. *Diagram of the percentage reduction in components of transient myocardial ischemia during the study in placebo patients (plac, open bars) and in pravastatin patients (prava, hatched bars). *P=0.017 and **P=0.0058. Adapted from [33].*

Plaque stability

Cholesterol lowering therapy is also able to increase stability of atherosclerotic plaques. Cholesterol lowering therapy with pravastatin has been shown to influence cholesterol metabolism in macrophages in vivo and in vitro [35]. Inhibition of cholesterol synthesis potentially reduces macrophage activation, foam cell formation and thrombogenicity of the plaques. It can also alter the lipid to cell ratio of the atherosclerotic lesion, which makes the plaque less vulnerable to rupture, possibly reducing acute coronary events. This is supported by reduction of acute coronary events observed in the large cholesterol lowering trials.

Endothelial function

Applying cholesterol lowering therapies Treasure et al. and Anderson et al. showed improved endothelium mediated responses on coronary angiography in coronary arteries of patients with atherosclerosis after treatment with lovastatin and lovastatin and antioxidant respectively [36,37]. Endothelial dysfunction can also result in decreased tissue perfusion. Pitkanen et al. demonstrated with PET imaging that in patients with familial hypercholesterolemia coronary flow reserve was impaired and that coronary vascular resistance was elevated compared to normal volunteers [38]. Hasdai et al. demonstrated myocardial perfusion defects with ^{99m}Tc-sestamibi SPECT in CAD patients with non-significant coronary artery stenosis (<50%) during infusion of acetylcholine [39]. However improved endothelial function might result in an increased flow and increased myocardial perfusion. In forearm blood flow studies cholesterol lowering therapy results in increased perfusion by restoration of endothelial derived NO synthesis [40] and enhanced endothelial vasodilatation [41]. The latter study demonstrated the beneficial effect after one month on simvastatin therapy indicating that improved endothelial function might be a short term effect of cholesterol lowering therapies. Measuring myocardial flow with PET, Gould et al. showed that size and severity of perfusion defects was reduced after 3 months of cholesterol lowering therapy [42]. Results from a recent PET study demonstrated that fluvastatin therapy increases coronary flow reserve after 6 months, but not after 2 months [43]. If cholesterol lowering therapy results in an improved endothelial function and subsequently increases myocardial flow and perfusion, it is very likely that intensity and frequency of cardiac, ischemic episodes can be reduced.

Vascular thrombosis

In acute coronary events plaque stability and vascular thrombosis play a significant role. Thrombogenicity is increased in patients with high cholesterol levels. Therefore a reduction of thrombosis might result in a reduction of ischemic events. Applying cholesterol lowering therapy in familial hypercholesterolemic patients the hemostatic balance is influenced positively [44]. Lovastatin therapy in hypercholesterolemic patients reduced serum fibrinogen levels and adenosine-diphosphate-induced aggregation[45]. Pravastatin reduced platelet aggregation in hypercholesterolemic CAD patients possibly due to decreased thromboxane production [46]. Cholesterol lowering also diminishes the interaction of fibrinogen and platelets as this is increased in hypercholesterolemia. The precise mechanism for reduction of thrombosis is still unclear but there might be an important role for endothelium derived NO which can reduce platelet adhesion and aggregation.

Inflammation
From transplant patients it is known that statin therapy also has anti-inflammatory effects. HMG-CoA reductase inhibitors reduce progression of CAD and decrease incidence of major rejection periods 1 year after transplantation [47]. HMG-CoA reductase inhibitors depress expression and function of leukocyte cell surface molecules required for monocytes to adhere to confluent endothelial monolayers [48] and reduce the response of monocytes to chemotactic stimuli [49]. When monocyte migration through the endothelium is prevented the atherosclerotic plaque contains less macrophages and less foam cells will be formed. As a result, also less cytokines and enzymes will be produced. The mechanism by which HMG-CoA reductase inhibitors modulate monocyte function is mediated by an increased generation of mevalonate. It is also reported that cytotoxicity of natural killer cells is reduced by statin therapy in in-vivo and in-vitro experiments [50]. Thus HMG-CoA reductase inhibitors directly interfere with the mechanisms by which leukocytes mediate the inflammatory response involved in the process of atherosclerosis.

Future directions

Since cholesterol lowering therapy enhances clinical outcome and influences the process of atherosclerosis by various mechanisms, HMG-CoA reductase inhibitors in ischemic heart disease are very promising. New HMG-CoA reductase inhibitors and higher dosages of established statins are more powerful in reducing LDL cholesterol. Since beneficial effects of cholesterol lowering therapy in perfusion studies are reported within 6 months, it is hypothesized that immediate aggressive statin therapy using a high dose and/or a more powerful statin results in better clinical outcome. Studies are performed which evaluate the effect of immediate aggressive statin therapy in post-myocardial infarction patients and in patients with unstable angina pectoris.

In our institution two studies are currently performed. The first compares the effect of aggressive cholesterol lowering with the effect of percutaneous coronary angioplasty (PTCA) procedure. In this study PET myocardial perfusion responses after 6 months on statin therapy are compared with perfusion responses 6 months after PTCA. The second study concerns endothelial dysfunction as an early atherosclerotic phenomenon. Can cholesterol lowering therapy improve or even reverse endothelial dysfunction in a primary prevention setting? With PET imaging we are studying perfusion responses in hypercholesterolemic asymptomatic patients before and on cholesterol lowering therapy. Preliminary results show that perfusion response to cold pressor test (an endothelial function test) increases on cholesterol lowering therapy (figure 2), suggesting improvement of endothelial function. However final results are not yet available and the effect of primary prevention on clinical outcome remains to be assessed.

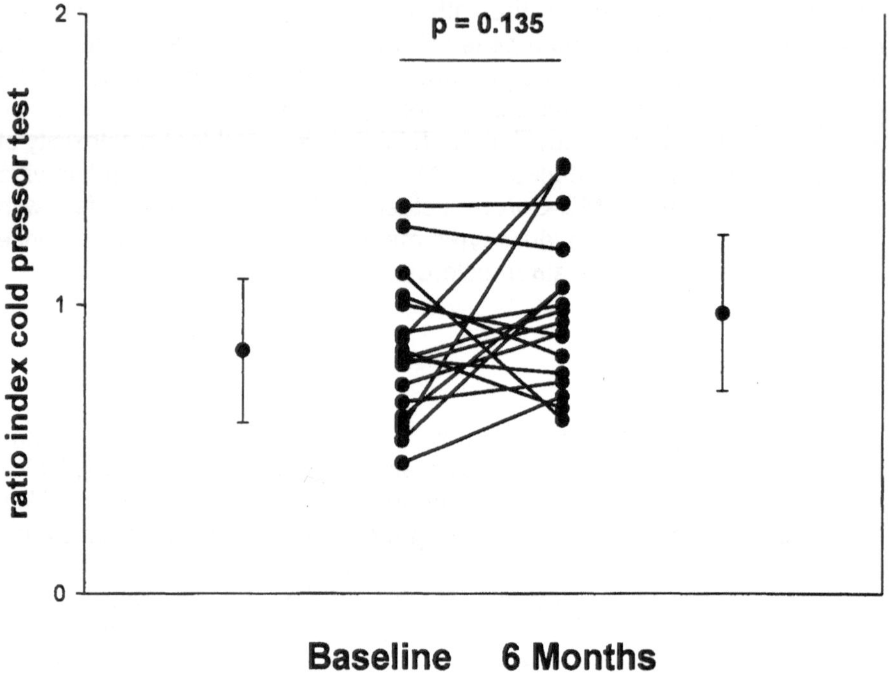

Figure 2. *Effect of 6 months cholesterol lowering therapy on PET myocardial perfusion response to cold pressor test corrected for rate pressure product in hypercholesterolemic asymptomatic non CAD patients.*

References

1. Gotto AM, D, Gorry GA, Thompson JR, et al. Relationship between plasma lipid concentrations and coronary artery disease in 496 patients. Circulation 1977;56:875-83.
2. Kannel WB Range of serum cholesterol values in the population developing coronary artery disease. Am J Cardiol 1995;76:69C-77C.
3. Frick MH, Elo O, Haapa K, et al. Helsinki Heart Study: primary-prevention trail with gemfibrozil in middle-aged men with dyslipidemia. Safety of treatment, changes in risk factors, and incidence of coronary heart disease. N Engl J Med 1987;317:1237-45.
4. Randomised trial of cholesterol lowering in 4444 patients with coronary heart disease: the Scandinavian Simvastatin Survival Study (45). Lancet 1994;344:1383-9.
5. Shepherd J, Cobbe SM, Ford I, et al. Prevention of coronary heart disease with pravastatin in men with hypercholesterolemia. West of Scotland Coronary Prevention Study Group. N Engl J Med 1995;333:1301-7.
6. Witztum JL. The oxidation hypothesis of atherosclerosis. Lancet 1994;344:793-5.
7. Gerrity RG. The role of monocyte in atherogenesis: I Transition of blood-borne monocytes into foam cells in fatty lesions. Am J Pathol 1981;103:181-90.
8. Ross R, Raines EW, Bowen-Pope DF. The biology of platelet derived growth factor. Cell 1986;46:155-69.
9. Ambrose JA, Tannenbaum MA, Alexopoulos D, et al. Angiographic progression of coronary artery disease and the development of myocardial infarction. J Am Coll Cardiol 1988;12:56-62.
10. Little WC, Constantinescu M, Applegate RJ, et al. Can coronary angiography predict the site of a subsequent myocardial infarction in patients with mild-to-moderate coronary artery disease? Circulation 1988;78:1157-66.
11. Brown BG, Zhao XG, Sacco DE, Albers JJ. Lipid lowering and plaque regression. New insights into prevention of plaque disruption and clinical events in coronary disease. Circulation 1993;87:1781-91.
12. Fuster V. Elucidation of the role of plaque instability and rupture in acute coronary events. Am J Cardiol 1995;76:24C-33C.
13. Felton CV, Crook D, Davies MJ, Oliver MF. Relation of plaque lipid composition and morphology to the stability of human aortic plaques. Atheroscler Thromb Vasc Biol 1997;17:1337-45.
14. Galis ZS, Sukhova GK, Lark MW, Libby P. Increased expression of matrix metalloproteinases and matrix degrading activity in vulnerable regions of human atherosclerotic plaques. J Clin Invest 1994;94:2493-503.
15. Buikema JH. Endothelial dysfunction in cardiovascular disease [dissertation]. Groningen: University of Groningen; 1995.
16. Hasdai D, Gibbons RJ, Holmes DR Jr, Higano ST, Lerman A. Coronary endothelial dysfunction in humans is associated with myocardial perfusion defects. Circulation 1997;96:3390-95.
17. Vita JA, Treasure CB, Nabel EG, et al. Coronary vasomotor response to acetylcholine relates to risk factors for coronary artery disease. Circulation 1990;81:491-7.
18. Steinberg HO, Bayazeed B, Hook G, Johnson A, Cronin J, Baron AD. Endothelial dysfunction is associated with cholesterol levels in the high normal range in humans. Circulation 1997;96:3287-93.

19. Hein TW, Kuo L. Oxidized LDL specifically impairs nitric oxide-mediated dilation of coronary arterioles [abstract]. Circulation 1997 (8 Suppl):I114.
20. Zeiher AM, Drexler H, Wollschlager H, Just H. Endothelial dysfunction of the coronary microvasculature is associated with impaired coronary blood flow regulation in patients with early atherosclerosis. Circulation 1991;84:1984-92.
21. Badimon JJ, Badimon L, Turitto VT, Fuster V. Platelet deposition at high shear rates is enhanced by high plasma cholesterol levels: In vivo study in the rabbit model. Arterioscler Thromb 1991;11:395-402.
22. DiMinno G, Silver MJ, Cerbone AM, Rainone A, Postiglione A, Mancini M. Increased fibrinogen binding to platelets from patients with familial hypercholesterolemia. Arteriosclerosis 1986;6:203-11.
23. Lacoste L, Lam JY, Hung J, Letchakovsky G, Solymoss CB, Waters D. et al. Hyperlipidemia and coronary disease. Correction of the increased thrombogenic potential with cholesterol reduction. Circulation 1995;92:3172-77.
24. Armstrong ML, Megan MB. Arterial fibrous proteins in cynomolgos monkeys after atherogenic and regression diets. Circ Res 1975;36:256-61.
25. Clarkson TB, Bond MG, Bullock BC, Marzetta CA. A study of atherosclerosis regression in Macaca mulatta. IV. Changes in coronary arteries from animals with atherosclerosis induced for 19 months and then regressed for 24 or 48 months at plasma cholesterol concentrations of 300 or 200 mg/dl. Exp Mol Pathol 1981;34:345-68.
26. Candipan RC, Wang BY, Buitrago R, Tsao PS, Cooke JP. Regression or progression. Dependency on vascular nitric oxide. Aterioscler Thromb Vasc Biol 1996;16:44-50.
27. Sacks FM, Pfeffer MA, Moye LA, et al.The effect of pravastatin on coronary events after myocardial infarction in patients with average cholesterol levels. Cholesterol and Recurrent Events Trial investigators. N Engl J Med 1996;335:1001-9.
28. Design features and baseline characteristics of the LIPID (Long Term Intervention with Pravastatin in Ischemic Disease) Study: a randomized trial in patients with previous acute myocardial infarction and/or unstable angina pectoris. Am J Cardiol 1995;76:474-9.
29. Waters D, Higginson L, Gladstone P, et al. Effects of monotherapy with an HMG-CoA reductase inhibitor on the progression of coronary atherosclerosis as assessed by serial quantitative arteriography. The Canadian Coronary Atherosclerosis Intervention Trial. Circulation 1994;89:959-68.
30. Jukema JW, Bruschke AV, Van Boven AJ, et al. Effects of lipid lowering by pravastatin on progression and regression of coronary artery disease in symptomatic men with normal to moderately elevated serum cholesterol levels. The Regression Growth Evaluation Statin Study (REGRESS). Circulation 1995;91:2528-40.
31. Effect of simvastatin on coronary atheroma: the Multicentre Anti-Atheroma Study (MAAS) [published erratum appears in Lancet 1994;344:762]. Lancet 1994;344:633-8.
32. Brown BG, Zhao XG, Sacco DE, Albers JJ. Lipid lowering and plaque regression. New insights into prevention of plaque disruption and clinical events in coronary disease. Circulation 1993;87:1781-91.
33. Van Boven AJ, Jukema JW, Zwinderman AH, Crijns HJ, Lie KI, Bruschke AV. Reduction of transient myocardial ischemia with pravastatin in addition to the conventional treatment in patients with angina pectoris. REGRESS Study Group. Circulation 1996;94:1503-5.

34. Andrews TC, Raby K, Barry J, et al. Effect of cholesterol reduction on myocardial ischemia in patients with coronary disease. Circulation 1997;95:324-8.
35. Keidar S, Aviram M, Moar I, Oiknine J, Brook JG. Pravastatin inhibits cellular cholesterol synthesis and increases low density lipoprotein receptor activity in macrophages: in vitro and in vivo studies. Br J Clin Pharmacol 1994;38:513-9.
36. Treasure CB, Klein JL, Weintraub WS, et al. Beneficial effects of cholesterol lowering therapy on the coronary endothelium in patients with coronary artery disease. N Engl J Med 1995;332:481-7.
37. Anderson TJ, Meredith IT, Yeung AC, Frei B, Selwyn AP, et al. The effect of cholesterol lowering and antioxidant therapy on endothelium dependent coronary vasomotion. N Engl J Med 1995;332: 488-493.
38. Pitkanen OP, Raitakari OT, Niinikoski H, et al. Coronary flow reserve is impaired in young men with familial hypercholesterolemia. J Am Coll Cardiol 1996;28:1705-11.
39. Hasdai D, Gibbons RJ, Holmes DR et al. Coronary endothelial dysfunction in humans is associated with myocardial perfusion defects. Circulation 1997;96:3390-5.
40. Stroes ES, Koomans HA, De Bruin TW, Rabelink TJ. Vascular function in the forearm of hypercholesterolaemic patients off and on lipid-lowering medication. Lancet 1995;346:467-71.
41. O'Driscoll G, Green D, Taylor RR. Simvastatin, an HMG-coenzyme a reductase inhibitor, improves endothelial function within 1 month. Circulation 1997;95:1126-31.
42. Gould KL, Martucci JP, Goldberg DI, et al. Short term cholesterol lowering decreases size and severity of perfusion abnormalities by positron emission tomography after dipyridamole in patients with coronary artery disease. A potential marker of healing coronary endothelum. Circulation 1994;89:1530-8.
43. Guethlin M, Kasel AM, Coppenrath K, Ziegler S, Delius W, Schwaiger M. Longterm effects of cholesterol lowering therapy with fluvastatin in patients with hypercholesterolemia and moderate coronary artery disease [abstract]. Circulation 1997;96 (8 Suppl):I68.
44. Jerling JC, Vorster HH, Oosthuizen W, Vermaak WJ, et al. Effect of simvastatin, a 3-hydroxy-3-methylglutaryl coenzyme A reductase inhibitor, on the haemostatic balance of familial hypercholesterolaemic subjects. Fibrinolysis Proteolysis 1997;11:91-6.
45. Mayer J, Eller T, Brauer P, et al. Effects of long-term treatment with lovastatin on the clotting system and blood platelets. Ann Hematol 1992;64:196-201.
46. Lacoste L, Lam LY, Hung J, et al. Hyperlipidaemia and coronary disease: correction of the increased thrombogenic potential with cholesterol reduction. Circulation 1995;92:3172-77.
47. Kobashigawa JA, Katznelson S, Laks H et al. Effect of pravastatin on outcomes after cardiac transplantation. N Engl J Med 1995;333:621-7.
48. Weber C, Erl W, Weber KS, Weber PC. HMG-CoA reductase inhibitors decrease CD11b expression and CD11b-dependent adhesion of monocytes to endothelium and reduce increased adhesiveness of monocytes isolated from patients with hypercholesterolemia. J Am Coll Cardiol 1997;30:1212-7.
49. Kreuzer J, Bader J, Jahn L, Hautmann M, Kubler W, Von Hodenberg E. Chemotaxis of the monocyte cell line U937: dependence on cholesterol and early mevalonate pathway products. Atherosclerosis 1991;90:203-9.

50. McPherson R, Tsoukas C, Baines MG, et al. Effects of lovastatin on natural killer cell function and other immunological parameters in man. J Clin Immunol 1993;13:439-44.

Chapter 8

MYOCARDIAL ISCHEMIA AND PAIN

Gert J. ter Horst

Myocardial ischemic events, arising from an unfavorable supply and demand of oxygen, are the most frequent cause of angina pectoris or heart pain. Angina pectoris can be treated effectively either with medication that improves blood supply to the ischemic myocardium, or with coronary artery bypass grafting surgery. In a relatively small number of patients these treatments remain ineffective and in such cases neurostimulation (transient electrical nerve stimulation, TENS) or dorsal spinal cord stimulation (SCS) may bring relief. The mechanisms responsible for the effects of TENS and SCS are unknown but it may involve both cardiac and central nervous system mediated effects.

Mechanisms underlying the effect of SCS were the subject of investigation in clinical trials and preclinical experiments conducted by members of our group. For the interpretation of preclinical and human neuro-imaging studies we have first characterized the nervous pathways that participate in cardiovascular regulation and pain perception in the rat. Pain perception pathways were studied in a conscious rat model of acute cardiac pain that is based on infusion of capsaicin and putative algogenic substances in the pericardial sac. Factors contributing to nociceptor activation during cardiac ischemic events, cardiac pain pathways, and cerebral structures participating in pain modulation, are some examples of poorly characterized mechanisms in angina pectoris. Only recently, Rosen and co-workers have presented the first neuro-imaging study in which forebrain regions were characterized that participate in perception of cardiac pain in human cardiac artery disease patients during experimentally generated myocardial ischemia (see chapter by Rosen).

Van der Wall et al. (eds.),
Advanced Imaging in Coronary Artery Disease, 121-136.

Chemical mediators of angina

The neurochemical mechanisms underlying activation of the cardiac nociceptors during ischemia have not yet been identified. Ischemic conditions induce release of various compounds that each have the capability to activate and/or sensitize nociceptors. Adenosine, bradykinin, serotonin, histamine, lactate, potassium, prostaglandines, and free radicals are examples of putative algogenic substances in cardiac nociceptive mechanisms [1]. It has been demonstrated that adenosine production is increased during myocardial ischemia [2] and that intravenous injections of adenosine cause angina-like pain in patients suffering from angina [3,4].

However, only large concentrations of adenosine that exceed the physiological or pathophysiological range provoke such angina-like pain [3,4] and adenosine could not activate the spinal cardiac afferent nerves in animal studies [5]. Bradykinin is the most widely examined putative chemical mediator in cardiac ischemia. Very small concentrations of bradykinin activate the cardiac nociceptors [5,6]; an effect that is potentiated by prostaglandines, serotonin and histamine [6]. The content of bradykinin in coronary artery sinus blood has been found to increase during and after experimental coronary artery occlusion[7]. Intracoronary injections of bradykinin cause vocalization and pseudo-affective responses in conscious dogs and cats in the first few days after thoracic surgery [8].

Such behavioral effects, suggesting pain sensation, were not found in animals that had recovered from the thoracic surgery[8]. Likewise, intracoronary or left ventricular injections of serotonin (5-HT) and histamine caused pain behavior in lightly anaesthetized dogs [9].

While the administration of the putative chemical mediators of cardiac ischemia has been shown to excite and/or sensitize the nociceptors, it has been reported that the application of a mixture of these substances is capable of activating a much larger proportion of polymodal nociceptors [6].

This effect of the so-called inflammatory soup is much more potent than the effect of any single substance. Moreover, it is probably physiologically more relevant because bradykinin, adenosine, histamine, 5-HT and prostaglandines are all released during ischemia produced in experimental animals and in humans during angina [1], although the concentrations in the mixture and the time-scales of the release are unknown. It has been accepted now that these substances act simultaneously to produce pain.

Cardiac bradykinin-receptors and anginal pain

We investigated whether altered cardiac bradykinin receptor expression - bradykinin being one of the most potent endogenous algogenic substances of the ischemic cascade - can explain changing perception of ischemic cardiac pain with increasing age. The bradykinin B2 receptor subtype has been associated with nociceptor activation and the B1 subtype with induction of hyperalgesia [10]. The subjective perception of anginal pain and the expression in the myocardium of a conserved part of the bradykinin receptor mRNA (base pairs 150-800) [11] were studied in 15 patients of different ages (11 male, age 38-75 years), using questionnaires and semi-quantitative Reverse Transcriptase Polymerase Chain Reactions (RT-PCR). Tissue was isolated from the right atrium during coronary artery bypass surgery. After the removal of the tissue it was immediately frozen in liquid nitrogen and grounded for the extraction of total mRNA with RNAzol (Campro Scientific). Expression of the mRNA of the housekeeping protein b-actin was assessed for normalization. The age of patients reporting constricting and discomfort-like sensations was significantly different and respectively 70±2 and 52±4 years (p=0.03). Normalized optical density units (ODU) of cardiac bradykinin receptor mRNA correlated with age (r= -0.694; p=0.004) (figure 1A), but not with medication, gender, and duration of the disease. A positive correlation between the normalized bradykinin receptor mRNA ODU and the pain intensity scores (r=0.631; p=0.037) was found in male patients (figure 1B).

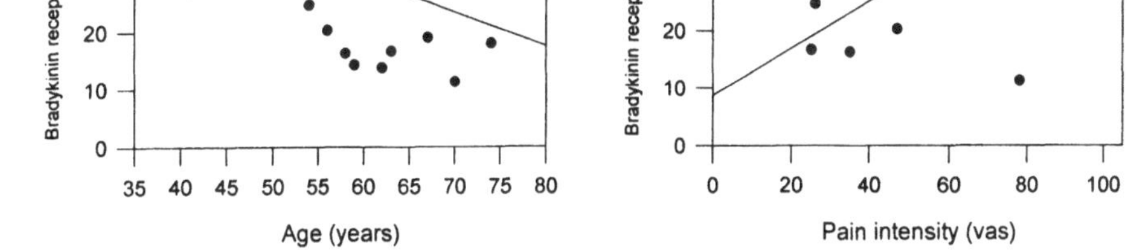

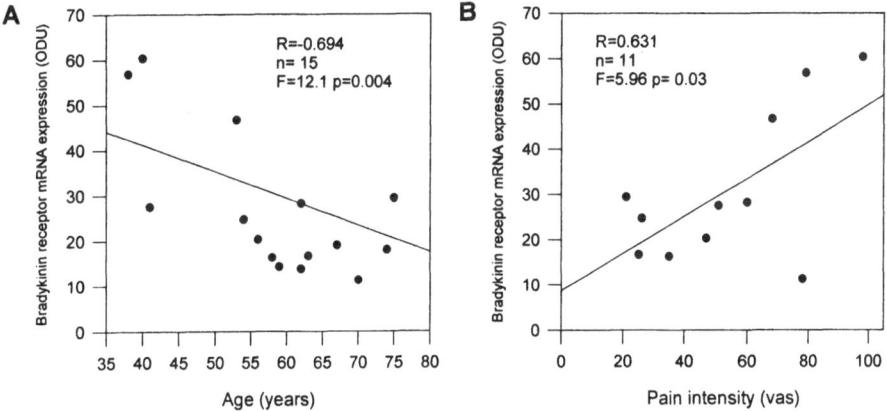

Figure 1. *Scatter diagrams showing the correlation's between normalized cardiac bradykinin receptor mRNA expression and the age of coronary artery bypass surgery patients **(A)**, and subjective pain intensity scores of the male patients **(B)**. Levels of mRNA are expressed in Optical Density Units (ODU)*

Age and normalized adenosine A1-receptor mRNA expression, which also has been implicated as mediator of cardiac pain [12], were not correlated. The findings support the conclusion that the level of cardiac bradykinin receptor expression determines characteristics of anginal pain perception.

Nervous pathways

Pain pathways have been studied predominantly in anaesthetized animals[6]. Angina for example was most often investigated in open thorax models. In such models, putative algogenic substances are applied topically on the myocardium or on the afferent nerves to activate the nervous circuitry [5]. However, pain modulation can not occur in this experimental setup because important modulators of nociception like adaptive behavior and stress-induced analgesia are prevented by the anesthetic. The behavioral response of the animal could be a valuable indication for occurrence of anginal pain and of its intensity. These aspects stimulated us to explore anginal pain pathways, pain behavior and cardiovascular responses to pain in a conscious rat model [6,13]. Acute heart pain was generated in chronically instrumented rats by infusion of capsaicin and other algogenic substances into the pericardial sac. The cardiovascular responses to anginal pain were monitored with telemetric blood pressure recording devices (Data Sciences Int) and pain pathways were studied with c-fos immunocytochemistry after the animal was sacrificed.

C-fos has been used as a marker of neuronal activity [14, 15]. This protein product of immediate early gene expression accumulates in neurons that respond to noxious stimuli. However, c-fos is not a selective marker for the nociceptive pathways in the brain since this protein accumulates in all cells that become activated during the painful stimulation of the heart. Behavioral responses, stress, cardiovascular activity, etc all will induce their own characteristic patterns of cerebral c-fos expression. Control experiments and anatomical data about nervous circuitry for cardiovascular regulation, stress and motor control are of utmost importance for interpretation of c-fos studies. Cerebral c-fos expression generated by stressful events is studied intensively [16].

The anatomy of neuronal networks participating in cardiovascular regulation, however, is less well known. Using a novel neuroanatomical tract tracing method we have analyzed the morphology of these networks before starting with characterization of anginal pain perception pathways and mechanisms underlying effects of TENS and SCS.

Structures in the brain that participate in cardiovascular regulation have been studied already for a long time with various neuroanatomical and neurophysiological techniques in animals, and recently also with neuro-imaging in humans. While the resolution of the latter method limits the detailed neuroanatomical characterization of structures involved, the experimental studies in animals were handicapped by the fact that putative relay stations in the brain could not be linked anatomically to the innervation of the heart. The retrograde transneuronal viral labeling techniques, which were introduced in the 1980's for neuroanatomical tract tracing [17], do not have this limitation. After regional infection of the myocardium with Pseudo Rabies Virus (PRV) solution the central nervous system showed infected nerve cells from the spinal to the cortical level [18]. Moreover, the method was used for identification of the parasympathetic forebrain circuitry for cardiovascular regulation in spinal cord transected animals.

Cardiovascular regulation

Injections of small amounts of a PRV solution into the various parts of the heart were used to characterize the nervous pathways for cardiovascular regulation in the rat. Virus infected nerve cells could be identified at all levels of the neuraxis (figure 2) after infection of the myocardium [18,19]. The PRV-infected preganglionic sympathetic cells were located bilaterally in the intermediolateral cell group of thoracic level 1 to 11 (T1-T11). The largest number of these infected preganglionic cells was found at levels T1 through T7. Of the PRV-infected preganglionic parasym-pathetic cells approximately 20% was situated in the dorsal motor vagus nucleus and the rest was located in the peri-ambiguus area in the ventral medulla oblon-gata. A myocardiotopy was evident both in the peri-ambiguus area and the ventral reticular formation [19]; a region that may be considered as an intermediate area in the nervous circuitry for cardiovascular regulation and maintenance of vasomotor tone in particular. The ventral reticular formation also participates in the baroreceptor reflex and receives information from the carotid baroreceptors through vagal afferents that terminate in the nucleus of the solitary tract (NTS) [20]. The NTS, the - serotonergic - raphe nuclei, the parabrachial region, the periaqueductal gray, various nuclei of the hypothalamus, the amygdala and the cortex all contained virus infected cells after the myocardial inoculations and thus it may be assumed that they all participate somehow in cardiovascular control. The virus infections of the cortex were restricted to parts of the anterior cingulate gyrus, the dysgranular insular cortex, and the frontal, the prelimbic, and the infralimbic area [19]. All infections were bilateral but most abundant at the right side of the brain.

The circuitry that is connected to the parasympathetic innervation of the heart was characterized selectively with spinal cord transections at T1. Most regions labeled in the healthy rats showed PRV immunoreactive cells in the transected animals too, although that the patterns of the infections deviated[19,21]. Clearly different patterns of infection were identified in the ventral reticular formation, the raphe nuclei, the peri-aqueductal gray, and in the ventral and the perifornical hypothalamus. The rostral insular and frontal cortexes were not infected at all in the spinal cord transected animals. Therefore, most likely these latter areas are only connected to the sympathetic heart innervation.

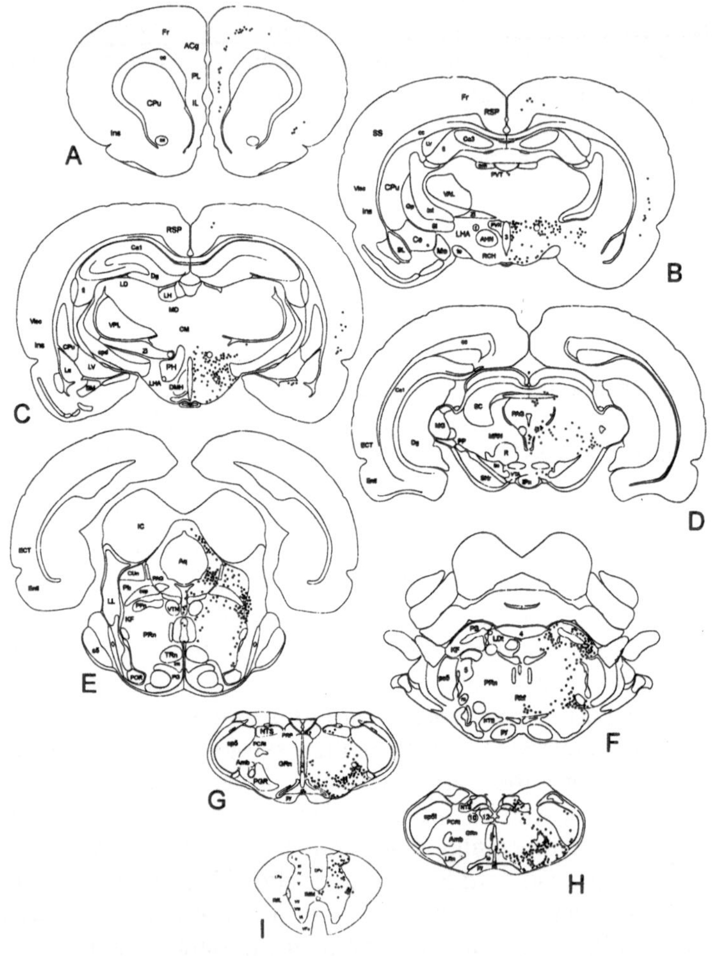

*Figure 2. Series of coronal sections of the rat brain from rostral **(A)** to caudal **(I)**, illustrating the locations of Pseudo Rabies Virus-infected cells after inoculation of the left ventricular myocardium. The infections were bilateral with no apparent lateralization*

Pain pathways

To characterize nervous pathways that participate in transmission of angina we have analyzed the cerebral c-fos expression patterns after infusion of the algogenic substances bradykinin and capsaicin into the pericardial sac of conscious rats. A strong behavioral (figure 3A) and cardiovascular response (figure 3C,D) was observed during infusions of capsaicin (50 µl of 10 µM capsaicin) [13] whereas bradykinin (50 µl of 250 nM bradykinin) triggered a modest behavioral and cardiovascular response. Capsaicin infusions into the pericardium induced an immediate active pain behavior [22] that consisted of vigorous scratching of the chest, forepaws and neck. After approximately 2 minutes this active pain behavior ceased and was followed by a long-lasting immobilization in which the rats extended both the fore- and hindlegs, meanwhile firmly pressing the chest to the bottom of the cage. Most animals remained in this position for about 40 minutes and thereafter they cautiously resumed the natural behavior. Characteristic for the cardiovascular response during the capsaicin infusions was an immediate bradycardia and hypertension, which was followed by a long-lasting tachycardia and hypotension 20 minutes after the start of the infusion (figure 3C,D).

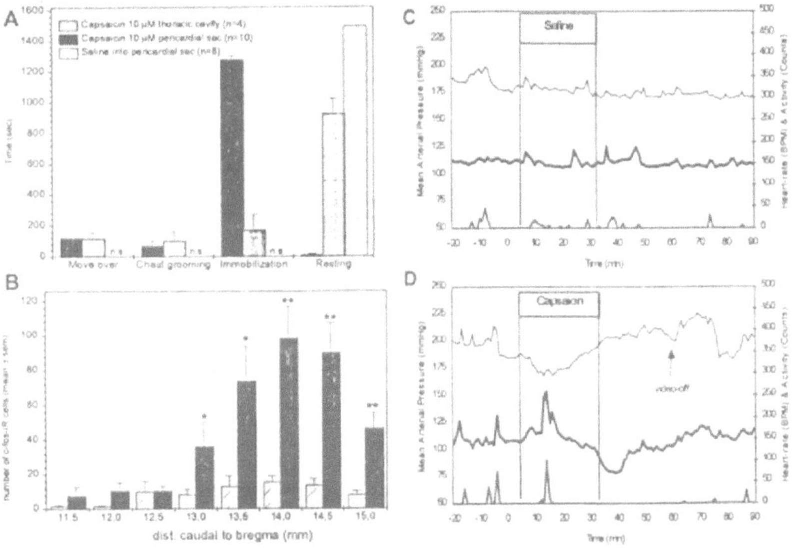

Figure 3. *Histograms illustrating the behavioral* ***(A)*** *and cardiovascular responses of conscious rats after infusions of saline* ***(C)*** *and* ***(D)*** *capsaicin (10 µM 50 µl) into the pericardial sac. The number of c-fos-IR cells at various rostro-caudal levels in the nucleus of the solitary tract is shown in* ***B****. Note that the rostral – orofacial - levels were not affected by the treatment.*

Infusions of bradykinin into the pericardial sac of conscious rats induced a different behavioral and cardiovascular response. Immediately after the bradykinin reached the pericardial space the animals became restless and thereafter they immobilized albeit in a different position than the animals that had received capsaicin. These bradykinin-treated animals remained immobile in a natural pose that resembled most the position shown during waking. As might be expected also the cardiovascular response was less strong. Immobilization was never observed in animals that received infusions of saline into the pericardial sac. Moreover, sometimes these control animals slept during the experiment.

The most important and also unexpected observation was that capsaicin-induced heart pain did not affect the pattern of c-fos expression in the dorsal laminae of the upper thoracic level (T2/T3) [22]. Infusions of bradykinin, on the other hand, almost doubled the number of c-fos immunoreactive cells at these thoracic levels. The c-fos positive cells were located in laminae I, II, III, and IV, and occupied positions there that were previously identified as sites of origin of the spinothalamic tract. C-fos immunoreactivity could be induced in the thoracic spinal segments with subcutaneous injections of capsaicin. These observations showed that spinal cardiac afferents are not responding to capsaicin and that the effects of capsaicin are mediated by the vagal afferents. This could be substantiated by the dose-response effect of c-fos expression in the caudal part of the nucleus of the solitary tract (figure 3B); the target area of the vagal cardiac afferent nerve fibers [1, 20]. The rostral parts of the NTS were not affected by the treatment since this area is involved in transmission of taste information [23]. The effects of bradykinin infusions in the pericardial sac on c-fos expression in the NTS were much less impressive but also in these animals the number of c-fos immunoreactive cells in the caudal NTS was significantly increased compared to infusions of saline. In many other areas of the central nervous system increased expression of c-fos was found and many nuclei showed differences that were restricted to selective regions [22]. Acute heart pain affected the c-fos expression in the peri-ambiguus area, the parabrachial complex, the periaqueductal gray, the dorsomedial and posterior ventral thalamus, various nuclei of the hypothalamus, the central amygdala, and some cortical areas, in particular the caudal anterior cingulate and insular cortexes.

The global pattern of c-fos expression is illustrated in figure 4. Many of the affected areas somehow are related to the limbic system and may show increased neuronal activation due to the adaptive response of the animal to pain. Painful stimuli can be considered as stressors, which trigger cardiovascular and behavioral responses and cerebral c-fos expression in various regions associated to the limbic system, in particular the hypothalamus, the amygdala, and the anterior cingulate cortex [16]. Also, hypotension may cause similar cerebral c-fos expression patterns [24].

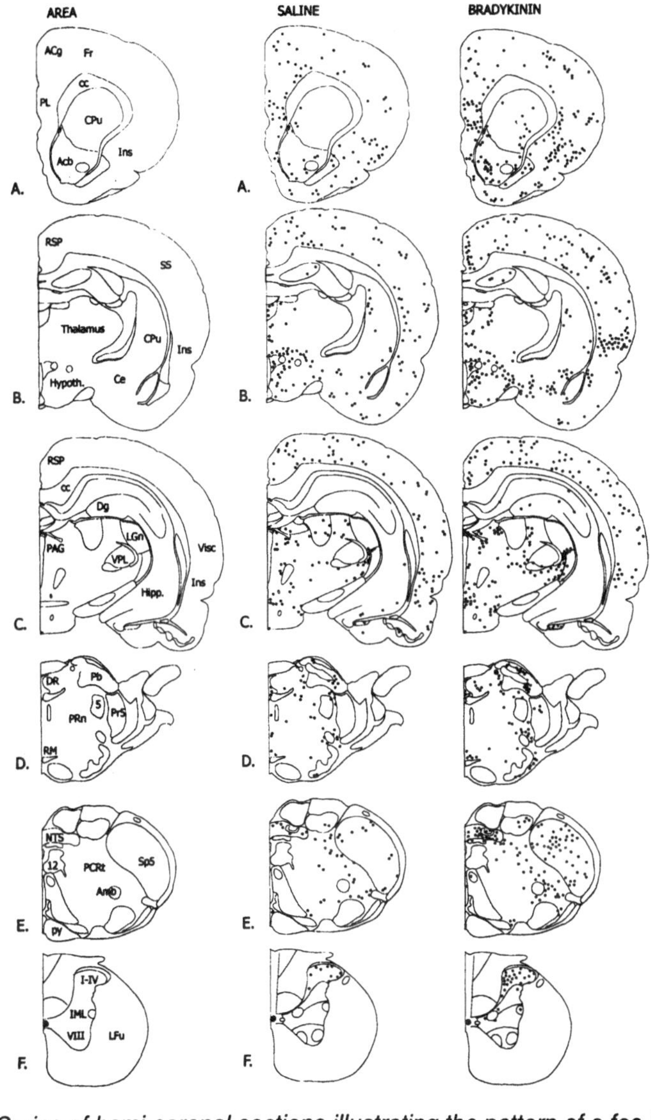

Figure 4. *Series of hemi-coronal sections illustrating the pattern of c-fos-IR at various rostro-caudal levels **(A-F)** of the neuraxis after infusion of saline and bradykinin (50 μl 250 nM) into the pericardial sac of conscious rats. The left set of brain sections shows the nomenclature of the various affected regions.*

The peri-aqueductal gray, the locus coeruleus, the parabrachial complex and the ventral reticular formation mediate output of the limbic system [25] and this may explain the increased c-fos expression in these areas. However, the parabrachial complex and the peri-aqueductal gray have long been associated with transmission of pain [26]. The dorsomedial and ventral posterior thalamus most likely are intermediate relay areas in pain transmission pathways since they have been related to activity of the spinothalamic tract [27]. Both thalamic nuclei have elaborate cortical projection fields in among other regions the anterior cingulate and insular cortexes. In the bradykinin experiments in particular a very abundant and selective expression of c-fos was found in a small part of the dysgranular insular cortex. This area and the ventral posterior thalamic region were never c-fos positive in saline treated rats. In the capsaicin treated animals the number of c-fos positive cells was increased in the same cortical area but in these cases it was less distinct due to the more abundant c-fos expression in all adjacent cortical fields. From these observations we conclude that the dysgranular insular cortex may serve a role in the conscious experience of heart pain.

The comparable behavioral responses and the similar patterns of c-fos expression found after capsaicin- and bradykinin-induced heart pain suggest that the role of the vagal afferents in transmission of visceral nociceptive information have been underestimated. Capsaicin-induced heart pain did not generate a spinal c-fos expression but all animals treated with this algogenic substance exhibited a very strong pain response. If we accept cerebral c-fos expression as a reliable marker of neuronal activity we must come to the conclusion that sensory information that was mediated by the vagal cardiac afferent nerves triggered the behavioral response to cardiac pain. Moreover, tract-tracing studies have provided additional information regarding the projection patterns of the caudal – visceral – NTS [28]. This part of the NTS selectively innervates the reticular formation, the parabrachial area, the periaqueductal gray and the mediodorsal thalamic nuclei. The reticular and midbrain areas have direct connections with the ventral posterolateral thalamus and through these structures visceral nociceptive signals mediated by the caudal NTS could be relayed to the target area of the spinothalamic tract cells. In fact, this would support the concept that at least three different ascending pathways conduct pain signals from the spinal cord to the thalamus; the spino-thalamic, the spino-reticular-thalamic, and the spino-mesencephalo-thalamic pathways. Basically, the caudal – visceral – NTS has a similar set of ascending connections, which may support a role of the caudal NTS in perception of visceral pain.

Spinal cord stimulation

The mechanisms underlying effects of spinal cord stimulation in patients with untractable angina pectoris are not known but both the central nervous system and the heart may be affected by the treatment. Cardiologists have shown that SCS increases exercise capacity and reduces both the frequency of the anginal attacks and the electrocardiographic signs of myocardial ischemia [22]. Studying regional myocardial blood flow in patients treated with SCS it could be demonstrated that the method generates a homogenization of myocardial blood flow [29]. This redistribution of coronary blood flow between the ischemic and unaffected myocardial regions will defer the moment at which the critical imbalance between oxygen demand and supply is reached.

In parallel studies we have investigated the effects of spinal cord stimulation on the central nervous system. Using differential cerebral c-fos expression patterns in SCS and sham stimulated rats the affected regions could be identified [22]. In patients, the effects of SCS on the central nervous system were studied with PET-imaging, comparing patterns of regional cerebral blood flow (rCBF) during stimulator on and off conditions [30]. Finally, we investigated whether spinal cord stimulated animals can experience acute heart pain during infusions of capsaicin into the pericardial sac [22].

Spinal cord stimulation in rats induced moderate behavioral effects (figure 5A). Stimulated animals showed significantly more waking which may be a sign of increased alertness. Furthermore, sham stimulated animals slept during the experiment, a behavior that was not shown in the SCS group. The increased alertness of the animals is dictated most likely by the stimulation conditions since we set the intensity of the stimulation to 75% of the stimulus strength that induced a clear motor activity in the forelimb area. It was argued that this stimulus strength probably was not painful but it may cause unrecognized paresthesias in the forelimbs. Paresthesias also are a common side effect of SCS in patients [22]. Analysis of the cerebral c-fos expression patterns showed that SCS triggered increased neuronal activity at various levels of the neuraxis. The dorsal laminae of the thoracic spinal cord (figure 5B), the peri-ambiguus area (figure 5D), the caudal parts of the peri-aqueductal gray (PAG), the dorsomedial thalamic area, the central amygdala and the dorsal hypothalamus, in particular the paraventricular nucleus (figure 5C), showed a significantly increased number of c-fos immunoreactive cells after SCS. The preganglionic sympathetic cells of the thoracic cord were labeled in sham but not after spinal cord stimulation, which may be indicative of a decrease of the sympathetic drive. Moreover, the preganglionic parasympathetic cardiomotor areas in the brainstem showed an increased c-fos expression after SCS, as did the ventrolateral part of the caudal PAG. The latter area is known for induction of bradycardia and hypotension [26].

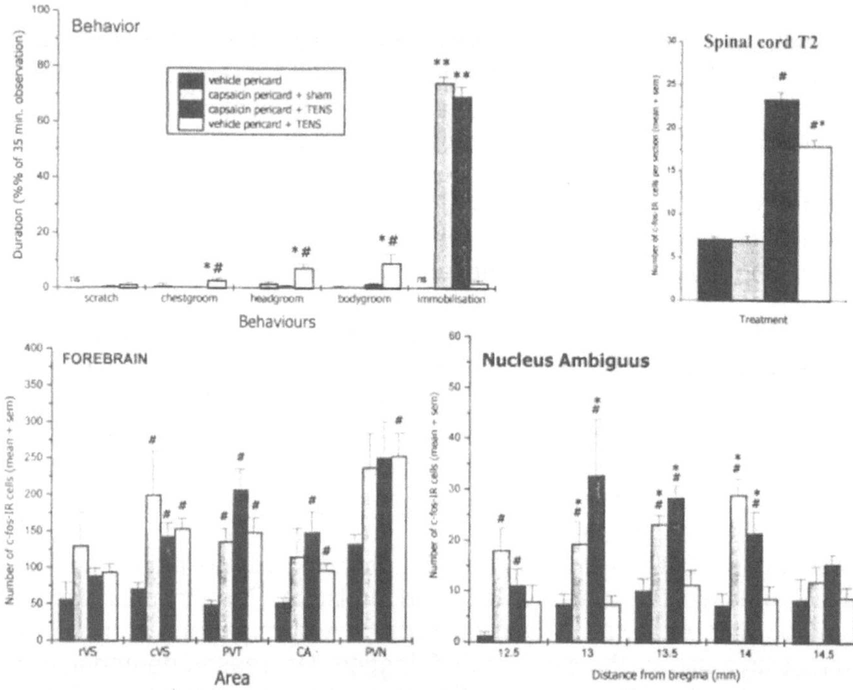

Figure 5. *The effect of spinal cord stimulation (TENS) in conscious rats on behavior (A) and c-fos-IR in various parts of the brain (B-D) after pericardial infusion of saline or capsaicin-induced angina. The number of c-fos-IR cells was quantified in the upper thoracic segments at T2; in the forebrain, in the rostral and caudal visceral sensory cortex (rVS and cVS), the paraventricular thalamic nucleus (PVT), the central amygdala (CA) and in the paraventricular hypothalamic nucleus (PVN); and at various levels in the peri-ambiguus area. (p<<0.05 was considered significant; legend: A: * compared to capsaicin+sham-TENS, # to capsaicin+TENS; B: * to capsaicin+TENS, # to sham-TENS; C,D: * to vehicle+TENS, # to vehicle).*

Using telemetric cardiovascular monitoring it could be established that indeed SCS significantly reduced the heart rate, however, it did not affect blood pressure. The general conclusion drawn from these c-fos studies is that 1) our model can be used for investigating mechanisms of spinal cord stimulation and that 2) spinal cord stimulation affects neuronal activity in regions of the brain that participate in cardiovascular regulation and transmission of pain. Regional cerebral blood flow (rCBF) changes, comparing active spinal cord stimulation and the off condition, were studied with $H_2{}^{15}O$ PET-imaging (labeled water) in nine patients that were equipped with stimulators for the treatment of angina pectoris [30]. Increased rCBF was observed in the left ventrolateral PAG, the medial prefrontal cortex (Brodmann Area (BA) 9/10), the dorsomedial thalamus, the left medial temporal gyrus (BA 21), the left pulvinar thalamic nucleus, bilateral in the posterior caudate nucleus, and the posterior cingulate gyrus (BA 30). Relative decreases in rCBF were noticed bilaterally in the insular cortex (BA 20/21 and BA 38), the right inferior temporal (BA 19/37), inferior frontal (BA 45), and anterior cingulate gyri (BA 24), and in the left inferior parietal lobe (BA 40), and the medial temporal gyrus (BA 39). In conclusion, it was demonstrated that both areas participating in cardiovascular regulation and nociception are affected by the treatment. The duration of the cerebral activity changes after SCS needs to be established. It is conceivable that SCS reconfigures the cardiovascular control system in such a way that the setpoints of the cardiovascular tone shift towards an increased parasympathetic drive. Also, we should consider the possibility that SCS alters the thalamo-cortical processing of pain. Increased strength of gating mechanisms either at the thalamic or spinal/brainstem level, may reduce the perception of pain and in turn stress that is associated with myocardial ischemia. Such a mechanism also would contribute to a shift of the cardiovascular tone towards an increased parasympathetic drive and subsequently a reduced myocardial oxygen demand. Finally, we investigated whether subcutaneous stimulation on the chest could reduce or prevent the perception of capsaicin-induced acute heart pain in conscious animals. The behavioral, cardiovascular and cerebral c-fos expression patterns (figure 5) all indicated that the stimulation did not abolish sensation of heart pain [22]. Thus, most likely, therefore SCS does not deprive patients with coronary artery disease of a warning signal.

Acknowledgements:
The contribution of Mike De Jongste, Raymond Hautvast, Ysbrand Van der Werf, Martin Muurling, Mirian Brink, Wim Dik, Bart-Jan Arkies, Folkert Postema and Jakob Korf was appreciated.

References

1. Meller ST, Gebhart GF. A critical review of the afferent pathways and the potential chemical mediators involved in cardiac pain. Neuroscience 1992; 48: 501-24.
2. Delyani JA, Van Wylen DG. Endocardial and epicardial interstitial purines and lactate during graded ischemia. Am J Physiol 1994 ; 266: H1019-26.
3. Crea F, Pupita G, Galassi A, et al. Role of adenosine in pathogenesis of anginae pain. Circulation 1990; 81: 164-72.
4. Sylven C, Beemann B, Jonzon B, Brandt R. Angina pectoris-like pain provoked by intravenous adenosine in healthy volunteers. Br Med J 1986; 293: 227-30.
5. Pan HL, Longhurst JC. Lack of a role of adenosine in activation of ischemically sensitive cardiac sympathetic afferents. Am J Physiol 1995; 269: H106-13.
6. Euchner-Wamser I, Meller ST, Gebhart GF. A model of cardiac nociception in chronically instrumented rats: behavioral and electrophysiological effects of pericardial administration of algogenic substances. Pain 1994; 58: 117-28.
7. Eldar M, Hollander G, Schulhoff N, et al. Bradykinin level in the great cardiac vein during balloon angioplasty of the left anterior descending coronary artery. Am J Cardiol 1992; 70: 1621-3.
8. Malliani A, Pagani M, Pizzinelli P, Furlan R, Guzzetti S. Cardiovascular reflexes mediated by sympathetic afferent fibers. J Auton Nerv Syst 1983; 7: 295-301.
9. Guzman F, Braun C, Lim KS. Visceral pain and the pseudoaffective response to intra-arterial injection of bradykinin and other algesic agents. Arch Int Pharmacodyn Ther 1962; 136: 353-84.
10. Dray A, Perkins M. Bradykinin and inflammatory pain. Trends Neurosci 1993; 16: 99-104.
11. Yang X, Polgar P. Genomic structure of the human bradykinin B1 receptor gene and preliminary characterization of its regulatory regions. Biochem Biophys Res Comm 1996; 222: 718-25.
12. Gaspardone A, Crea F, Tomai F, et al. Muscular and cardiac adenosine-induced pain is mediated by A1 receptors. J Am Coll Cardiol 1995; 25: 251-7.
13. Ter Horst GJ, Arkies BJ, Postema F, Hautvast RW, De Jongste MJ. Cerebral Meeting c-fos expression in unaesthetized rats experiencing capsaicin-induced acute cardiac pain. Anna Soc Neurosci Abstr 1996; 22: 869.
14. Hunt SP, Pini A, Evan G. Induction of c-fos-like protein in spinal cord neurons following sensory stimulation. Nature 1987; 328: 632-4.
15. Morgan JI, Curran T. Stimulus-transcription coupling in the nervous system: involvement of the inducible proto-oncogenes fos and jun. Annu Rev Neurosci 1991; 14: 421-51.
16. Cullinan WE, Herman JP, Battaglia DF, Akil H, Watson SJ. Pattern and time course of immediate early gene expression in rat brain following acute stress. Neuroscience 1995; 64: 477-505.
17. Card JP, Rinaman L, Lynn RB, et al. Pseudorabies virus infection of the rat central nervous system: ultrastructural characterization of viral replication, transport and pathogenesis. J Neurosci 1993; 13: 2515-39.
18. Ter Horst GJ, Van den Brink A, Homminga SA, et al. Transneuronal viral labelling of rat heart left ventricle controlling pathways [published erratum appears in Neuroreport 1994;5:531]. Neuroreport 1993; 4: 1307-10.
19. Ter Horst GJ, Hautvast RW, De Jongste MJ, Korf J. Neuroanatomy of cardiac activity-regulating circuitry: a transneuronal retrograde viral labelling study in the rat. Eur J Neurosci 1996; 8: 2029-41.

20. Spyer KM. Neural mechanisms involved in cardiovascular control during affective behaviour. Trends Neurosci 1989; 12: 506-13.
21. Ter Horst GJ, Postema F. Forebrain parasympathetic control of heart activity: retrograde transneuronal viral labeling in rats. Am J Physiol. In press 1997.
22. Hautvast RWM. Spinal cord stimulation for chronic refractory angina pectoris [dissertation]. Groningen: University of Groningen: 1997.
23. Ter Horst GJ, De Boer P, Luiten PG, Van Willigen JD. Ascending projections from the solitary tract nucleus to the hypothalamus. A Phaseolus vulgaris lectin tracing study in the rat. Neuroscience 1989; 31: 785-97.
24. Graham JC, Hoffman GE, Sved AF. C-Fos expression in brain in response to hypotension and hypertension in conscious rats. J Auton Nerv Syst 1995; 55: 92-104.
25. Luiten PG, Ter Horst GJ, Steffens AB. The hypothalamus, intrinsic connections and outflow pathways to the endocrine system in relation to the control of feeding and metabolism. Prog Neurobiol 1987; 28: 1-54.
26. Clement CI, Keay KA, Owler BK, Bandler R. Common patterns of increased and decreased fos expression in midbrain and pons evoked by noxious deep somatic and noxious visceral manipulations in the rat. J Comp Neurol 1996; 366: 495-515.
27. Hobbs SF, Chandler MJ, Bolser DC, Foreman RD. Segmental organization of visceral and somatic input onto C3-T6 spinothalamic tract cells of the monkey. J Neurophysiol 1992; 68: 1575-88.
28. Ter Horst GJ, Streefland C. Ascending projections of the solitary tract nucleus. In: Barraco IRA, editor. Nucleus of the solitary tract. Boca Raton: CRC Press: 1994: 93-103.
29. Hautvast RW, Blanksma PK, De Jongste MJ, Pruim J, Van der Wall, Vaalburg W. Effect of spinal cord stimulation on myocardial blood flow assessed by positron emission tomography in patients with refractory angina pectoris. Am J Cardiol 1996; 77: 462-7.
30. Hautvast RW, Ter Horst GJ, De Jong BM, et al. Relative changes in regional cerebral blood flow during spinal cord stimulation in patients with refractory angina pectoris. Eur J Neurosci 1997; 9: 1178-83.

Abbreviations:

10: dorsal motor vagus nucleus; 5: trigeminal motor nucleus; ac: anterior commissure; ACg: anterior cingulate gyrus; AHN: anterior hypothalamic area; Amb: nucleus ambiguus; BL: basolateral amygdala; BM: basomedial amygdala; cc: corpus callosum; Ce: central amygdala; CM: central-medial thalamic nucleus; CPu: caudate putamen; Dg: dentate gyrus; DMH: dorsomedial hypothalamic nucleus; Fr: frontal cortex; IC: colliculus inferior; IL: infralimbic cortex; IML: intermediolateral autonomic cell group; Ins: insula; int: internal capsule; KF: Kölliker-Fuse nucleus; La: lateral amygdala; LD: laterodorsal thalamic nucleus; LFu: lateral funiculus; LH: lateral habenula; LHA: lateral hypothalamic nucleus; LRn: lateral reticular nucleus; LV: lateral ventricle; MD: mediodorsal thalamic nucleus; Me: medial amygdala; MRN: midbrain reticular nucleus; NTS: nucleus of the solitary tract; PAG: periaqueductal gray; Pb: parabrachial region; PCRt: parvocellular reticular nucleus; PH: posterior hypothalamic nucleus; PL: prelimbic cortex; PP: peripeduncular area; PRn: pontine reticular nucleus; PVN: paraventricular hypothalamic nucleus; PVT: paraventricular thalamic nucleus; py: pyramidal tract; R: red nucleus; RCH: retrochiasmatic area; RM: raphe magnus; RSP: retrosplenial cortex; SC: superior colliculus; sm: stria medullaris; SNr: substantia nigra reticular part; VAL: anterior ventral thalamic nucleus; Visc: visceral cortex; VPL: ventral posterior thalamic nucleus; Zi: zona incerta. (Only the most relevant abbreviations are listed here.).

Chapter 9

FUNCTIONAL NEUROIMAGING OF ANGINA PECTORIS

Stuart D. Rosen

Introduction

The origins of myocardial ischemia

In the normal heart, both intrinsic mechanisms (such as coronary vascular autoregulation and Starling mechanical properties) and extrinsic (mainly neurohumoral) influences allow adaptation to a wide range of demand for output of blood [1]. Even under resting conditions, oxidative metabolism is crucial to function of the heart, indeed mitochondria comprise 1/3 of the mass of the myocardial cells. Oxygen extraction is near maximal even under resting conditions at 60-70%, and is only increased to 80% with severe exercise. Therefore the increased oxygen required during exercise has to be obtained from an increase in myocardial blood flow (MBF) [2]. In circumstances of cardiac disease - especially (and in the West, most commonly) - coronary artery disease (CAD), the limits of adaptation are much more closely confined. Critical stenosis of an epicardial artery, whether such a stenosis is static or dynamic, sharply reduces coronary vasodilator reserve (CVR, the ratio of maximal MBF/resting MBF) in the myocardial territory supplied by the stenosed vessel[3]. (With respect to vulnerability to reduction in perfusion or to increase in demand, it is well established that the subendocardium is at greater risk than the subepicardium; this issue has been reviewed in extenso by Hoffman [4] and will not be discussed further here). MBF and therefore oxygen supply cannot increase adequately to satisfy the increased myocardial demand and aerobic metabolism can no longer be sustained downstream. Regional contractile function is compromised.

Van der Wall et al. (eds.),
Advanced Imaging in Coronary Artery Disease, 137-161.

At the tissue level, ischemia has a number of consequences. These include:
1) a build up of adenosine from the breakdown of ATP, as well as the products of anaerobic metabolism, in particular hydrogen ions;
2) altered function of ionic transport mechanisms, increasing intracellular calcium loading and allowing leak of intracellular potassium ions and
3) changed local mechanical forces, which are presumably most acute in the border zone between ischemic and non-ischemic myocardium [1]. All these factors combine to stimulate undifferentiated nerve endings within the myocardium (there are no known specific nociceptive nerve endings in the myocardium) and generate an increase in afferent nerve traffic [4].

The registration of myocardial ischemia through the neuraxis

Afferent nerve traffic evoked by myocardial ischemia is carried by the cardiac sympathetic and vagal nerve fibres These pathways, as determined from animal studies, have been reviewed in detail [5-7]. (The main methods used in these studies have been recording with microelectrodes in very specific brainstem and cortical sites to register the effect of discrete peripheral stimuli; retrograde neuronal transport techniques have also been employed, using agents such as horse radish peroxidase). In summary, the sympathetic afferent fibres travel predominantly via the dorsal columns to the ventral posterior lateral (VPL) thalamus. Neurones in VPL also receive visceral afferent inputs via the spinothalamic tracts. Vagal fibres mainly connect to the nucleus of the solitary tract and thence to the parabrachial nucleus (in the pons) and to the parvocellular region ventral to the ventral posterior thalamus. Beyond the thalamus, cardiopulmonary inputs have been shown to activate neurones in the ventral and caudal (agranular) zone of insular cortex. The latter is also connected to medial prefrontal cortical regions and to the contralateral agranular insular cortex. Altogether, the physiological and anatomic evidence is consistent with the idea that the insula is involved in monitoring common visceral sensations and in modifying and integrating autonomic responses. In addition to the above, there are projections to the ventrolateral orbital cortex and to the primary somatosensory cortex. The parabrachial nuclei also have efferent connections to the hypothalamus and amygdala.

Studies in man

The pathways described are thought to participate in regulation of the cardiovascular system in response to changes in physiological demand e.g. during orthostatic change or exercise. For obvious ethical reasons, the afferent neural pathways from the heart have not been directly amenable to investigation *in vivo* in man, although a number of indirect studies of cardiac neural activity have been performed in man, many centred upon the baroreflex [8-10]. In addition to physiological adaptation, the pathways are also assumed to be involved in compensation for pathological events or processes e.g. in the maintenance of cardiac output during myocardial ischemia. Although for obvious reasons cardiac pain has not been studied so extensively in experimental animal models, the higher projections described would also constitute appropriate neural substrate for the perception of pain from the heart and for the mediation of the effects of mental stress upon autonomic drive to the heart.

Central nervous system activation during myocardial ischemia

From the clinical point of view there has been interest in heart->brain neural pathways for many years, in relation to the symptom of angina pectoris [11]. Francois-Franck described the role of sympathetic afferents in cardiac nociception more than a century ago and cervical sympathectomy was advocated in the treatment of intractable angina [12] in the days before surgical revascularization of the heart (and later percutaneous transluminal coronary angioplasty (PTCA)) addressed the problem by dealing directly with the underlying cause, namely myocardial ischemia. More recently, for inoperable CAD patients with angina, spinal cord stimulation has also had its proponents as a useful treatment [13].

Our own group has, in the last few years, recognized that

1) there appears to be only very limited correlation between perceived chest pain and objective measurements of myocardial performance [14];

2) improved knowledge of the central processing of myocardial ischemia would be of particular value in understanding painless ('silent') myocardial ischemia, a condition in which the absence of an 'early warning system' of pain may be associated with a worse prognosis;

3) from a wider perspective, angina pectoris may serve as a model for the study of the neurophysiology of visceral pain in general [7].

We have adopted the method of measuring regional cerebral blood flow (rCBF) using PET with $H_2{}^{15}O$ to study brain activation during myocardial ischemia [15,16]. In most circumstances, rCBF is a highly reliable index of cerebral glucose consumption, which rises when a given cerebral territory is activated [17,18]. The glucose consumption is, in turn, coupled with Na/K dependent ATPase and therefore with neuronal firing rates [19]. rCBF measurements had previously largely been confined to neurological studies to investigate, for example, brain responses to various motor tasks or auditory or visual stimuli [20].

Central neural correlates of angina pectoris

In our first study, we sought to define the functional central nervous pathways activated by angina pectoris [14]. To achieve this, we employed dynamic PET with $H_2{}^{15}O$ to measure rCBF changes during an episode of drug-induced angina in patients with symptomatic CAD.

Study population

The study population comprised 12 dextral patients (age 60 (9) years, mean (SD); 9 male and 3 female). All patients developed typical angina with ischemic changes (>0.1mV downsloping or rectilinear ST segment depression 80ms after the J point) on the stress electrocardiogram (ECG). At angiography, all had significant single vessel CAD (i.e. stenoses > 50% of luminal diameter). The diseased coronary artery was the left anterior descending in 7 patients and the right in 5. None of the patients was diabetic or had any systemic disease. For each patient, dynamic PET using $H_2{}^{15}O$ (from inhaled oxygen-15 labeled carbon dioxide ($C^{15}O_2$)) was employed to make six rCBF measurements. As previously reported [21,22] for each measurement, a 30 second background frame was recorded, then scanning was continued for a further 2 minutes, during which $C^{15}O_2$ was administered at 500 $ml.min^{-1}$ and 6$MBq.ml^{-1}$ activity.The scanner was an ECAT 931-08/12 positron tomograph (CTI-Siemens, Knoxville, TN, USA), the characteristics of which have been described previously [23]. Angina was provoked by means of the increase in cardiac work caused by infusion of the β_1 agonist dobutamine, a drug which does not cross the blood-brain barrier [24] and which has a short half life (2.4 min) [25].

PET imaging protocol

The following sequence of scans was performed:

1-Baseline one: subject lying on the scanner couch in dimly lit circumstances with eyes closed;

2-Placebo: after 6 minutes of a placebo infusion of saline. Patients were blind with respect to knowing the identity of the infused substance and were warned of the possibility of chest pain due to the infusion, which was continued throughout the scan. The placebo scan was included to control for possible rCBF changes due to anticipation of pain;

3-Baseline two;

4-Low dose dobutamine: during infusion of low dose dobutamine, the dose being 5 $\mu g.kg^{-1}.min^{-1}$ for 3 min and then 10 $\mu g.kg^{-1}.min^{-1}$ or 3 minutes, the latter continued throughout the scan. Patients were again blind with respect to knowing the identity of the infused substance and were warned of the possibility of chest pain. This infusion was to control for effects of dobutamine upon rCBF at doses insufficient to cause myocardial ischemia and angina;

5-High dose dobutamine: during infusion of high dose dobutamine, from 20 $\mu g.kg^{-1}.min^{-1}$ up to 35 $\mu g.kg^{-1}.min^{-1}$, increased by 5 $\mu g.kg^{-1}.min^{-1}$ increments every 3 min until angina was produced. From the onset of angina, the infusion was continued at the same concentration (i.e. angina-provoking dose) for the 2.5 minutes of imaging. Immediately after this, the infusion was stopped. Typical chest pain was produced in all patients and the development of myocardial ischemia was confirmed electrocardiographically;

6-Baseline 3: after angina had ceased and the ECG had returned to baseline. This was performed 13 min after stopping dobutamine, allowing for complete clearance of the drug.

Analysis of PET images

PET images were transformed into a standard stereotactic space defined by Talairach and Tournoux [26,27]. Comparisons of rCBF were made between the different stages of the study by carrying out a series of t tests (more precisely a blocked design ANCOVA) on a voxel by voxel basis by Statistical Parametric Mapping (SPM, MRC Cyclotron Unit, Hammersmith Hospital, London, UK) [21,22,27]. The magnitude of rCBF changes induced by angina were compared to the mean of baselines 2 and 3. (The reason for the combination of baselines 2 and 3 was to limit order effects upon the changes in rCBF). Subsequently, these results were tested further by analysis of the interaction: angina minus baseline compared to non-specific arousal (placebo minus baseline). In addition, we explored the rCBF changes induced by placebo and low dose dobutamine compared to baseline. Finally, as it is known that myocardial metabolic changes can persist for hours after ischemia [28], we also compared rCBF in the post anginal phase (baseline 3) to baselines 1 and 2 combined. These analyses permitted the construction of statistical parametric maps for the description of significant changes in rCBF between the different test stages. Significant changes were identified by applying a statistical threshold of 0.05, corrected for multiple non-independent comparisons [27]. Quantification of changes in rCBF equivalents (δrCBF) between angina and baseline were performed according to the formula:

$$\delta CBF = \frac{rCBF_{angina} - (rCBF_{baseline\ 2} + rCBF_{baseline\ 3})/2}{(rCBF_{baseline\ 2} + rCBF_{baseline\ 3})/2} \times 100\%$$

NB *Due to the nature of the statistical analysis in this study and the silent ischemia study (below), the results are considered in the form of pooled data sets for each patient group. Intra- and inter-individual comparisons are not feasible within the methodology of the present study.*

Ethical considerations
These projects were approved by the Research Ethics Committee, Hammersmith Hospital and UK Administration of Radioactive Substances Advisory Committee (ARSAC).

Results

Clinical observations
No chest pain or other sensations of note were reported during the baseline scans, the placebo infusion or the low dose dobutamine infusion. During the high dose dobutamine infusion, all patients experienced typical angina pectoris in the form of retrosternal chest pain only; in two patients, there was a slight radiation of the pain to the left arm. All patients reported that it was the sensation of chest pain which occupied their attention during the high dose dobutamine image, rather than any awareness of a fast or unusually powerful heart beat. In all cases, the angina was accompanied by ischemic changes on the ECG. The final image, Baseline 3, was performed in all cases after the complete cessation of pain or any other unusual sensation in the chest and when the ECG had returned to baseline.

Hemodynamic effects of the high dose dobutamine infusion
The mean heart rate increased from 65 (7) beats/min at rest to 99 (21) beats/min ($p<0.001$) at peak effect of the dobutamine infusion. Systolic blood pressure correspondingly rose from a mean of 139 (13)mmHg to 160 (32) mmHg ($p<0.05$). The diastolic blood pressure was unchanged (86 (24) mmHg versus 81 (8) mmHg; p=NS). The heart rate systolic pressure product (RPP) increased from 9110 (1689) to 15840 (4982) mmHgxbeats per minute ($p<0.001$) (Table 1).

PET findings
During angina, rCBF was significantly increased in the hypothalamus, periaquaductal grey and bilaterally in the thalamus as well as bilaterally in the prefrontal cortex (BA 10, 47 and BA 44/6) and in the left inferior anterocaudal cingulate cortex (BA 25) (Figure 1, Table 2).

Reduction in rCBF was observed bilaterally in the mid-rostrocaudal cingulate cortex (BA 24) and fusiform gyrus (BA 28/35) and in the right posterior cingulate (BA 31) and left parietal cortex (BA 40). The detailed results of the rCBF changes during angina compared to baseline are presented in Table 2 and the regions in which the interaction test corroborated the primary data are marked. There were no differences in rCBF either between the placebo infusion and the resting state or between low dose dobutamine and the resting state. When Baseline 3, the image subsequent to angina, was compared with the previous baseline image, thalamic but not cortical rCBF was noted to remain significantly increased (Figure 2).

The enigma of silent ischemia

Soon after Heberden's classical description of angina pectoris [29], the discrepancy between the extent of anatomical coronary artery disease and patients' symptoms was noted [30]. Indeed, it has subsequently been recognized that myocardial ischemia and infarction can occur in the absence of pain, infarction being either discovered in life on the electrocardiogram or myocardial ischemia being assumed retrospectively after post mortem demonstration of significant coronary artery disease [31-33]. Reversible silent myocardial ischemia has been investigated in particular, by means of ambulatory electrocardiographic monitoring [34-36] and is a common finding. Up to 70% of episodes of myocardial ischemia in patients with coronary artery disease patients may be asymptomatic; for acute myocardial infarction, the incidence of painless events is estimated at ~30%[32-36]. Silent ischemia often co-exists with painful ischemia in the same patient; this common observation precludes any simple explanation related to the particular characteristics of an individual patient.

Clinically, silent myocardial ischemia is important because of its association with a poor prognosis e.g. after an episode of unstable angina [33-37] or myocardial infarction [38,39]. Most dramatically, silent ischemia has been assumed in patients in whom sudden cardiac death is the first presentation of coronary artery disease [40]. Silent ischemia has also been found during exercise in cardiac arrest survivors and in patients with life-threatening arrhythmias [41].

The pathophysiological basis of silent ischemia has not been established. From the observation [35] that in stable angina the number of painless episodes of ST segment depression can far exceed the number of painful ones, it was hypothesized that silent myocardial ischemia represented less severe ischemia [33,35,36,42,43]. A recent study [44], however, which assessed the significance of chest pain in coronary artery disease patients with a high *a priori* likelihood of inducible ischemia, found that the differences in objective measurements of ischemia (using ambulatory ECG monitoring and thallium-201 SPECT exercise testing) between patients with angina and silent ischemia patients were insignificant. The higher incidence in diabetics[45] implicated peripheral neuropathy in the process; differences in autonomic nerve function have also been described in non-diabetic patients with silent myocardial ischemia [46]. Conversely, silent ischemia can be shown in many non-diabetics with no evidence of neuropathy. With the discovery of the brain's endogenous opiate system [47], a higher pain threshold due to enhanced central opiate activity offered an explanation for the silence of silent myocardial ischemia. However, the opiate studies to date have been equivocal [42,48-53], often having been based on plasma endorphin measurements. In addition, psychological and personality factors may play a role in the perception of angina [54].

With this background, we proceeded to study a series of patients with 'pure' silent myocardial ischemia (i.e. no pain experienced despite reproducible ECG and echo signs of ischemia) according to the same study protocol as for our angina study (see above). A particular aspect of the angina study which encouraged us towards the study of patients with silent ischemia was the finding of persistence of thalamic activation after the cessation of the symptoms and signs of myocardial ischemia, inviting the hypothesis that gating [55] of painful signals may occur at the thalamic level.

Central neural correlates of silent myocardial ischemia

Study population

Nine right-handed male patients (age 62 (7) years) with significant (i.e. at least one stenosis > 50% of luminal diameter) coronary artery disease at angiography were studied. Five patients had three vessel disease, two patients had two vessel disease and two patients had undergone previous coronary bypass grafting, but had recently developed occlusion of important grafts. Eight of the patients were identified during the investigation of exertional breathlessness; in two of these cases, this symptom (breathlessness) was found in patients who had previously undergone coronary artery bypass surgery for breathlessness, mild angina and reduced effort tolerance. One patient had previously sustained an inferior myocardial infarction. All exhibited painless myocardial ischemia demonstrable by the development of ischemic electrocardiographic changes and new regional wall motion abnormalities during dobutamine stress echocardiography in the complete absence of chest pain. As mentioned above, none of the 9 silent ischemia patients displayed a 'mixed' clinical picture (i.e. of angina on some occasions and painless ischemia on others). Resting ventricular function was normal in all patients except the one who had sustained the infarct; in him, inferolateral hypokinesia could be seen. No patient in either group was diabetic nor had any systemic disease.

PET imaging protocol

The same protocol as that described above was employed to make the same six rCBF measurements. However, because of the absence of pain accompanying the ECG changes as an indication of myocardial ischemia, we were particular to include stress echocardiography during the imaging sequence as a means of demonstrating unequivocal ischemia in this patient group. A brief echocardiogram (Challenge 7000, Esaote Biomedica, Florence, Italy) was recorded before the start of PET imaging and optimal echocardiographic views were chosen on the basis of the previous stress echocardiogram as those which best showed the development of a new wall motion abnormality. An echocardiogram was performed before each image to allow for the effects of pressure of the transducer on the anterior chest wall. During the dobutamine infusion ischemia was confirmed electrocardiographically and echocardiographically. In all silent ischemia patients, chest pain was obligatorily absent, however, awareness of an increase in heart rate and/or force of contraction was no obstacle to inclusion in the study.

Analysis of PET images

This was performed as for the angina study above. The magnitude of rCBF changes induced by silent myocardial ischemia were compared to the mean of baselines 1 and 2. In addition, the rCBF changes induced by placebo and low dose dobutamine were compared to baseline and, finally, rCBF in the post ischemic phase (baseline 3) was compared to baselines 1 and 2 combined.

Results

Clinical observations

No chest pain or other sensations of note were reported during the baseline scans, the placebo infusion or the low dose dobutamine infusion. During the high dose dobutamine infusion, 7 of the silent ischemia patients were aware of a rapid and more forceful heart beat, one patient experienced slight warmth of the chest wall and one experienced no unusual sensations at all. All of the patients denied that any of the sensations they felt were in any way painful or uncomfortable. In all cases, the occurrence of silent myocardial ischemia was confirmed electrocardiographically and by the development of a new regional wall motion abnormality during real time two-dimensional echocardiography. The final image, Baseline 3, was performed in all cases after the complete return of the echocardiogram and electrocardiogram to baseline.

Hemodynamic effects of the high dose dobutamine infusion

The silent ischemia patients received comparable doses of intravenous dobutamine for the induction of myocardial ischemia to those administered to the angina patients. There were significant increases in heart rate, systolic blood pressure and product of heart rate and systolic blood pressure (rate-pressure product) in the silent ischemia patients, but the changes were comparable to those in the angina patients. The time to significant ischemic electrocardiographic changes and the extent of such changes were also comparable between the silent ischemia patients and the earlier group of patients with angina pectoris. The data are presented in detail in Table 1.

PET findings

During myocardial ischemia, rCBF increased bilaterally in the brainstem, thalamus, left hippocampal gyrus (Brodmann area 30) and, to a lesser extent, the right and left dorsal and right lateral basal frontal cortical areas (Brodmann areas 6 and 47 respectively). (Figure 1 and Table 3). The low dose dobutamine infusion, although not producing echocardiographic or electrocardiographic changes of myocardial ischemia, was associated with a small increase in rCBF bilaterally in the thalami (Z scores 4.7 (left) and 4.3 (right)) and in the left hippocampal (Brodmann area 19) and right anterior cingulate (Brodmann area 24) cortices (Z scores 4.7 and 3.9 respectively). The placebo infusion produced a small activation in the right frontal cortex [Brodmann area 46; Z score 3.8)]. A comparison of the post-ischemic scan, Baseline 3, to the previous baseline scans, showed persistent increases in left thalamic and dorsal frontal cortical (Brodmann area 6) rCBF (Z scores 3.8 and 3.9 respectively) (Figure 2).

Differences between angina pectoris and silent ischemia.

After separate analysis of the PET data from the 2 patient groups, a direct comparison of the silent ischemia and angina pectoris data was performed. Differences between the two patient groups with respect to the areas of increased rCBF during myocardial ischemia were computed as interactions between the between-group factors: (angina versus silent ischemia) and the within-group conditions (myocardial ischemia versus baselines 1 and 2). As the interaction effect could be predicted by the main effect (myocardial ischemia - baselines 1 and 2) in each group, a less harsh statistical threshold ($p<0.01$, without Bonferroni correction) was used for the statistical maps.

An overall comparison of the results for myocardial ischemia/angina versus baseline in the two patient groups showed that angina was associated with greater rCBF increases bilaterally in the anterior and ventral cingulate cortex (Brodmann areas 24/32 and 25), mesial orbitofrontal and basal frontal cortex (Brodmann areas 10 and 11) and left temporal pole (Brodmann areas 28). (Figures 1 and 2 and Table 4).

Discussion

We believe that the areas identified in the angina study constitute the central components mediating perception of pain from the heart. An important finding was that thalamic but not frontal cortical activity persisted through the post-angina image, possibly indicating that the thalamus continues to receive inputs from the heart after angina ceases to be felt. However, although the thalamus is active, this less intense signal is not transmitted to the cerebral cortex and consequently conscious perception of angina does not occur. The silent ischemia study showed that during silent myocardial ischemia, significant rCBF increases are observed in subcortical structures but that the degree and extent of cortical activation in silent ischemia is slight, compared to overt cardiac pain. In the latter, a much more extensive pattern of activation was observed, especially at the cortical level in the ventral cingulate and basal frontal cortices. In the silent ischemia patients, as in those with angina pectoris, thalamic activity persisted through the post-ischemic image.

These findings - that an equivalent stress upon the hearts of silent ischemia patients produced the same degree of thalamic activation, but significantly less cortical activation, especially with respect to the anterior and ventral cingulate and basal frontal cortices - show that afferent stimuli from the heart *do* reach the central nervous system in patients with silent ischemia absence of sensation of chest pain is unlikely to be due to failure of transmission by the peripheral nerves. The results point to a difference in the central nervous handling of the afferent signals from the heart in the silent ischemia patients. One hypothesis to account for this would be gating[55] of afferent stimuli at the thalamic level.

The differences between the silent ischemic and angina patients were, principally, the absence of activation of the basal frontal and anterior and ventral cingulate cortices and left temporal pole. Now the two patient groups were closely matched with respect to resting ventricular function, dobutamine dose, hemodynamic changes due to dobutamine and time to onset of, and extent of, ischemia. It might therefore be reasonable to suggest that, as far as could be determined, the threshold for myocardial ischemia was similar in both groups. For this reason, we propose that the cerebral areas just described represent specific cortical projections of a pathway mediating the perception of pain from the heart.

The anterior cingulate has been associated with emotional responses to pain [56] and it has documented connections to the nucleus of the solitary tract [57], dorsal motor nucleus of the vagus and to the sympathetic thoracic intermediolateral cell column [58]. In addition, it is known from studies in the rhesus monkey, that there are connections between the frontal cortex and the anterior cingulate [59,60]. That perception of chest pain involves the cingulate cortex is therefore entirely consistent with current neuroanatomical data. A potential regulatory role for the frontal cortex - modifying the emotional response to angina in the light of previous subjective experience of it - is also possible.

Investigation of both patient groups indicated that the thalamus continues to receive inputs from the heart after the cessation of myocardial ischemia, consistent with the observation that metabolic disturbances continue in the heart hours after ischemia has apparently resolved [28]. Presumably, the less intense signal is not transmitted further since it is below the necessary threshold (the Z scores for thalamic activation at this stage were substantially lower than during myocardial ischemia).

One hypothesis concerning silent ischemia referred to above [33,35,36,42,43] is that silent myocardial ischemia is merely milder than that which produces angina pectoris. This is not supported by our data, in which the silent ischemia patients had coronary artery disease of comparable if not greater severity (more vessels were diseased per patient) than the angina pectoris group. The maximal dobutamine dose and the increase in cardiac work produced by the latter were equivalent for the two patient groups. Finally, the fact that in the silent ischemia patients, even low dose dobutamine infusion evoked a significant bilateral increase in thalamic rCBF, might suggest that there was a ready induction of myocardial ischemia in this patient group.

Our findings suggest that a stimulus of comparable intensity can induce myocardial ischemia which, in certain circumstances (i.e. those which make the ischemia silent) may or may not be associated with a painful sensation. We are clearly far from being able to predict the code of afferent stimuli which represents an adequate algogenic signal. This absence of predictability might reflect a complex pattern of afferent impulses related to mechanical and/or chemical stimulation rather than the relatively simple involvement of a specific nociceptive pathway [61]. It could still be claimed that the afferent signals which reach the thalamus during myocardial ischemia in silent ischemia patients (and which we assume to be gated from further transmission), are not painful signals but are proprioceptive inputs from mechanoceptors in the myocardium. In addition, as far as is known, there are no nerve endings in the myocardium whose specific function is the mediation of pain signals [61]. If it were the case that proprioceptive inputs to the heart can be shown to be increased during silent myocardial ischemia, it would give further support to the argument that cardiac nociception depends upon the intensity of general afferent signals from the heart rather than a specific pain pathway (the 'intensity' rather than the 'specificity' theory of cardiac pain mediation [61]). Our study does not address the precise mechanism of operation of the gating which we hypothesise to occur in the thalamus. Further research at the neurotransmitter level might elucidate this.

There are important differences between the findings in our angina study and those for somatic pain [62,63]. In the latter, increases in rCBF were found in the contralateral dorsal cingulate cortex (BA 24 and 32), thalamus and lenticular nucleus, as well as the prefrontal (BA 9 and 10), contralateral insular and prefrontal cortices (BA 45 and 46). In contrast, angina evokes a bilateral thalamic increase in rCBF with activation of the periaquaductal grey and hypothalamus, but with *reduction* in dorsal cingulate cortical flow bilaterally. Connections have been demonstrated between the pre-frontal and dorsal cingulate cortices [64]. There is also evidence that the dorsal cingulate cortex (BA 24) is involved in the avoidance of noxious stimuli [65]. Since there is no appropriate withdrawal reaction from angina, avoidance of movement by inhibition of the dorsal cingulate may be the most useful response. (This clinical situation has been elegantly described by Keefer and Resnick [66]: "It is characteristic of angina pectoris that when pain develops the patient stops and usually maintains absolute quiet until the paroxysm has disappeared. Such absolute quiet is not often present in cases of acute coronary obstruction; and with good reason. The patient with angina is brought to a halt by his pain since he has learned from experience that the less he moves, the more rapidly will his pain disappear.")

As for somatic pain, bilateral prefrontal cortical activation could be demonstrated. The topographical differences in the activation of the cingulate cortex between somatic and visceral pain may also represent somatotopic differences of the pain pathways.

Limitations of the study

The above technique is an attractive one, being an *in vivo* approach and one which is repeatable within and between subjects and conditions However, there are, unfortunately, some important limitations.

1) Despite good spatial resolution (~8 mm), the temporal resolution of the technique is limited. Essentially, the regional activation data acquired is the sum of the changes in rCBF (compared to resting conditions) summed into a single 30 second frame. The method therefore does not permit a distinction between those brain regions activated afferently and those activated efferently.
2) We employed only one method for the induction of myocardial ischemia. Exercise would have been impractical because of the need to keep the patient's position constant for optimal scan acquisition. As far as other pharmacological stressors were concerned, dipyridamole and adenosine both cause cerebral vasodilation, which could have confounded the rCBF measurements. Pacing stress was feasible, but was felt to be excessively invasive.
3) Cerebral regions not involved in pain perception could have been activated, but, averaging across subjects, the inclusion of the additional baseline scans and the uniformity of scanning circumstances (eyes closed and dim lighting in the scanner room) should have minimized any effects on the results. The comparison of the two patient groups will also have reduced the possibility of false positive areas of activation.
4) Possible order effects in the scanning sequence are of methodological importance. Thus, the placebo and dobutamine infusions should ideally have been administered in a random sequence. We opted for the sequence described above because earlier evidence had demonstrated the long term persistence of the effects of myocardial ischemia [28]. Again, a direct comparison of the results in the two patient groups will have reduced the influence of order effects upon the final results.
5) It might be argued that the rCBF changes observed may merely have been a direct pharmacological effect of the dobutamine infusion, rather than reflecting a true neurophysiological response to angina. The current study, in which the maximum ischemia-inducing dose of dobutamine was

equivalent in both patient groups, despite the clear differences in their rCBF responses, refutes this criticism. However, we have subsequently studied a series of normal subjects to deal conclusively with this point.

6) It is theoretically possible that the cortical activation observed during angina pectoris is an epiphenomenon, a non-specific, secondary response to the pain and that the essential differences between the patient groups lies in differences in thalamic activation which cannot be spatially resolved by the methodology used. On purely experimental grounds it is not possible to distinguish which activation is a consequence of pain perception and which reflects the perceptual event per se. Such a distinction might be possible if one were to a study a group of patients with angina who perceived the pain but felt no affective response towards it (such as angina patients who had previously undergone a frontal leukotomy). However, the fact that when considering the areas of the interaction effect it was possible to identify cortical areas which are known on the basis of invasive experiments in primates to have direct specific visceral connections [e.g. the ventral cingulate (BA 25)] inclines us to believe that the cortical activations are more than incidental.

7) The greater extent of coronary artery disease in the silent ischemia patients, predominantly three vessel disease versus single vessel disease for the angina patients, might have affected the afferent signals from the heart. However, since as noted above, resting ventricular function, hemodynamic changes due to dobutamine and time to onset of, and extent of, ischemia were comparable, we supposed that the signals initiated in the hearts of the two patient groups would be equivalent. This would, though, require to be confirmed by other means.

8) The definition of silent ischemia for the purposes of this study excluded a "mixed pattern" i.e. of experience of painful myocardial ischemia on some occasions, but the latter being painless at other times. It is (at least theoretically) possible that the mechanism of the silence of myocardial ischemia in the mixed pattern is different from "pure" silent ischemia patients whom we studied. Ideally, our protocol would be repeated in the same subject under both conditions - painful and painless, although the feasibility of this is probably remote.

9) The silent ischemia patient group included two patients who had had coronary bypass surgery. It is just conceivable that the surgery could have led to afferent nerve fibres becoming divided, with an effect upon pain perception. However, omission of these patients made no significant difference to the data.

10) The present study would have yielded more information if the same patients had also been subjected to a somatic painful stimulus and a direct comparison made between the rCBF effects of the visceral and the somatic stimuli. However, the extra radiation exposure and discomfort which this would have occasioned were not considered acceptable on ethical grounds. Also, there would be no guarantee that any somatic pain provoked would not in turn provoke angina or silent myocardial ischemia. In addition, there may be differential thresholds for somatic and myocardial afferent pain signals [67].

Preliminary report on the central neural correlates of dobutamine stress in normal subjects and in patients with syndrome X [68,69]

Normal subjects

Ten normal controls have subsequently been studied with the same protocol as that described above for the angina and silent ischemia patients. In these, the dobutamine infusion produced an awareness of increased heartbeat in 9/10. a moderate increase in rCBF was noted bilaterally in the thalamus, but accompanied by only minor activation of the frontal cortex, more particularly the left insula.

Syndrome X

We have also studied 9 patients [7 female, age 56 (11)] with syndrome X according to the above protocol. Chest pain was induced with an equivalent dobutamine dose to that in the earlier brain activation studies. Chest pain occurred in response to low dose dobutamine in 4 of the syndrome X patients; during the high dose dobutamine infusion, chest pain was reported in all cases. Although the chest pain in syndrome X was associated with ischemic-like ECG changes in 8 patients, it occurred in the absence of correlates of myocardial ischemia such as left ventricular wall motion abnormality. Compared to the patients with angina due to coronary artery disease, the syndrome X patients showed greater rCBF increases in the midbrain, right thalamus and right insular cortex and bilaterally in the frontal and prefrontal cortices.

Conclusion

We conclude from these studies that, in the patients with coronary artery disease, the central structures activated in angina pectoris but not in silent ischemia constitute the pathways involved in the perception of anginal pain. It is also hypothesized that the thalamus may have a key role in the perception of pain from the heart, acting as a gate to afferent pain signals, with cortical activation being necessary for the sensation of pain. From the silent ischemia study, it might be concluded that altered central nervous handling of afferent signals from the heart (an 'overactive gate') contributes to the lack of perception of chest pain in this group of patients. In contrast, (possibly due to an 'underactive thalamic gate') the study of patients with syndrome X suggests that the brain areas activated in them but not in angina due to coronary artery disease, might represent the central neural substrate of abnormal pain perception in syndrome X.

References

1. Opie LH. The heart: physiology and metabolism. 2nd ed. New York: Raven Press; 1991 p. 52-66.
2. Hoffman JI. Transmural myocardial perfusion. Prog Cardiovasc Dis 1987;29:429-64.
3. Uren NG, Melin JA, De Bruyne B, Wijns W, Baudhuin T, Camici PG. Relation between myocardial blood flow and the severity of coronary artery stenosis. N Engl J Med 1994;330:1782-8.
4. Malliani A. The conceptualisation of cardiac pain as a non-specific and unreliable alarm system. In: Gebhart GF, editor. Visceral pain. Seattle: IASP Press; 1995. p. 63-74.
5. Spyer KM. Central nervous control of the cardiovascular system. In: Bannister R, Mathias CJ, editors. Autonomic failure: a textbook of clinical disorders of the autonomic nervous system. Oxford: Oxford University Press, Oxford 1992. p. 54-77.
6. Cechetto DF. Supraspinal mechanisms of visceral representation. In: Gebhart GF, editor. Visceral pain. Seattle: IASP Press; 1995. p. 261-90.
7. Meller ST, Gebhart GF. A critical review of the afferent pathways and the potential chemical mediators involved in cardial pain. Neuroscience 1992; 48: 501-24.
8. Mancia G, Mark AL. Arterial baroreflex in humans. In: Shepherd JT, Abboud FM, editors. Peripheral circulation and organ blood flow. New ed. Washington: American Physiological Society; 1983. p. 755-93.
9. Pagani M, Somers V, Furlan R, et al. Changes in autonomic regulation induced by physical training in mild hypertension. Hypertension 1988; 12:600-10.
10. Dampney RA. Functional organization of central pathways regulating the cardiovascular system. Physiol Rev 1994;74:323-64.
11. White JC. Cardiac pain: anatomic pathways and physiologic mechanisms. Circulation 1957;16:644-55.
12. Francois-Franck CA. Signification physiologique de la résection du sympathetique dans la maladie de Basedow, l'épilepsie, l'idiotie et le glaucome. Bull Acad Med Paris 1899; 41:565-74.
13. Spinal cord stimulation
14. Hill JA, Pepine CJ. Myocardial ischemia and chest pain: a misunderstood and oversimplified relationship? Cardiol Clin 1986; 4: 621-5.
15. Rosen SD, Paulesu E, Frith CD, et al. Central nervous pathways mediating angina pectoris. Lancet 1994; correlates of angina pectoris as a model of visceral pain. Lancet 1994;344:147-50.
16. Rosen SD, Paulesu E, Nihoyannopoulos P, et al. Silent ischemia as a central problem: regional brain activation compared in silent and painful myocardial ischemia. Ann Intern Med 1996; 124:939-49.
17. Fox PT, Raichle ME, Mintun MA, Dence C, et al. Nonoxidative glucose consumption during focal physiologic neural activity. Science 1988; 241:462-4.
18. Raichle M. Circulatory and metabolic correlates of brain function in normal humans In: Plum F, editor. Higher functions of the brain. New ed. Washington: American Physiological Society, 1987. p. 643-74.
19. Mata M, Fink DJ, Ganier H, et al. Activity-dependent energy metabolism in rat posterior pituitary primarily reflects sodium pump activity. J Neurochem 1980;34:213-5.

20. Friston KJ, Frackowiak RS. Imaging functional anatomy. In: Lassen NA, Ingvar DH, Raichle ME, Friberg L, editors. Brain work and mental activity. Copenhagen: Munksgaard; 1991. p. 267-79.
21. Friston KJ, Frith CD, Liddle PF, Dolan RJ, Lammertsma AA, Frackowiak RS. The relationship between global and local changes in PET scans. J Cereb Blood Flow Metab 1990;10:458-66.
22. Friston KJ, Frith CD, Liddle PF, Frackowiak RS. Comparing functional (PET) images: the assessment of significant change. J Cereb Blood Flow Metab 1991;11:690-9.
23. Spinks TJ, Jones T, Bailey DL, et al. Physical performance of a positron tomograph for brain imaging with retractable septa. Phys Med Biol 1992;37:1637-55.
24. Takao Y, Kamisaki Y, Itoh T. Beta adrenergic regulation of amine precursor amino acid transport across the blood-brain barrier. Eur J Pharmacol 1992;215:245-51.
25. Opie LH. Drugs for the heart. 3rd ed. Philadelphia: Saunders; 1991. p. 143.
26. Talairach J, Tournoux P. Co-planar stereotactic atlas of the human brain. Stuttgart: Thieme; 1988.
27. Friston KJ, Passingham RE, Nutt JG, Heather JD, Sawle GV, Frackowiak RS. Localisation in PET images: direct fitting of the intercommissural (AC-PC) line. J Cereb Blood Flow Metab 1989;9:690-5.
28. Camici P, Araujo LI, Spinks T, et al. Increased uptake of 18F-fluorodeoxyglucose in postischemic myocardium of patients with exercise-induced angina. Circulation 1986;74:81-8.
29. Heberden W. Some account of a disorder of the breast. Med Roy Coll Phys Lond 1772;2:59-67.
30. Warren J. Remarks on angina pectoris. N Engl J Med Surg 1812; 1:1-11.
31. Babey AM. Painless acute infarction of heart. N Engl J Med 1939; 220:410-2.
32. Kannel WB, Abbott RD. Incidence and prognosis of unrecognised myocardial infarction. An update on the Framingham study. N Engl J Med 1984;311:1114-7.
33. Epstein SE, Quyyumi AA, Bonow RO. Myocardial ischemia-silent or symptomatic. N Engl J Med 1988;318:1038-43.
34. Schang SJ Jr, Pepine CJ. Transient asymptomatic S-T segment depression during daily activity. Am J Cardiol 1977;39:396-402.
35. Deanfield JE, Maseri A, Selwyn AP, et al. Myocardial ischemia during daily life in patients with stable angina: its relation to symptoms and heart rate changes. Lancet 1983;2:753-8.
36. Quyyumi A, Mockus L, Wright C, Fox KM. Morphology of ambulatory ST segment changes in patients with varying severity of coronary artery disease. Investigation of the frequency of nocturnal ischemia and coronary spasm. Br Heart J 1985;53:186-93.
37. Gottlieb SO, Weisfeldt ML, Ouyang P, Mellits ED, Gerstenblith G. Silent ischemia as a marker for early unfavorable outcome in patients with unstable angina. N Engl J Med 1986;314:1214-9.
38. Tzivoni D, Gavish A, Zin D, et al. Prognostic significance of ischemic episodes in patients with previous myocardial infarction. Am J Cardiol 1988;62:661-4.
39. Gottlieb SO, Gottlieb SH, Achuff SC, et al. Silent ischemia on Holter monitoring predicts mortality in high-risk post- infarction patients. JAMA 1988; 259: 1030-5.

40. Warnes CA, Roberts WC. Sudden coronary death: relation of amount and distribution of coronary narrowing at necropsy to previous symptoms of myocardial ischemia, left ventricular scarring and heart weight. Am J Cardiol 1984;54:65-73.
41. Hong RA, Bhandari AK, McKay CR, Au PK, Rahimtoola SH. Life threatening ventricular tachycardia and fibrillation induced by painless myocardial ischemia during exercise testing. JAMA 1987; 257: 1937-40.
42. Glazier JJ, Chierchia S, Brown MJ, Maseri A. Importance of generalized defective perception of painful stimuli as a cause of silent myocardial ischemia in chronic stable angina pectoris. Am J Cardiol 1986; 58:667-72.
43. Chierchia S, Lazzari M, Freedman B, Brunelli C, Maseri A. Impairment of myocardial perfusion and function during painless myocardial ischemia. J Am Coll Cardiol 1983;1:924-30.
44. Klein J, Chao SY, Berman DS, Rozanski A. Is 'silent' myocardial ischemia really as severe as symptomatic ischemia? The analytical effect of patient selection biases. Circulation 1994; 89: 1958-66.
45. Langer A, Freeman MR, Josse RG, Steiner G, Armstrong PW. Detection of silent myocardial ischemia in diabetes mellitus. Am J Cardiol 1991; 67: 1073-8.
46. Shakespeare CF, Katritsis D, Crowther A, Cooper IC, Coltart JC, Webb-Peploe MW. Differences in autonomic nerve function in patients with silent and symptomatic myocardial ischemia. Br Heart J 1994; 71: 22-9.
47. Woolf CJ, Wall PD. Endogenous opioid peptides and pain mechanisms: a complex relationship. Nature 1983; 306: 739-40.
48. Sheps DS, Maixner W, Hinderliter AL. Mechanisms of pain perception in patients with silent myocardial ischemia. Am Heart J 1989; 119: 983-7.
49. Droste C, Roskamm H. Pain perception and endogenous pain modulation in angina pectoris. In: Kellerman JJ, Braunwald E, editors. Silent myocardial ischemia: a critical appraisal. Basel: Karger; 1990. p. 42-64.
50. Van Rijn T, Rabkin SW. Effect of naloxone on exercise-induced angina pectoris: a randomized double blind crossover trial. Life Sci 1986; 38: 609-15.
51. Ellestad MH, Kuan P. Naloxone and asymptomatic ischemia: failure to induce angina during exercise testing. Am J Cardiol 1984; 54: 982-4.
52. Heller GV, Garber CE, Connolly MJ, et al. Plasma beta-endorphin levels in silent myocardial ischemia induced by exercise. Am J Cardiol 1987;59:735-9.
53. Falcone C, Specchia G, Rondanelli R, et al. Correlation between beta-endorphin plasma levels and anginal symptoms in patients with coronary artery disease. J Am Coll Cardiol 1988;11:719-23.
54. Barsky AJ, Hochstrasser B, Coles NA, Zisfein J, O'Donnell C, Eagle KA. Silent myocardial ischemia. Is the person or the event silent? JAMA 1990;264:1132-5.
55. Wall PD. The gate control theory of pain mechanisms. A re-examination and a re-statement. Brain 1978;101:1-18.
56. Neafsey EJ, Terreberry RR, Hurley KM, Ruit KG, Frysztak RJ. Anterior cingulate cortex in rodents: connections, visceral control functions and implications for emotion. In: Vogt BA, Gabriel M, editor. Neurobiology of cingulate cortex and limbic thalamus. Boston: Birkhâuser; 1993. p. 206-23.
57. Terreberry RR, Neafsey EJ. Rat medial frontal cortex: a visceral motor region with a direct projection to the solitary nucleus. Brain Res 1983; 278:245-9.
58. Hurley KM, Herbert H, Moga MM, Saper CB. Efferent projections of the infralimbic cortex of the rat. J Comp Neurol 1991; 308: 249-76.

59. Vogt BA, Pandya DN. Cingulate cortex of the rhesus monkey: II. Cortical afferents. J Comp Neurol 1987;262:271-89.
60. Van Hoesen GW, Morecraft RJ, Vogt BA. Connections of the monkey cingulate cortex. In: Vogt BA, Gabriel M, editor. Neurobiology of cingulate cortex and limbic thalamus. Boston: Birkhâuser; 1993:249-84.
61. Malliani A. Pathophysiology of ischemic cardiac pain. In: von Arnim T, Maseri A, editor Silent ischemia. Darmstadt: Steinkopff; 1987. p. 19-24.
62. Jones AKP, Brown WD Friston KJ, Qi LY, Frackowiak RS. Cortical and subcortical localization of response to pain in man using positron emission tomography. Proc R Soc Lond Biol Sci 1991; 244:39-44.
63. Talbot JD, Marrett S, Evans AC, Meyer E, Bushnell MC, Duncan GH. Multiple representations of pain in human cerebral cortex. Science 1991;251:1355-8.
64. Morecraft RJ, Geula C, Mesulam MM. Cytoarchitecture and neural afferents of orbitofrontal cortex in the brain of the monkey. J Comp Neurol 1992;323:341-58.
65. Gabriel M, Kubota Y, Sparenborg S, Straube K, Vogt BA. Effects of cingulate cortical lesions on avoidance learning and training-induced unit activity in rabbits. Exp Brain Res 1991;86:585-600.
66. Keefer CS, Resnik WH. Angina pectoris: a syndrome caused by anoxemia of the myocardium. Arch Intern Med 1928; 41:769-807.
67. Ahn J, Jarmukli NF, Iranmanesh A, Russell DC. Modulation of beta-endorphin levels alters peripheral pain threshold but not anginal threshold in patients with stable angina [abstract]. Circulation 1994; 90 (4 pt.2): I57.
68. Rosen SD, Paulesu E, Frackowiak RS, Camici PG. Central neural correlates of chest pain in syndrome X [abstract]. Circulation 1995; 92 (Suppl 1): I651.
69. Rosen SD, Paulesu E, Tousoulis D, Foale RA, Camici PG. Role of the thalamus and cerebral cortex in the perception of cardiac symptoms [abstract]. Circulation 1997; 96 (8 Suppl): I761.

a) Silent ischaemia

Patient	Age	Sex	Angio	ECG (rest)	ECG (dob)	HR (rest)	HR (dob)	SBP (rest)	SBP (dob)	DBP (rest)	DBP (dob)	RPP (rest)	RPP (dob)	Max dose dob	RWMA
1	75	M	3 V	√T in III, aVF	√ST V3-5	55	105	140	150	65	60	7700	15750	30	antero-lateral
2	57	M	3V, CABG, new R occ	Old inf Qs	√ST V4	70	110	160	225	90	85	11200	24750	20	antero-apical
3	60	M	3V	Part RBBB	√ST V4	64	100	140	160	80	80	8960	16000	30	inferior
4	64	M	3V	Normal	√ST V5, 6	57	110	165	175	90	75	9405	19250	20	infero-basal
5	61	M	Cx and RCA (stenosis)	Normal	√ST V4, 5	50	66	135	165	65	65	6750	10890	25	lateral
6	66	M	3V	Normal	√ST II, V5, 6	52	86	120	155	70	70	6240	13330	35	infero-lateral
7	59	M	3V	Partial RBBB	√ST II, III, V5,6	60	120	145	170	85	80	8700	20400	30	inferior
8	51	M	CABG (4), 2 grafts occ	Normal	√ST II, III, V3-5	65	140	150	200	95	105	9750	28000	25	inferior
9	63	M	LAD and RCA stenoses	Normal	√ST V4-6	74	130	145	150	70	65	10730	19500	30	postero-septal

b) Angina pectoris

Patient	Age	Sex	Angio	ETT	ECG (rest)	ECG (dob)	HR (rest)	HR (dob)	SBP (rest)	SBP (dob)	DBP (rest)	DBP (dob)	RPP (rest)	RPP (dob)	Max dose dob
1	53	M	LAD (stenosis)	+	Normal	√ST II, V5	58	90	150	205	85	95	8700	18450	20
2	64	F	LAD (stenosis)	+	Partial RBBB	√ST II, III, VF	65	93	135	155	75	75	8775	14420	20
3	66	M	RCA (stenosis)	+	Normal	√ST II, III, VF	60	75	130	165	75	75	7800	12380	30
4	59	M	RCA (occlusion)	+	Old inf Qs	√ST V4,5	68	102	140	170	80	85	9520	17340	25
5	48	M	LAD (stenosis)	+	Normal	√ST V4	60	108	130	160	85	75	7800	9180	25
6	72	M	LAD (stenosis)	+	Normal	√ST II, III, VF	60	70	115	160	70	80	6900	11200	30
7	61	M	LAD/Cx (occlusion)	+	Normal	√ST V4,5	65	99	140	160	85	80	9100	15840	25
8	60	F	LAD/diag (stenosis)	+	Normal	√ST II, V4	80	145	155	200	85	90	12400	29000	20
9	65	M	RCA (stenosis)	+	√T inferolat	LBBB	70	110	160	220->160	80	90	11200	17600	25

***Table 1**. Patients' characteristics and hemodynamic findings. M - male; F - female; CAD - coronary artery disease shown at angiography; RCA - right coronary artery; LAD - left anterior descending coronary artery; Cx - left circumflex coronary artery; diag - diagonal branch of LAD; 3V - three vessel coronary artery disease; new R occ - new occlusion of the right coronary artery; CABG - coronary artery bypass grafting; ETT - exercise treadmill test; + - ETT positive for ischemic changes; ECG - electrocardiogram; RBBB - right bundle branch block; old inf Qs - old inferior lead Q waves; dob - at peak effect of dobutamine infusion; √ST - ST segment depression; √T - T wave inversion; inferolat - inferolateral; LBBB - left bundle branch block; HR - heart rate; SBP - systolic blood pressure; DBP - diastolic blood pressure; RPP - heart rate x systolic pressure product; Max dose dob - maximal dose of dobutamine; RWMA - echocardiographic regional wall motion abnormality.*

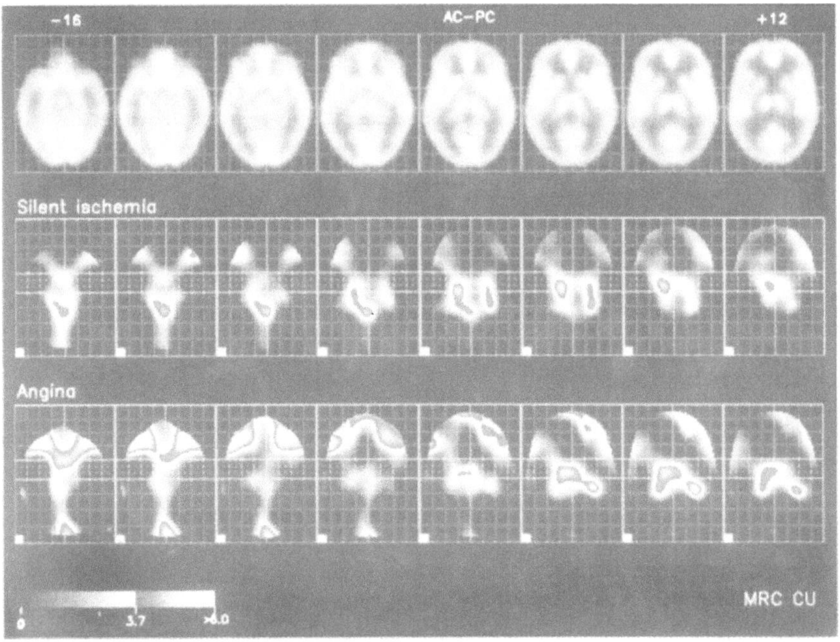

Figure 1. *Cerebral areas activated during angina pectoris and silent ischemia. The top row shows averaged blood flow maps from all subjects and all conditions normalised into a standard stereotactic space. These pictures can be used for anatomical localisation of the activation foci. The latter are displayed as statistical parametric maps in the same stereotactic anatomical space shown in the above averaged blood flow maps. Results for the silent ischemia patients are shown in the middle row and results for the angina pectoris patients are shown in the bottom row. The magnitude of the Z scores is displayed for both patients groups according to the same linear colour scale (threshold for significance: 3.7). AC-PC: this indicates the inter-commissural plane. Distances are expressed in millimetres from this reference (AC-PC) plane.*

(See also Colour Plates, p. 341)

		LEFT							RIGHT				
Brodmann Area		x	y	z	∂ rCBF	Z score		x	y	z	∂ rCBF	Z score
47	*	-32	26	-16		6.2		22	26	-8		5.7
17								2	-94	-12		5.3
10		-8	56	0		4.6		8	54	-4		4.2
25		-14	8	-20		4.3	*	12	6	-16		4.4
Thalamus	*	-10	-18	4		4.7		28	-38	8		5.2
Hypothalamus		-6	-2	-20		4.7						

Table 2. *Co-ordinates of loci of maximal increases in rCBF during angina pectoris. Table 3 reports the co-ordinates in the x, y and z axes, of the significant rCBF increases with reference to the stereotactic space defined by the atlas of Talairach and Tournoux [38]. Statistical magnitudes are expressed as Z scores. * - Those regions where a significant change in rCBF was present in the interaction: (angina - baseline 2) - (placebo - baseline 1). In addition to the loci presented, an additional brainstem locus, [-8 -36 -20], Z score 3.5 was found when the data were analysed according to omnibus significance with 0.01 threshold. It was not included in the main table as it did not reach significance at the Bonferroni level. BA - Brodmann area; δrCBF - change in regional cerebral blood flow equivalents.*

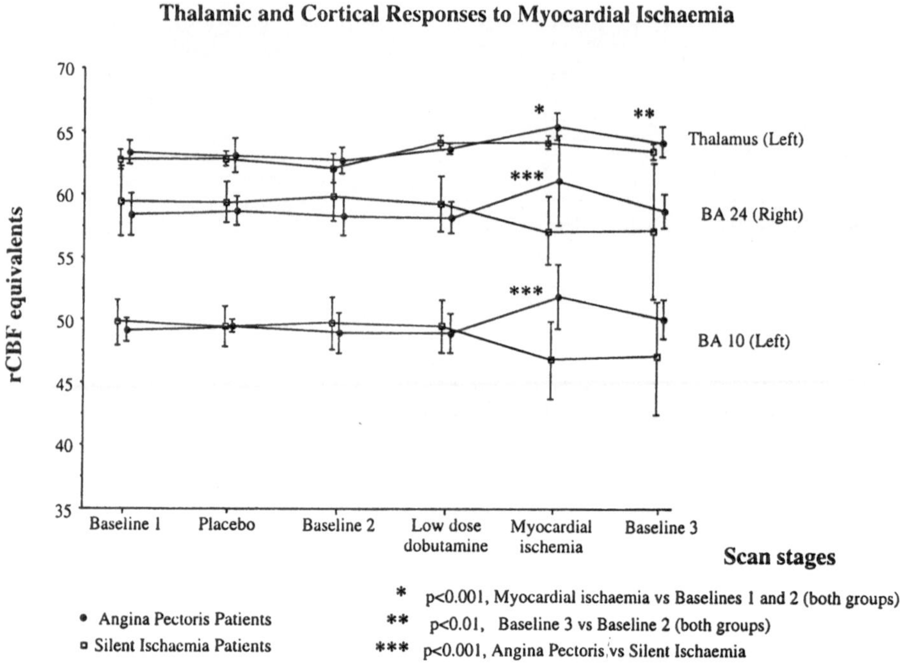

***Figure 2**. Time course of rCBF changes in selected regions. Changes over time in rCBF in the left thalamus, right Brodmann area 24 and the left Brodmann area 10 are shown. These areas have been selected to illustrate the difference in frontal activation between the silent ischemia and angina pectoris patients as well as the difference in time course of activation of the frontal areas compared to the thalami. Thus, i) the rCBF changes in Brodmann area 24 and Brodmann area 10 during myocardial ischemia are significantly greater in the angina pectoris patients than in the patients with silent ischemia; and ii) although the rCBF increases in Brodmann area 24 and Brodmann area 10 have entirely resolved by baseline 3, thalamic rCBF is seen to remain increased in both patient groups during the post-ischemic scan. Angina patients - black circles; silent ischemia patients - open squares.*

	LEFT					RIGHT				
Brodmann Area	x	y	z	∂ rCBF	Z score	x	y	z	∂ rCBF	Z score
47						36	24	-12		4.3
36	-2	-48	-8		4.5					
30	-14	-40	0		3.9					
6	-2	-2	52		4.9					
Thalamus	-16	-20	4		4.9	24	-40	4		4.3

***Table 3**. Co-ordinates of loci of maximal increases in rCBF during silent myocardial ischemia. Table 2 reports the co-ordinates in the x, y and z axes, of the significant rCBF increases, with reference to the stereotactic space defined by the atlas of Talairach and Tournoux [38]. Statistical magnitudes are expressed as Z scores. BA - Brodmann area; δrCBF - change in regional cerebral blood flow equivalents.*

Brodman Area	LEFT x	y	z	Z score	RIGHT x	y	z	Z score
10	-6	50	-4	3.2				
11	-4	18	-20	2.9				
24	-16	42	-4	2.8	6	42	-4	3.4
25	-12	22	-16	2.9	12	28	-12	2.6
28	-36	10	-20	3.4				
36	-54	-44	-20	2.4				

NB In this table, Z>2.3 reflects p<0.01.

Table 4. *Co-ordinates of loci of significant differences in maximal rCBF increases during myocardial ischemia between patients with angina pectoris and patients with silent myocardial ischemia. Table 4 reports the co-ordinates in the x, y and z axes, of the significant differences in rCBF increases between the patient groups. (Coordinates refer to the atlas of Talairach and Tournoux [38]). Statistical magnitudes are expressed as Z scores. NB In this table, Z>2.3 reflects p<0.01. The table includes the BA 28 locus, not included in table 3 because although the omnibus significance of the result was p<0.001, this did not withstand the more rigorous Bonferroni correction employed for all the other loci. It has been included in Table 4 because of the adequate significance of its result according to the interaction test.[(angina - baseline 2) - (placebo - baseline 1)]. BA - Brodmann area; δrCBFang - change in regional cerebral blood flow equivalents during angina pectoris; .δrCBFsi - change in regional cerebral blood flow equivalents during silent myocardial ischemia.*

Chapter 10

Clinical Relevance of Myocardial Viability

Frans C. Visser, Jeroen J. Bax, Lucas J. Klein, William Wijns and Cees A. Visser

Introduction

The morphologic characterization of the dysfunctional myocardium [1-3] has led to further insight into the mechanisms that determine the presence or absence of functional recovery after revascularization. Contractile dysfunction may be caused by necrotic myocardium or by jeopardized but viable myocardium. If the dysfunction is due to fibrosis, no recovery can be expected after revascularization; if the dysfunction is due to jeopardized but viable myocardium, recovery can occur in some patients [3-5]. Although the exact pathophysiology of dysfunctional but viable myocardium remains controversial[5-8], the potential for functional recovery has clinical relevance. Indeed, whatever the exact mechanism of reversible dysfunction, reperfusion in the acute stage of ischemic syndromes or revascularization in the chronic stage is required for functional recovery.

The awareness that even severely dyssynergic myocardium in patients with coronary artery disease (CAD) may show an improvement in functional state after revascularization [6] has resulted in a tremendous amount of research for identifying viable tissue and for the optimal diagnostic approach to identify areas with recoverable dysfunction [9].

Viability detection can be used for a number of clinical issues: 1) preoperative detection of functional recovery after revascularization in patients with chronic depressed left ventricular (LV) function, 2) perioperative risk

Van der Wall et al. (eds.),
Advanced Imaging in Coronary Artery Disease, 163-183.

assessment in patients undergoing revascularization, 3) determination of prognosis in patients with chronic CAD, 4) prediction of reversal of LV function after acute myocardial infarction, and 5) determination of prognosis after myocardial infarction.

Methods to assess viability

Several techniques have been developed to identify dysfunctional but viable myocardium, but the most commonly used are positron emission tomography (PET) with F-18 FDG, Tl-201 stress-redistribution-reinjection, Tl-201 rest-redistribution, Tc-99m MIBI SPECT and low dose dobutamine echocardiography (LDDE).

F-18 FDG. Since the original observation by Marshall et al. [10] in 1981, considerable evidence has accumulated to show that F-18 FDG in combination with PET can detect viable myocardium [11,12]. F-18 FDG is a glucose analogue that traces exogenous glucose uptake by the myocardium. Viable myocardium is characterized by preserved F-18 FDG uptake in an area with depressed LV function.

Tl-201 scintigraphy. The initial uptake of Tl-201 by myocytes is mainly determined by regional perfusion, whereas the integrity of the cell membrane is predominantly important for delayed imaging of tracer retention. Although different Tl-201 protocols have been described [9], mainly Tl-201 stress-redistribution-reinjection and Tl-201 rest-redistribution are currently used. Several studies have shown [13-15] that reinjection of 37 MBq (1 mCi) of Tl-201 after 3- to 4-h redistribution imaging detects viability in 31% to 49% of segments deemed irreversibly damaged because they showed a fixed defect on conventional stress-redistribution Tl-201 imaging. Bonow et al. [16] showed concordance between Tl-201 stress-redistribution-reinjection and F-18 FDG PET for the presence or absence of viable myocardium in 88% of segments. It also appears that semiquantitation of Tl-201 activity is important. The majority of mild to moderate (Tl-201 activity $\geq$50% of normal) fixed defects on redistribution [16] and reinjection images [17] were viable on F-18 FDG PET.

Whereas Tl-201 stress-redistribution-reinjection scintigraphy provides information on both exercise-induced ischemia and viability, Tl-201 rest-redistribution provides information on viability only. Two studies [18,19] compared Tl-201 stress-redistribution-reinjection with Tl-201 rest-redistribution imaging and showed a concordance between the two techniques of 80%, at least when defect reversibility was considered an indicator of viability. When the severity of Tl-201 activity in irreversible defects was considered, the concordance increased to 94% [18]. In addition, Dilsizian et al. [18] showed that F-18 FDG PET and Tl-201 rest-redistribution imaging yielded comparable information regarding viability when the Tl-201 rest-redistribution studies were analyzed semiquantitatively.

Tc-99m MIBI. Myocardial uptake of Tc-99m MIBI parallels regional perfusion and provides adequate information for the detection of CAD [20]. The uptake and retention of Tc-99m MIBI is also dependent on cell membrane integrity and mitochondrial function (membrane potential) [21-23] and thus may reflect cellular viability. Many studies have compared Tc-99m MIBI imaging with other scintigraphic modalities, including Tl-201 stress-redistribution-reinjection [24,25], Tl-201 rest [26-29], Tl-201 rest-redistribution [28,30-32] and F-18 FDG PET [31,33-38]. These concordance studies were consistent in showing that Tc-99m MIBI was less accurate in the detection of myocardial viability. However, as discussed below, specificity of Tc-99m MIBI is higher than of Tl-201 stress-redistribution-reinjection and Tl-201 rest-redistribution in detecting absence of functional recovery after revascularization.

Low-dose dobutamine echocardiography. Echocardiography during the infusion of low dose dobutamine (5 to 15 ug/kg body weight per min) has been proposed as an alternative method for assessing myocardial viability in patients with chronic ischemic heart disease [39]. The hallmark of viability is improved contraction of a dyssynergic segment after adrenergic stimulation. Several studies have compared LDDE with other imaging modalities to assess viability, including F-18 FDG PET [40-42], Tl-201 stress--redistribution-reinjection [43-48], Tl-201 rest-redistribution [26,49-52] and Tc-99m MIBI [26], showing good agreement in most studies.

Pre-operative detection of functional recovery after revascularization in patients with chronic depressed LV function

Reversal of myocardial dysfunction is particularly relevant in patients with depressed ventricular function because surgical revascularization improves long-term survival in such patients [53,54]. However, surgical intervention is associated with a higher risk for perioperative complications and mortality in the same patient subset [55]. Thus, it becomes critical to identify and select those patients who may benefit from a revascularization procedure. All above mentioned techniques have successfully demonstrated the ability to predict improvement of regional and global function after revascularization.

Data on regional function are discussed below. More importantly, Tillisch et al. [56] were one of the first who demonstrated that the LVEF improved on average from 30% to 45% in patients with three or more viable, dysfunctional segments on F-18 FDG PET, whereas the LVEF did not improve in the patients with two or less viable, dysfunctional segments. Comparable findings have been recently reported [4,57,58] using the same technique. With Tl-201 scintigraphy Bax et al. [43] evaluated 17 patients with Tl-201 reinjection imaging to assess improvement of global function after revascularization. Tl-201 reinjection identified five of six patients who demonstrated improvement in LVEF of at least 5%. Of the 11 patients with no improvement in global function, Tl-201 reinjection identified nonviable myocardium in six patients. Vanoverschelde et al. [46] recently reported a sensitivity of 72% and a specificity of 73% for Tl-201 reinjection imaging in predicting improved global LV function. Similar data were found by Iskandrian et al. [59] and others using Tl-201 rest-redistribution [60,61]. Using LDDE, Meluzin et al. [62] showed that the LVEF increased on average from 38% to 42% after revascularization in patients with contractile reserve but did not improve in patients without contractile reserve. Moreover, the improvement in LVEF was linearly related to the number of segments with contractile reserve on LDDE, indicating that the amount of viable tissue determines the magnitude of improvement of LV function [62]. Several studies[43,46,63] have now confirmed these findings. Important from a patient point of view are the findings of Marwick et al. [64] and Di Carli et al. [65] that revascularization of viable tissue was associated with an improvement of exercise capacity and quality of life. Thus, viability assessment has proved to be clinical successful in predicting outcome after revascularization.

Peri-operative risk assessment in patients undergoing revascularization

Not only is viability assessment useful for the long-term outcome after revascularization, but it may also be used for perioperative risk assessment. Haas et al. [66] studied 84 patients with advanced CAD who underwent coronary artery bypass surgery (CABG). Of these patients 43 underwent CABG on basis of clinical and angiographic data, while 41 also underwent FDG PET imaging. Patients without viability assessment had a significantly higher low output syndrome (14%) and mortality (12%) compared to patients with viability assessment (2% and 0%, respectively). Although this was a retrospective study in which the reasons for performing FDG PET, the presence of viable tissue and the decision process for accepting patients are not given, the data suggest that if cardiac surgeons include viability data in their patient management, perioperative outcome may be better than without the use of viability data. Larger, prospective studies are needed to confirm these findings.

Determination of prognosis in patients with chronic CAD

In addition to the prediction of functional recovery after revascularization, F-18 FDG PET imaging may also provide prognostic information on morbidity and mortality. Four retrospective studies [67-70] have been published, indicating that the presence of a mismatch pattern in patients who are treated medically is associated with a higher morbidity and mortality. Tamaki et al. [67] showed in 158 stable patients with a previous myocardial infarction, that the mismatch pattern was the best predictor of future cardiac events, among all clinical, angiographic and Tl-201 stress-redistribution variables. The studies by Eitzman et al. [68] and Di Carli et al. [69] evaluated mortality in a total of 175 patients with severely depressed ventricular function who underwent F-18 FDG PET imaging; patients were followed for an average of 12 and 13.6 months respectively. Eighty-three patients were revascularized and 92 patients were treated medically. The patients were subsequently divided into 4 groups: depending on the therapy and on the presence or absence of a mismatch pattern (figure 1).

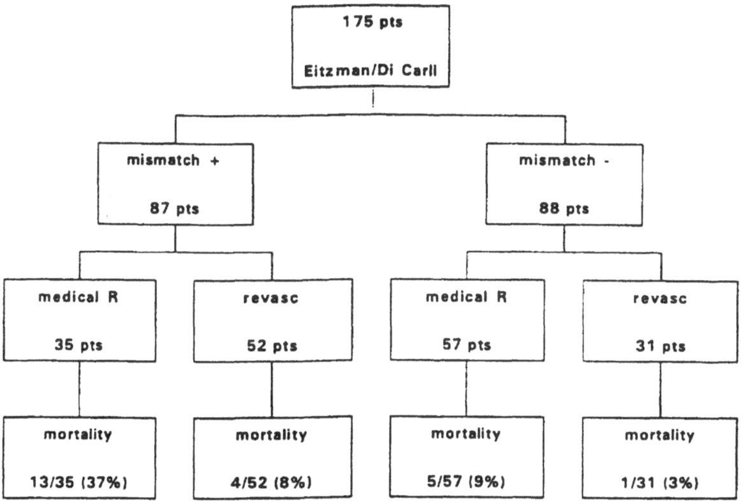

Figure 1. *Flow-chart illustrating the increased mortality in patients with viability, who are treated medically. In contrast, all other groups showed a low mortality (Data based on studies by Eitzman et al. [68] and Di Carli et al. [69]. Medical R = medical therapy, revasc = revascularization.*

The highest mortality was observed in the group of patients with a mismatch pattern who were treated medically (37% versus 3%, 8%, and 9% in the other groups (figure 1). Lee et al. [70] evaluated 129 patients with a mean LVEF of 38±16% over a mean follow-up of 17±9 months. The frequency of non-fatal ischemic cardiac events was 48% in the group of patients with a mismatch who were treated medically versus 8% in the group with a mismatch who were revascularized. Recently, similar results were published with Tl-201 rest-redistribution imaging. Gioia et al. [71] studied the prognosis of patients with severe LV dysfunction, who were treated medically. During a mean follow-up of 31 months, there were 11 cardiac deaths in patients with no redistribution (26%) on Tl-201 rest-redistribution imaging and 22 in patients with redistribution (58%), and multivariate Cox survival analysis on important clinical, angiographic, and thallium variables showed that the presence of redistribution was an independent predictor of death.

The results of these studies suggest that viability provides information not only in the prediction of improvement of contractile function, but also in the prediction of survival. It should be stated however, that all these studies were based on retrospective analyzes of data obtained in patients with poor LV function who were often referred for viability imaging. Prospective studies are required to confirm these findings.

Prediction of reversal of LV function after acute myocardial infarction

The presence of viability in patients with an acute myocardial infarction is associated with improvement of LV function during follow-up. Schwaiger et al. performed in 1986 a study in which patients underwent F-18 FDG imaging within 3 days after myocardial infarction [72]. They found that viable segments showed improvement of regional function during follow-up in 50%, in contrast to non-viable segments which showed no improvement al all. These FDG findings were confirmed by Huitink et al. [73] Also LDDE has been successfully employed to predict functional recovery after acute myocardial infarction [74-78]. Using LDDE and PET, Piérard et al. [74] studied 17 patients with acute anterior infarction, treated with thrombolysis. Functional recovery during follow-up was observed in all patients with normal perfusion and LDDE viable segments. In patients with increased FDG uptake and contractile recovery during LDDE recovery of function during follow-up was observed in a minority of patients, whereas patients without signs of viability with both techniques showed no recovery. This study implicates that viable tissue with increased FDG uptake indicates jeopardized myocardium that frequently loses viability if no revascularization intervention is done. Indeed,

Barilla et al. [75] demonstrated that acute infarct patients with viable tissue, who underwent coronary revascularization showed a better LV function improvement during follow-up than infarct patients with viable tissue who were treated medically.

Thus, viability in the infarct area is associated with spontaneous improvement of LV function and the absence of viability is strongly predictive of absence of recovery. However, the initial data suggest that viable infarct areas with increased FDG uptake are at risk for deterioration. Probably, these patients merit revascularization for improvement of LV function and thus prognosis. This needs confirmation in a prospective trial.

Determination of prognosis after myocardial infarction

Data regarding the effect of viability on prognosis after myocardial infarction are conflicting. The small study of Yoshida and Gould using PET [79] and mainly the study of Carlos et al. [80] using LDDE showed that viability, together with a small infarct size and absence of ischemia was associated with a good prognosis after myocardial infarction (figure 2). In contrast, a number studies observed the opposite i.e. a worse prognosis in patients with viability. Brown et al. [81] found that patients with reversible perfusion defects in the infarct area, defined as viability, had a higher risk of cardiac events. Similarly, Basu et al. [82] found in infarct patients treated with thrombolysis that the event-free survival of patients with reversible perfusion defects, detected by stress/nitroglycerine-enhanced rest Tl-201 imaging was significantly lower than patients without reversible perfusion defects (figure 3). Strikingly, Tl-201 stress-redistribution imaging did not discriminate between event and event-free patients. At our institution two prognostic studies in patients admitted with an acute myocardial infarction were performed. Huitink et al. [83] performed planar FDG imaging and followed the infarct patients for mean 47 month. Patients with a mismatch pattern had a 49% event rate in contrast to patients with a match pattern 7% ($p<0.009$). Nijland et al.[84] studied the in-hospital event rate of admitted patients. Viability was assessed by LDDE early after myocardial infarction. They found in patients with viability an in-hospital event rate of 32% versus 10% in patients without viability; ($p<0.05$). Thus, most of the data on infarct patients relate the presence of viability with an adverse prognosis which is in line with prognosis data in patients with chronic CAD. The data of Carlos et al. [80] are quite opposite and the differences in clinical outcome of viability in this patient group need further studies.

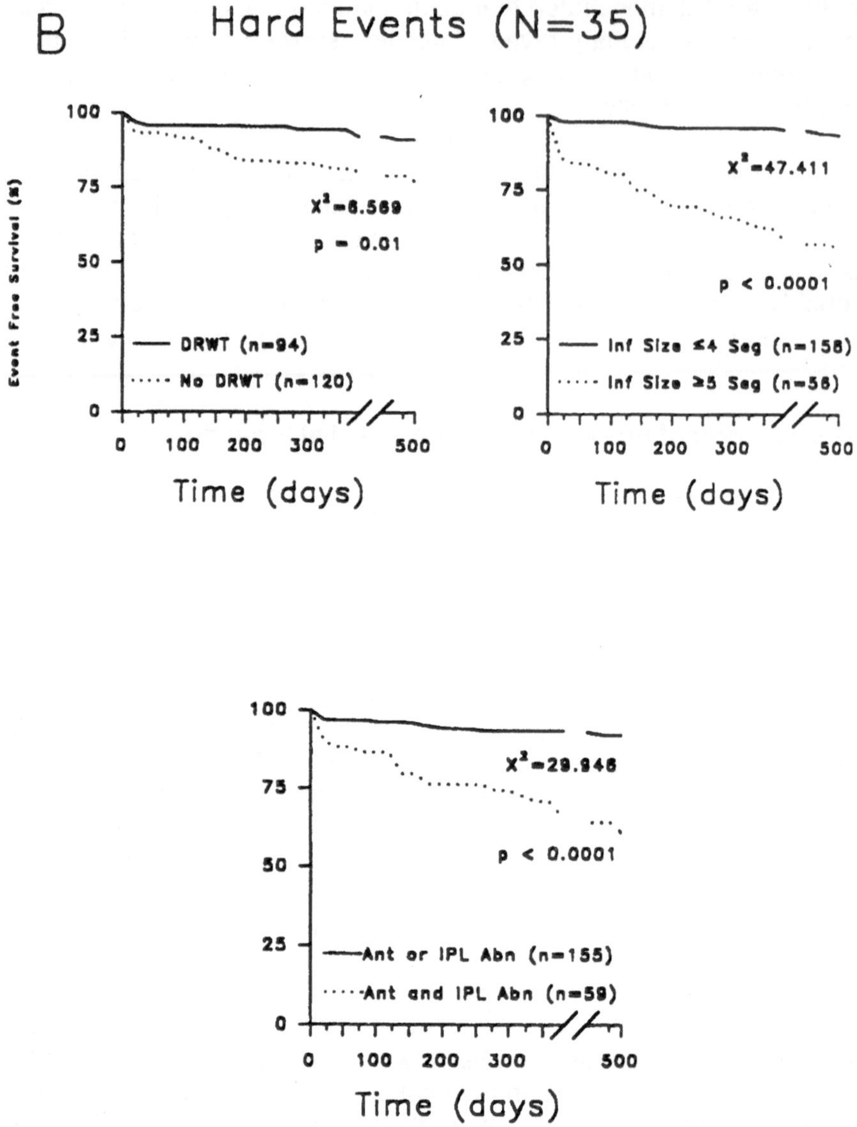

Figure 2. Kaplan-Meier life table curves of hard event-free survival on the basis of dobutamine responsive wall thickening (DRWT) at low dose, infarct size (inf size) and remote ischemia/infarction (from Carlos et al. [80], printed with permission).

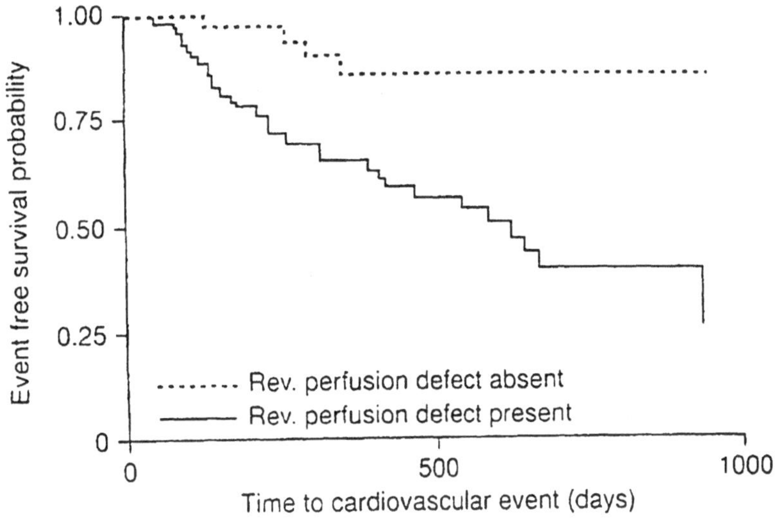

Figure 3. Kaplan-Meier event-free survival curve of patients with and without reversible (Rev) perfusion defects by stress/nitroglycerin-enhanced rest Tl-201 imaging (hazard ratio 8.1; 95% CI 2.7 to 23.8; p<0.001). (From Basu et al. [82]*, printed with permission)*

Which technique for assessment of viability

To assess the relative diagnostic value of these techniques we performed a pooled data analysis of the presently available reports for the prediction of functional recovery. For this purpose a search of the MEDLINE data base was conducted. Moreover a manual search of eight cardiology and nuclear medicine journals was carried out and the reference lists of the reports obtained through these searches were screened. Only articles in English were considered, and reviews or abstracts were discarded. The study had to be prospective and evaluated one or more techniques for functional outcome after revascularization, assessed during follow-up in patients with chronic, stable LV dysfunction. The studies had to contain sufficient details to calculate the sensitivity and specificity for predicting improvement in regional LV function. From the pooled data, weighted sensitivities and specificities were calculated. The 95% confidence intervals (CI) of the weighted sensitivities and specificities were also calculated [85] and the individual intervals were compared. The majority of the studies in patients undergoing revascularization concentrated on changes in regional contraction. Although for the individual patient, improvement in global LV function is the most clinically relevant factor, available data on global function improvement were too limited for calculating accurate sensitivities/specificities. The search strategy yielded 396 reports, of which only 37 fulfilling the inclusion criteria. Most of the 396 studies were excluded because of absence of revascularization (n=275).

Results

	no of pts	mean LVEF (%)	Range LVEF (%)	Sens (%) Sens (%)	CI	Spec (%)	CI Spec (%)	DA %
F-18 FDG PET	332	40	32-53	88	84-91	73	69-77	80
Tl-201 reinjection	209	36	31-46	86	83-89	47	43-51	63
Tl-201 RR	145	35	27-39	90	87-93	54	49-60	74
Tc-99m MIBI	207	43	34-52	83	78-87	69	63-74	76
LDDE	448	36	26-46	84	82-86	81	79-84	83

CI = 95% confidence intervals, DA = diagnostic accuracy, LDDE = low dose dobutamine echocardiography, LVEF = LV ejection fraction, Sens = sensitivity, Spec = specificity, Tl-201 RR = Tl-201 rest-redistribution

Table 1. *Weighted sensitivity and specificity for the different imaging techniques*

F-18 FDG PET. Many studies have used F-18 FDG PET to predict functional recovery in patients undergoing revascularization [33,40,41,56,86-93]. The results from these studies are summarized in Table 1. Reanalysis of the original data (obtained in 332 patients) showed that the sensitivity ranged from 71% to 100%, with a weighted mean of 88%. Specificity ranged from 38% to 91%, with a weighted mean of 73%.

Tl-201 stress-redistribution-reinjection.
Seven studies [13,15,43-46,93], including 209 patients, have evaluated the diagnostic accuracy of Tl-201 stress-redistribution-reinjection for assessing improvement in regional function after revascularization. The available data revealed that Tl-201 stress-redistribution-reinjection imaging has a high sensitivity (average 86%) but a relatively low specificity (average 47%). These results suggest an overestimation of potential recovery by Tl-201 stress-redistribution-reinjection imaging.

Tl-201 rest-redistribution

Eight studies [26,27,49-52,60,61] evaluated the use of Tl-201 rest-redistribution imaging in revascularization patients. In these studies the average sensitivity and specificity were 90% and 54%, also suggesting some overestimation of recovery by Tl-201 rest-redistribution imaging.

Tc-99m MIBI

The results of studies that evaluated Tc-99m MIBI imaging with regard to functional outcome after revascularization are summarized in table 1 [26,27,33,94-97]. All studies reported a high sensitivity, whereas specificity varied considerably from 35% to 86%. Recently, the administration of nitrates before Tc-99m MIBI imaging has been described [98-100]. Three studies that have used this approach clearly showed improved specificity.

Low dose dobutamine echocardiography

The results of the available studies indicate that LDDE [26,40-44,46,49-52,63,101-104] adequately detects recovery of contractile function after revascularization, with a mean sensitivity of 84% and a mean specificity of 81%. It is worth mentioning that all studies with low dose dobutamine have used echocardiography, rather than an independent technique, to assess improvement of regional wall motion.

This review revealed that sensitivity for predicting improved regional contractile function after revascularization is high for all techniques analyzed; however specificity varied greatly for all techniques and was lowest for Tl-201 stress-redistribution-reinjection and Tl-201 rest-redistribution. Although the specificities were lower compared to the other techniques, the question is how clinically relevant this low specificity is. Because of the high sensitivities, the negative predictive value for functional outcome is high (assuming a balanced division between recoverable and non-recoverable regions in the study population).Thus, patients are probably correctly denied revascularization if no viable tissue is present and the cardiologist/cardiac surgeon may take the risk of absence of functional recovery because patients are usually proposed for revascularization because of complaints. Moreover, we have recently studied the diagnostic value of rest-redistribution Tl-201 SPECT for the prediction of global LV function recovery after revascularization. The specificity for detecting absence of global function improvement (defined as an improvement of at least 5 ejection fraction units) was 76%. [105] This implicates that the Tl-201 techniques are adequate for the more clinically relevant global function improvement after revascularization. Finally, the presence of viable myocardium may have implications for and long-term effects on clinical factors that are independent from the rest functional state of the left ventricle[68-70]. These factors include prognosis, the response during stress[106], exercise capacity [64] and quality of life [65]. At present, the relative merits of the different viability techniques for the prediction of these clinical factors are largely unknown and should be prospectively evaluated in a large patient cohort.

This analysis of the published data reveals some of the weaknesses of the currently available evidence. The inclusion criteria may vary considerably from one study to the other, particularly with respect to the severity of baseline dysfunction. Ideally, only patients with a global ejection fraction <30-35% should be studied because these patients are both likely to benefit from and to have a greater risk during revascularization. Most studies included only a limited number of patients, suggesting inclusion bias. The majority of studies do not provide evidence of vessel or graft patency; reocclusion may prohibit viable segments from recovering, thereby underestimating the true specificity of all techniques. The optimal moment for the assessment of functional follow-up after revascularization is uncertain. Currently, follow-up is frequently performed 3 months after revascularization. However, preliminary data [107] have demonstrated that full recovery should not be expected to occur before 6 or even 12 months after revascularization. Importantly, global and regional function should be evaluated by an independent technique. Studies of LDDE have invariably used echocardiograms to evaluate the effect of revascularization. The use of an internally consistent standard may contribute in part to the excellent predictive value of this technique. In addition, the acquisition and interpretation of echocardiograms strongly depends on operator experience. There are data for predicting improvement in global rest function; however, the number of available studies remains too small to compare their respective accuracy.

In practice, the choice between imaging modalities also depends on local availability and expertise, which is particularly critical for the acquisition and interpretation of LDDE.

Conclusion

Assessment of myocardial viability can be used in patients to detect functional outcome in acute and chronic ischemic syndromes and for risk assessment in different clinical settings. However, it is obvious that the viability tests are not perfect (table 1), and that the tests do not have equivalent performance characteristics. Possibly, complementary techniques could be combined to obtain an more optimal clinical result. Then strategies can be developed for a cost-effective use of tests in a sequential manner [108].

References

1. Flameng W, Suy R, Schwarz F, et al. Ultrastructural correlates of left ventricular contraction abnormalities in patients with chronic ischemic heart disease: determinants of reversible segmental asynergy postrevascularization surgery. Am Heart J 1981;102:846-57.
2. Borgers M. Structural correlates of regional myocardial dysfunction in patients with critical coronary artery stenosis: chronic hibernation? Cardiovasc Pathol 1993;2:237-45.
3. Depré C, Vanoverschelde JL, Melin JA, et al. Structural and metabolic correlates of the reversibility of chronic left ventricular ischemic dysfunction in humans. Am J Physiol 1995;268:H1265-75.
4. Maes A, Flameng W, Nuyts J, et al. Histological alterations in chronically hypoperfused myocardium. Correlation with PET findings. Circulation 1994;90:735-45.
5. Vanoverschelde JL, Wijns W, Depré C, et al. Mechanisms of chronic regional postischemic dysfunction in humans. New insights from the study of noninfarcted collateral-dependent myocardium. Circulation 1993;87:1513-23.
6. Rahimtoola SH. The hibernating myocardium. Am Heart J 1989;117:211-21.
7. Bolli R. Myocardial 'stunning' in man. Circulation 1992;86:1671-91.
8. Vanoverschelde JL, Wijns W, Borgers M, et al. Chronic myocardial hibernation in humans. From bedside to bench. Circulation 1997;95:1961-71.
9. Dilsizian V, Bonow RO. Current diagnostic techniques of assessing myocardial viability in patients with hibernating and stunned myocardium. [published erratum appears in Circulation 1993;87:2070]. Circulation 1993;87:1-20.
10. Marshall RC, Tillisch JH, Phelps ME, et al. Identification and differentiation of resting myocardial ischemia and infarction in man with positron computed tomography, 18F-labeled fluorodeoxyglucose and N-13 ammonia. Circulation 1983;67:766-78.
11. Schwaiger M, Hicks R. The clinical role of metabolic imaging of the heart by positron emission tomography. J Nucl Med 1991;32:565-78.
12. Schelbert HR. Positron emission tomography for the assessment of myocardial viability. Circulation 1991;84 (3 Suppl):I122-31.
13. Dilsizian V, Rocco TP, Freedman NM, Leon MB, Bonow RO. Enhanced detection of ischemic but viable myocardium by the reinjection of thallium after stress-redistribution imaging. N Engl J Med 1990;323:141-6.
14. Tamaki N, Ohtani H, Yonekura Y, et al. Significance of fill-in after thallium-201 reinjection following delayed imaging: comparison with regional wall motion and angiographic findings. J Nucl Med 1990;31:1617-23.
15. Ohtani H, Tamaki N, Yonekura Y, et al. Value of thallium-201 reinjection after delayed SPECT imaging for predicting reversible ischemia after coronary artery bypass grafting. Am J Cardiol 1990;66:394-9.
16. Bonow RO, Dilsizian V, Cuocolo A, Bacharach SL. Identification of viable myocardium in patients with chronic coronary artery disease and left ventricular dysfunction. Comparison of thallium scintigraphy with reinjection and PET imaging with 18F-fluorodeoxyglucose. Circulation 1991;83:26-37.
17. Dilsizian V, Freedman NM, Bacharach SL, Perrone-Filardi P, Bonow RO. Regional thallium uptake in irreversible defects. Magnitude of change in thallium activity after reinjection distinguishes viable from nonviable myocardium. Circulation 1992;85:627-34.

18. Dilsizian V, Perrone-Filardi P, Arrighi JA, et al. Concordance and discordance between stress-redistribution-reinjection and rest-redistribution thallium imaging for assessing viable myocardium. Comparison with metabolic activity by positron emission tomography. Circulation 1993;88:941-52.
19. Galassi AR, Centamore G, Fiscella A, et al. Comparison of rest-redistribution thallium-201 imaging and reinjection after stress-redistribution for the assessment of myocardial viability in patients with left ventricular dysfunction secondary to coronary artery disease. Am J Cardiol 1995;75:436-42.
20. Berman DS, Kiat H, Van Train K, Garcia E, Friedman J, Maddahi I. Technetium 99m sestamibi in the assessment of chronic coronary artery disease. Semin Nucl Med 1991;21:190-212.
21. Beanlands RS, Dawood F, Wen WH, et al. Are the kinetics of technetium-99m methoxyisobutyl isonitrile affected by cell metabolism and viability? Circulation 1990;82:1802-14.
22. Piwnica-Worms D, Kronauge JF, Chiu ML. Uptake and retention of hexakis (2-methoxyisobutyl isonitrile) technetium(I) in cultured chick myocardial cells. Mitochondrial and plasma membrane potential dependence. Circulation 1990;82:1826-38.
23. Freeman I, Grunwald AM, Hoory S, Bodenheimer MM. Effect of coronary occlusion and myocardial viability on myocardial activity of technetium-99m-sestamibi. J Nucl Med 1991;32:292-8.
24. Cuocolo A, Pace L, Ricciardelli B, chiariello M, Trimario B, Salvatore M. Identification of viable myocardium in patients with chronic coronary artery disease: comparison of thallium-201 scintigraphy with reinjection and technetium-99m-methoxyisobutyl isonitrile. J Nucl Med 1992;33:505-11.
25. Dilsizian V, Arrighi JA, Diodati JG, et al. Myocardial viability in patients with chronic coronary artery disease. Comparison of 99mTc-sestamibi with thallium reinjection and [18F]fluorodeoxyglucose [published erratum appears in Circulation 1995;91:3026]. Circulation 1994;89:578-87.
26. Marzullo P, Parodi O, Reisenhofer B, et al. Value of rest thallium-201/technetium-99m sestamibi scans and dobutamine echocardiography for detecting myocardial viability. Am J Cardiol 1993;71:166-72.
27. Udelson JE, Coleman PS, Metherall J, et al. Predicting recovery of severe regional ventricular dysfunction. Comparison of resting scintigraphy with 201Tl and 99mTc-sestamibi. Circulation 1994;89:2552-61.
28. Dondi M, Tartagni F, Fallani F, et al. A comparison of rest sestamibi and rest-redistribution thallium single photon emission tomography: possible implications for myocardial viability detection in infarcted patients. Eur J Nucl Med 1993;20:26-31.
29. Maurea S, Cuocolo A, Pace L, et al. Rest-injected thallium-201 redistribution and resting technetium-99m methoxyisobutylisonitrile uptake in coronary artery disease: relation to the severity of coronary artery stenosis. Eur J Nucl Med 1993;20:502-10.
30. Cuocolo A, Maurea S, Pace L, et al. Resting technetium-99m methoxyisobutylisonitrile cardiac imaging in chronic coronary artery disease: comparison with rest-redistribution thallium-201 scintigraphy. Eur J Nucl Med 1993;20:1186-92.

31. Rossetti C, Landoni C, Lucignani G, et al. Assessment of myocardial perfusion and viability with technetium-99m methoxyisobutylisonitrile and thallium-201 rest redistribution in chronic coronary artery disease. Eur J Nucl Med 1995;22:1306-12.
32. Kauffman GJ, Boyne TS, Watson DD, Smith WH, Beller GA. Comparison of rest thallium-201 imaging and rest technetium-99m sestamibi imaging for assessment of myocardial viability in patients with coronary artery disease and severe left ventricular dysfunction. J Am Coll Cardiol 1996;27:1592-7.
33. Maes AF, Borgers M, Flameng W, et al. Assessment of myocardial viability in chronic coronary artery disease using technetium-99m sestamibi SPECT. Correlation with histologic and positron emission tomographic studies and functional follow-up. J Am Coll Cardiol 1997;29:62-8.
34. Altehoefer C, Kaiser HJ, Dorr R, et al. Fluorine-18 deoxyglucose PET for assessment of viable myocardium in perfusion defects in 99mTc-MIBI SPET: a comparative study in patients with coronary artery disease. Eur J Nucl Med 1992;19:334-42.
35. Altehoefer C, vom Dahl J, Biedermann M, et al. Significance of defect severity in technetium-99m-MIBI SPECT at rest to assess myocardial viability: comparison with fluorine-18-FDG PET. J Nucl Med 1994;35:569-74.
36. Sawada SG, Allman KC, Muzik O, et al. Positron emission tomography detects evidence of viability in rest technetium-99m sestamibi defects. J Am Coll Cardiol 1994;23:92-8.
37. Soufer R, Dey HM, Ng CK, Zaret BL. Comparison of sestamibi single-photon emission computed tomography with positron emission tomography for estimating left ventricular myocardial viability. Am J Cardiol 1995;75:1214-9.
38. Lucignani G, Landoni C, Mengozzi G, et al. Relation between dobutamine trans-thoracic echocardiography, 99Tcm-MIBI and 18FDG uptake in chronic coronary artery disease. Nucl Med Commun 1995;16:548-57.
39. Cigarroa CG, deFilippi CR, Brickner ME, Alvarez LG, Wait MA, Grayburn PA. Dobutamine stress echocardiography identifies hibernating myocardium and predicts recovery of left ventricular function after coronary revascularization. Circulation 1993;88:430-6.
40. Gerber BL, Vanoverschelde JL, Bol A, et al. Myocardial blood flow, glucose uptake, and recruitment of inotropic reserve in chronic left ventricular ischemic dysfunction. Implications for the pathophysiology of chronic myocardial hibernation. Circulation 1996;94:651-9.
41. Baer FM, Voth E, Deutsch HJ, et al. Predictive value of low dose dobutamine transesophageal echocardiography and fluorine-18 fluorodeoxyglucose positron emission tomography for recovery of regional left ventricular function after successful revascularization. J Am Coll Cardiol 1996;28:60-9.
42. Baer FM, Voth E, Deutsch HJ, Schneider CA, Schicha H, Sechtem U. Assessment of viable myocardium by dobutamine transesophageal echocardiography and comparison with fluorine-18 fluorodeoxyglucose positron emission tomography. J Am Coll Cardiol 1994;24:343-53.
43. Bax JJ, Cornel JH, Visser FC, et al. Prediction of recovery of myocardial dysfunction after revascularization. Comparison of fluorine-18 fluorodeoxyglucose/thallium-201 SPECT, thallium-201 stress-reinjection SPECT and dobutamine echocardiography. J Am Coll Cardiol 1996;28:558-64.

44. Arnese M, Cornel JH, Salustri A, et al. Prediction of improvement of regional left ventricular function after surgical revascularization. A comparison of low-dose dobutamine echocardiography with 201Tl single-photon emission computed tomography. Circulation 1995;91:2748-52.
45. Haque T, Furukawa T, Takahashi M, Kinoshita M. Identification of hibernating myocardium by dobutamine stress echocardiography: comparison with thallium-201 reinjection imaging. Am Heart J 1995;130:553-63.
46. Vanoverschelde JL, D'Hondt AM, Marwick T, et al. Head-to-head comparison of exercise-redistribution-reinjection thallium single-photon emission computed tomography and low dose dobutamine echocardiography for prediction of reversibility of chronic left ventricular ischemic dysfunction. J Am Coll Cardiol 1996;28:432-42.
47. Panza JA, Dilsizian V, Laurienzo JM, Curiel RV, Kafsiyiannis PT. Relation between thallium uptake and contractile response to dobutamine. Implications regarding myocardial viability in patients with chronic coronary artery disease and left ventricular dysfunction. Circulation 1995;91:990-8.
48. Vanoverschelde JL, Gerber BL, D'Hondt AM, et al. Preoperative selection of patients with severely impaired left ventricular function for coronary revascularization. Role of low-dose dobutamine echocardiography and exercise-redistribution-reinjection thallium SPECT. Circulation 1995;92 (9 Suppl):II37-44.
49. Alfieri O, La Canna G, Giubbini R, Pardini A, Zogno M, Fucci C. Recovery of myocardial function. The ultimate target of coronary revascularization. Eur J Cardiothorac Surg 1993;7:325-30.
50. Charney R, Schwinger ME, Chun J, et al. Dobutamine echocardiography and resting-redistribution thallium-201 scintigraphy predicts recovery of hibernating myocardium after coronary revascularization. Am Heart J 1994;128:864-9.
51. Perrone-Filardi P, Pace L, Prastaro M, et al. Assessment of myocardial viability in patients with chronic coronary artery disease. Rest-4-hour-24-hour 201Tl tomography versus dobutamine echocardiography. Circulation 1996;94:2712-9.
52. Qureshi U, Nagueh SF, Afridi I, et al. Dobutamine echocardiography and quantitative rest-redistribution 201Tl tomography in myocardial hibernation. Relation of contractile reserve to 201Tl uptake and comparative prediction of recovery of function. Circulation 1997;95:626-35.
53. Alderman EL, Fisher LD, Litwin P, et al. Results of coronary artery surgery in patients with poor left ventricular function (CASS). Circulation 1983;68:785-95.
54. Pigott JD, Kouchoukos NT, Oberman A, Cutter GR. Late results of surgical and medical therapy for patients with coronary artery disease and depressed left ventricular function. J Am Coll Cardiol 1985;5:1036-45.
55. Mickleborough LL, Maruyama H, Takagi Y, Mohamed S, Sun Z, Ebisuzzaki L. Results of revascularization in patients with severe left ventricular dysfunction. Circulation 1995;92 (9 Suppl):II73-9.
56. Tillisch J, Brunken R, Marshall R, et al. Reversibility of cardiac wall-motion abnormalities predicted by positron tomography. N Engl J Med 1986;314:884-8.
57. Vom Dahl J, Eitzman DT, al-Aouar ZR, et al. Relation of regional function, perfusion, and metabolism in patients with advanced coronary artery disease undergoing surgical revascularization. Circulation 1994;90:2356-66.
58. Maes A, Flameng W, Borgers M, et al. Regional myocardial blood flow, glucose utilization and contractile function before and after revascularization and ultrastructural findings in patients with chronic coronary artery disease. Eur J Nucl Med 1995;22:1299-305.

59. Iskandrian AS, Hakki AH, Kane SA, et al. Rest and redistribution thallium-201 myocardial scintigraphy to predict improvement in left ventricular function after coronary arterial bypass grafting. Am J Cardiol 1983;51:1312-6.
60. Mori T, Minamiji K, Kurogane H, Ogawa K, Yoshida Y. Rest-injected thallium-201 imaging for assessing viability of severe asynergic regions. J Nucl Med 1991;32:1718-24.
61. Ragosta M, Beller GA, Watson DD, Kaul S, Gimple LW. Quantitative planar rest-redistribution 201Tl imaging in detection of myocardial viability and prediction of improvement in left ventricular function after coronary bypass surgery in patients with severely depressed left ventricular function. Circulation 1993;87:1630-41.
62. Meluzin J, Cigarroa CG, Brickner ME, et al. Dobutamine echocardiography in predicting improvement in global left ventricular systolic function after coronary bypass or angioplasty in patients with healed myocardial infarcts. Am J Cardiol 1995;76:877-80.
63. Perrone-Filardi P, Pace L, Prastaro M, et al. Dobutamine echocardiography predicts improvement of hypoperfused dysfunctional myocardium after revascularization in patients with coronary artery disease. Circulation 1995;91:2556-65.
64. Marwick TH, Nemec JJ, Lafont A, Salcedo EE, MacIntyre WJ. Prediction by postexercise fluoro-18 deoxyglucose positron emission tomography of improvement in exercise capacity after revascularization. Am J Cardiol 1992;69:854-9.
65. Di Carli MF, Asgarzadie F, Schelbert HR, et al. Quantitative relation between myocardial viability and improvement in heart failure symptoms after revascularization in patients with ischemic cardiomyopathy. Circulation 1995;92:3436-44.
66. Haas F, Haehnel C, Duvernoy C, et al. Improved mid-term survival and functional status after CABG in patients with congestive heart failure selected for revascularization based on viability assessment [abstract]. J Nucl Cardiol 1997;4:S43
67. Tamaki N, Kawamoto M, Takahashi N, et al. Prognostic value of an increase in fluorine-18 deoxyglucose uptake in patients with myocardial infarction: comparison with stress thallium imaging. J Am Coll Cardiol 1993;22:1621-7.
68. Eitzman D, al-Aouar Z, Kanter HL, et al. Clinical outcome of patients with advanced coronary artery disease after viability studies with positron emission tomography. J Am Coll Cardiol 1992;20:559-65.
69. Di Carli MF, Davidson M, Little R, et al. Value of metabolic imaging with positron emission tomography for evaluating prognosis in patients with coronary artery disease and left ventricular dysfunction. Am J Cardiol 1994;73:527-33.
70. Lee KS, Marwick TH, Cook SA, et al. Prognosis of patients with left ventricular dysfunction, with and without viable myocardium after myocardial infarction. Relative efficacy of medical therapy and revascularization. Circulation 1994;90:2687-94.
71. Gioia G, Milan E, Giubbini R, De Pace N, Heo J, Iskandrian AS. Prognostic value of tomographic rest-redistribution thallium 201 imaging in medically treated patients with coronary artery disease and left ventricular dysfunction. J Nucl Cardiol 1996;3:150-6.

72. Schwaiger M, Brunken R, Grover-McKay M, et al. Regional myocardial metabolism in patients with acute myocardial infarction assessed by positron emission tomography. J Am Coll Cardiol 1986;8:800-8.
73. Huitink JM, Visser FC, Bax JJ, Van Lingen A, Visser CA. Course of impaired left ventricular function after acute myocardial infarction predicted with planar thallium-201 chloride and F18-fluorodeoxyglucose imaging. Int J Cardiol 1996;57:271-81.
74. Pierard LA, De Landsheere CM, Berthe C, Rigo P, Kulberhus HE. Identification of viable myocardium by echocardiography during dobutamine infusion in patients with myocardial infarction after thrombolytic therapy: comparison with positron emission tomography. J Am Coll Cardiol 1990;15:1021-31.
75. Barilla F, Gheorghiade M, Alam M, Khaja F, Goldstein S. Low-dose dobutamine in patients with acute myocardial infarction identifies viable but not contractile myocardium and predicts the magnitude of improvement in wall motion abnormalities in response to coronary revascularization. Am Heart J 1991;122:1522-31.
76. Smart SC, Sawada S, Ryan T, et al. Low-dose dobutamine echocardiography detects reversible dysfunction after thrombolytic therapy of acute myocardial infarction. Circulation 1993;88:405-15.
76. Previtali M, Poli A, Lanzarini L, Fetiveau R, Mussini A, Ferrario M. Dobutamine stress echocardiography for assessment of myocardial viability and ischemia in acute myocardial infarction treated with thrombolysis. Am J Cardiol 1993;72:124G-130G.
78. Watada H, Ito H, Oh H, et al. Dobutamine stress echocardiography predicts reversible dysfunction and quantitates the extent of irreversibly damaged myocardium after reperfusion of anterior myocardial infarction. J Am Coll Cardiol 1994;24:624-30.
79. Yoshida K, Gould KL. Quantitative relation of myocardial infarct size and myocardial viability by positron emission tomography to left ventricular ejection fraction and 3-year mortality with and without revascularization. J Am Coll Cardiol 1993;22:984-97.
80. Carlos ME, Smart SC, Wynsen JC, Sagar KB. Dobutamine stress echocardiography for risk stratification after myocardial infarction. Circulation 1997;95:1402-10.
81. Brown KA, Weiss RM, Clements JP, Wackers FJ. Usefulness of residual ischemic myocardium within prior infarct zone for identifying patients at high risk late after acute myocardial infarction. Am J Cardiol 1987;60:15-9.
82. Basu S, Senior R, Raval U, Lahiri A. Superiority of nitrate-enhanced ^{201}Tl over conventional redistribution ^{201}Tl imaging for prognostic evaluation after myocardial infarction and thrombolysis. Circulation 1997;96:2932-7.
83. Huitink JM, Visser FC, Bax JJ, et al. Predictive value of planar 18F-fluorodeoxyglucose imaging for cardiac events in patients after acute myocardial infarction: a 4 year follow-up study. Am J Cardiol. In press 1998.
84. Nijland F, Kamp O, Verhorst PM, De Voot WG, Carcagni A, Visser CA. Prognostic implications of low dose dobutamine echocardiography early after myocardial infarction [abstract]. Circulation 1996;94 (8 Suppl):I679.
85. Bax JJ, Wijns W, Cornel JH, Visser FC, Boersma E, Fioretti PM. Accuracy of currently available techniques for prediction of functional recovery after revascularization in patients with left ventricular dysfunction due to chronic coronary artery disease: comparison of pooled data. J Am Coll Cardiol 1997;30:1451-60.

86. Marwick TH, MacIntyre WJ, Lafont A, Nemec JJ, Salcedo JJ. Metabolic responses of hibernating and infarcted myocardium to revascularization. A follow-up study of regional perfusion, function, and metabolism. Circulation 1992;85:1347-53.
87. Tamaki N, Yonekura Y, Yamashita K, et al. Positron emission tomography using fluorine-18 deoxyglucose in evaluation of coronary artery bypass grafting. Am J Cardiol 1989;64:860-5.
88. Gropler RJ, Geltman EM, Sampathkumaran K, et al. Comparison of carbon-11-acetate with fluorine-18-fluorodeoxyglucose for delineating viable myocardium by positron emission tomography. J Am Coll Cardiol 1993;22:1587-97.
89. Tamaki N, Kawamoto M, Tadamura E, et al. Prediction of reversible ischemia after revascularization. Perfusion and metabolic studies with positron emission tomography. Circulation 1995;91:1697-705.
90. Knuuti MJ, Saraste M, Nuutila P, et al. Myocardial viability: fluorine-18-deoxyglucose positron emission tomography in prediction of wall motion recovery after revascularization. Am Heart J 1994;127:785-96.
91. Lucignani G, Paolini G, Landoni C, et al. Presurgical identification of hibernating myocardium by combined use of technetium-99m hexakis 2-methoxyisobutylisonitrile single photon emission tomography and fluorine-18 fluoro-2-deoxy-D-glucose positron emission tomography in patients with coronary artery disease. Eur J Nucl Med 1992;19:874-81.
92. Carrel T, Jenni R, Haubold-Reuter S, Von Schulthess G, Pasic M, Turina M. Improvement of severely reduced left ventricular function after surgical revascularization in patients with preoperative myocardial infarction. Eur J Cardiothorac Surg 1992;6:479-84.
93. Tamaki N, Ohtani H, Yamashita K, et al. Metabolic activity in the areas of new fill-in after thallium-201 reinjection: comparison with positron emission tomography using fluorine-18-deoxyglucose. J Nucl Med 1991;32:673-8.
94. Marzullo P, Sambuceti G, Parodi O, et al. Regional concordance and discordance between rest thallium 201 and sestamibi imaging for assessing tissue viability: comparison with postrevascularization functional recovery. J Nucl Cardiol 1995;309-16.
95. Gonzalez P, Massardo T, Munoz A, et al. Is the addition of ECG gating to technetium-99m sestamibi SPET of value in the assessment of myocardial viability? An evaluation based on two-dimensional echocardiography following revascularization. Eur J Nucl Med 1996;23:1315-22.
96. Marzullo P, Sambuceti G, Parodi O. The role of sestamibi scintigraphy in the radioisotopic assessment of myocardial viability. J Nucl Med 1992;33:1925-30.
97. Maublant JC, Citron B, Lipiecki J, et al. Rest technetium 99m-sestamibi tomoscintigraphy in hibernating myocardium. Am Heart J 1995;129:306-14.
98. Maurea S, Cuocolo A, Soricelli A, et al. Enhanced detection of viable myocardium by technetium-99m-MIBI imaging after nitrate administration in chronic coronary artery disease. J Nucl Med 1995;36:1945-52.
99. Bisi G, Sciagra R, Santoro GM, Fazzini PF. Rest technetium-99m sestamibi tomography in combination with short-term administration of nitrates: feasibility and reliability for prediction of postrevascularization outcome of asynergic territories. J Am Coll Cardiol 1994;24:1282-9.

100. Bisi G, Sciagra R, Santoro GM, Rossi V, Fazzini PF. Technetium-99m-sestamibi imaging with nitrate infusion to detect viable hibernating myocardium and predict postrevascularization recovery. J Nucl Med 1995;36:1994-2000.
101. Afridi I, Kleiman NS, Raizner AE, Zoghbi WA. Dobutamine echocardiography in myocardial hibernation. Optimal dose and accuracy in predicting recovery of ventricular function after coronary angioplasty. Circulation 1995;91:663-70.
102. Senior R, Glenville B, Basu S, et al. Dobutamine echocardiography and thallium-201 imaging predict functional improvement after revascularisation in severe ischaemic left ventricular dysfunction. Br Heart J 1995;74:358-64.
103. La Canna G, Alfieri O, Giubbini R, Gargano M, Ferrari R, Visioli O. Echocardiography during infusion of dobutamine for identification of reversibly dysfunction in patients with chronic coronary artery disease. J Am Coll Cardiol 1994;23:617-26.
104. DeFilippi CR, Willett DL, Irani WN, Eichhorn EJ. Velasio CE, Grayburn PA. Comparison of myocardial contrast echocardiography and low-dose dobutamine stress echocardiography in predicting recovery of left ventricular function after coronary revascularization in chronic ischemic heart disease. Circulation 1995;92:2863-8.
105. Bax JJ, Cornel JH, Visser FC, Fioretti PM, Elhendy A, Visser CA. Thaliium-201 rest-redistribution SPECT to predict improvement of global ventricular function after revascularization [abstract]. J Am Coll Cardiol 1997;29 (Suppl A):377A.
106. Kaul S. There may be more to myocardial viability than meets the eye. Circulation 1995;92:2790-3.
107. Vanoverschelde JL, Melin JA, Depré C, Borgers M, Dion R, Wijns W. Time-course of functional recovery of hibernating myocardium after coronary revascularization [abstract]. Circulation 1994;90:(4 pt 2):I378.
108. Gerber B, Vanoverschelde JL, Robert A, et al. Dobutamine echocardiography, 201-Thallium SPECT and positron emission tomography. Which test for the prediction of myocardial viability [abstract]. Circulation 1994;90 (4 pt 2):I134.

Chapter 11

PATHOPHYSIOLOGY OF ACUTE OR SHORT-TERM HIBERNATION

Tom J.C. Ruigrok, Xavier A. van Binsbergen and Cees J.A. van Echteld

Introduction

Myocardial hibernation refers to a clinical state of chronic regional contractile dysfunction characterized by a reduced regional myocardial blood flow, either persistently at rest [1,2] or repetitively during stress [3], that can be partially or completely restored to normal upon coronary revascularization. In hibernation, the observed reduction in function reflects preservation of viability rather than the occurrence of necrosis. Stress echocardiography using low-dose dobutamine infusion is at present the preferred initial approach for the selection of patients with hibernating or viable myocardium who would benefit from coronary revascularization [4]. Additional techniques to assess viability include fluorine-18(^{18F}) fluorodeoxyglucose positron emission tomography (FDG-PET), technetium-99m (^{99m}Tc) sestamibi single photon emission tomography (SPECT), or thallium-201 (^{201}Tl) rest-redistribution SPECT imaging. Although the concept of chronic adaptive reduction of contractile function in response to reduction in myocardial blood flow is straightforward and simple, the mechanisms responsible for the development and maintenance of hibernation are unclear at present. This is mainly due to a large distance between the available experimental models of (acute or short-term) hibernation and the clinical scenario of (chronic or long-term) hibernation. In this chapter an experimental model of short-term hibernation will be discussed that is based on the observation that the majority of patients with hibernating myocardium

Van der Wall et al. (eds.),
Advanced Imaging in Coronary Artery Disease, 185-198.

has a history of an acute ischemic insult (either in the form of a transmural myocardial infarction or prolonged ischemic pain) followed by hypoperfusion[5].

Perfusion-Contraction Matching

When the concept of hibernation was proposed, it was assumed that the observed contractile dysfunction that was restored upon revascularization must have reflected a situation of a reduced resting blood flow [1,2]. On the basis of experimental studies in which a proportionate reduction in regional myocardial blood flow and contractile function was demonstrated in response to graded reductions in coronary flow in dog hearts with maintained viability, the concept of perfusion-contraction matching was introduced and was assumed to be the basis of myocardial hibernation [6]. Subsequently, it was demonstrated that during an ongoing period of flow-reduction, aerobic myocardial metabolism recovered, pointing to the regulatory nature of perfusion-contraction matching [7-9]. It should be noted that the experimental studies demonstrating perfusion-contraction matching have thus far limited observation periods. It was therefore proposed to make a distinction between short-term hibernation, as observed in the experimental setting, and long-term hibernation, as seen in the clinical setting [6]. The existence of perfusion-contraction matching in long-term hibernation is, as yet, unproven.

Only a few experimental studies have been performed to investigate the transition from short-term hibernation to long-term hibernation. When resting regional myocardial blood flow was measured in these studies on chronically instrumented dogs and pigs, it was found to be either reduced, normal, or almost normal. However, with normal or almost normal resting blood flow, coronary reserve was consistently impaired [10-14]. The reduction of contractile function under these conditions of normal resting flow is most likely due to repetitive stunning as a consequence of repetitive periods of stress- or exercise-induced ischemia and reperfusion. It is generally agreed at present that blood flow must be reduced, either persistently at rest or repetitively during stress, for hibernation to develop.

A Possible Trigger for Hibernation

One of the questions and controversies in the field of hibernation that were recently identified [15] was: How does hibernation develop, and is a 'trigger' required? Possible factors determining the development of hibernation originate from experimental studies on short-term hibernation. These findings, however, may be relevant to the clinical situation because it is reasonable to assume that short-term hibernation, established by some means or other, is the precursor of long-term hibernation. One of the features emerging from a number of studies on short-term hibernation is the possibility that some trigger may be necessary to predispose a heart to hibernate during a sustained period of flow reduction.

In 1993, Ferrari et al. introduced an experimental protocol that was based on the observation that the majority of patients with hibernating myocardium has a history of an acute ischemic insult followed by hypoperfusion [5]. Short-term hibernation was induced by making isolated rabbit hearts totally ischemic for 10 minutes before the hearts were hypoperfused (10% of the pre-ischemic flow) for 4 hours. During total ischemia interstitial pH (measured by means of a needle electrode) decreased by 0.8 units, developed pressure decreased to zero and tissue phosphocreatine (PCr) and adenosine tri-phosphatase (ATP) decreased to 4% and 50%, respectively. Subsequent hypoperfusion resulted in an increase of PCr and ATP to 50% and 94% of pre-ischemic values; the hearts, however, remained akinetic and interstitial pH only increased by 0.3 units. Reperfusion caused normalization of interstitial pH, 86% recovery of developed pressure and no further changes in PCr and ATP. The authors concluded that a decrease of tissue pH may be involved in the down-regulation of mechanical function during short-term hibernation.

Data from an in situ pig heart model

The results obtained by Ferrari et al. [5] in isolated rabbit hearts, suggesting that an initial stimulus of no-flow ischemia is required to permit the development of short-term hibernation during sustained low-flow ischemia, prompted Schulz et al. to use a similar protocol in the in situ pig heart [16].

By blocking ATP-dependent potassium channels, these authors attempted to determine whether the increased tolerance to sustained low-flow ischemia by a preceding short period of no-flow ischemia is related to ischemic preconditioning or hibernation. In previous studies they had demonstrated that blockade of ATP-dependent potassium channels abolishes the protective effect achieved by preconditioning[17] but not that achieved by short-term hibernation [18]. Ischemic preconditioning refers to the reduction of infarct size resulting from sustained myocardial ischemia by one or more preceding short periods of ischemia and reperfusion [19].

In the anesthetized pigs, the left anterior descending coronary artery was cannulated and the anterior myocardial wall was hypoperfused for 90 minutes (group 1), or was made totally ischemic for 10 minutes and was subsequently hypoperfused for 80 minutes (group 2). In a third group of experiments, the ATP-dependent potassium channel blocker glibenclamide was administered before the 10-minute period of no-flow ischemia. Infarct size was determined in all groups after 120 minutes of reperfusion. Infarct size in group 2 was significantly smaller (6.8±6.0%) than in group 1 (13.2±9.8%) and group 3 (16.7±8.3%).

It was concluded that a brief period of no-flow ischemia without intermittent reperfusion increases the tolerance to sustained low-flow ischemia, and that this protective effect is mediated by activation of ATP-dependent potassium channels and as a consequence relates to preconditioning rather than to hibernation [16].

Data from an isolated rabbit heart model

In an extensive study on isolated rabbit hearts [20], Ferrari et al. elaborated their initial observation [5]. In one group of hearts, 10 minutes of no-flow ischemia were immediately followed by 230 minutes of low-flow ischemia, and 60 minutes of reperfusion. No-flow ischemia caused quiescence, a fall in interstitial pH (from 7.2±0.01 to 6.1±0.8), PCr (from 54.5±5.0 to 5.0±1.1 µmol/g dry weight), and ATP (from 25.0±1.9 to 15.3±2.5 µmol/g dry weight). Subsequent low-flow ischemia failed to restore myocardial function, but pH increased to 6.8±0.6 and PCr to 20.1±3.4 µmol/g dry weight. There was only a minor increase in the rate of lactate release. Reperfusion resulted in restoration of pH, developed pressure (to 92.3%), and NAD/NADH, and caused a slight washout of lactate and creatine kinase, with no alterations in mitochondrial function or oxidative stress.

In a second group, 240 minutes of low-flow ischemia were followed by 60 minutes of reperfusion. During low-flow ischemia, interstitial pH fell more slowly and to a lesser extent than in the first group. pH was 6.8±0.6 after 10 minutes and gradually fell to 6.2±0.7 after 240 minutes. Diastolic pressure increased to 34±5.6 mmHg, PCr and ATP became depressed, and oxidative stress occurred. Lactate release increased throughout low-flow ischemia, and was exacerbated by reperfusion. Reperfusion partially restored myocardial metabolism and function (47%).

It was concluded that a brief period of no-flow ischemia is important to maintain myocardial viability during a sustained period of low-flow ischemia. This protective effect may be the result of a resetting of metabolism with down-regulation of both energy need and production, or of preconditioning, or both. The authors suggested that similar sequences of coronary flow restriction may occur during development of hibernation [20].

Data from an isolated rat heart model

To examine in more detail the conclusion by Ferrari et al.[5] that a decrease of tissue pH during an initial period of no-flow ischemia may be involved in the down-regulation of mechanical function during short-term hibernation, ^{31}P NMR spectroscopy was used to follow the time course of high-energy phosphates and intracellular pH (calculated from the chemical shift of the intracellular inorganic phosphate peak relative to the PCr peak) in isolated rat hearts during no-flow ischemia, low-flow ischemia and reperfusion[21].

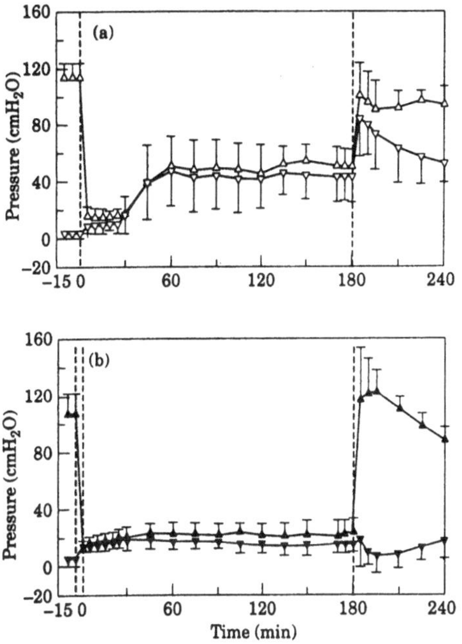

Figure 1. *Left ventricular pressure of isolated rat hearts, measured by means of a fluid-filled latex balloon, which was inserted through the mitral valve into the left ventricle and connected to a Statham P23dB pressure transducer. <1> and <2>: peak systolic pressure; <3> and <4>: end-diastolic pressure. Perfusion sequences: control group (a), 15 minutes of control perfusion (-15 to 0 minutes), 180 minutes of low-flow ischemia (0 to 180 minutes), 60 minutes of reperfusion (180 to 240 minutes); short-term hibernation group (**b**), 10 minutes of control perfusion (-15 to -5 minutes), 5 minutes of no-flow ischemia (-5 to 0 minutes), 180 minutes of low-flow ischemia (0 to 180 minutes), 60 minutes of reperfusion (180 to 240 minutes). Means ± S.D.; n=6 per group. Reproduced with permission from reference 21.*

Control hearts were subjected to 180 minutes of low-flow ischemia (10% of the pre-ischemic flow) and 60 minutes of reperfusion (group a). In the short-term hibernation group, low-flow was preceded by 5 minutes of no-flow ischemia (group b). In group (a), contracture developed during low-flow (figure 1). The time to onset of contracture was 51 minutes (range: 28 to 123 minutes). In group (b), contracture did not occur during low-flow ischemia; recovery of left ventricular developed pressure (i.e. the difference between peak systolic and end-diastolic pressure) and end-diastolic pressure were significantly better during the first 15 minutes of reperfusion.

In group (a), intracellular pH (pH_i) decreased from 7.06±0.04 to 6.64±0.14 during the first 30 minutes of low-flow. Between 5 and 10 minutes after the onset of contracture, splitting of the intracellular inorganic phosphate (P_i) peak was observed [figure 2(a), peak 2].

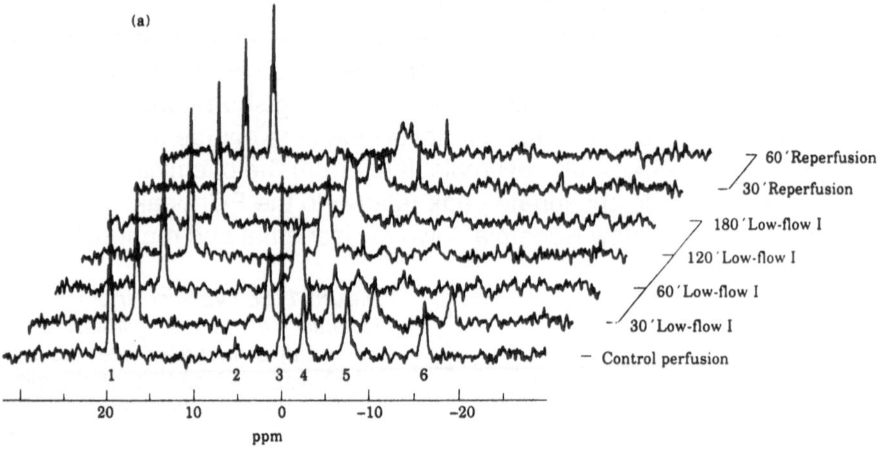

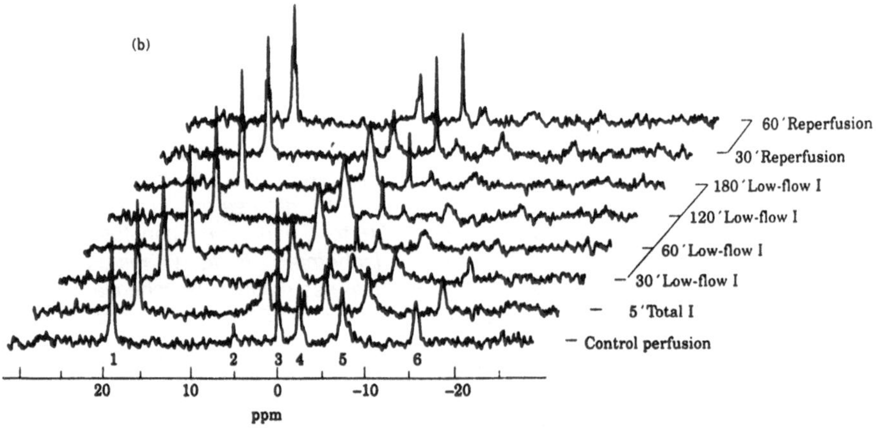

Figure 2. (a) *^{31}P NMR spectra of an isolated rat heart of group (a) during control perfusion, after 30, 60, 120 and 180 minutes of low-flow ischemia, and after 30 and 60 minutes of reperfusion. Numbered peaks are as follows: 1, methylene diphosphonate (external reference); 2, inorganic phosphate (P_i); 3, phosphocreatine (PCr); 4, 5 and 6, γ-, α- and β-phosphate group of ATP, respectively.* ***(b)*** *^{31}P NMR spectra of an isolated rat heart of group (b) during control perfusion, after 5 minutes of no-flow ischemia, after 30, 60, 120 and 180 minutes of low-flow ischemia, and after 30 and 60 minutes of reperfusion. See legend to figure 2(a) for peak identification. ^{31}P NMR spectra were acquired at 81.0 MHz on a Bruker MSL 200 spectrometer equipped with a 4.7 Tesla vertical 150 mm bore magnet. For each spectrum 128 free induction decays were accumulated, following 90° pulses at a repetition time of 2.34 seconds. The peak of β-ATP was used for the quantification of ATP. Intracellular pH (pH_i) values were calculated from the chemical shift of the intracellular inorganic phosphate (P_i) peak relative to the PCr peak. Zero ppm was assigned to Pcr. Reproduced with permission from reference 21.*

These multiple P_i peaks most likely represent myocardial areas with different pH_i values. From this point of time two pH_i values are given, corresponding with the highest and lowest chemical shift values of the P_i peaks present. The lower and higher pH_i values amounted to 6.33±0.15 and 6.86±0.05, respectively, at the end of low-flow ischemia [figure 3(a)]. During reperfusion a split P_i peak remained visible. In group (b), pH_i decreased from 7.08±0.03 to 6.55±0.03 during the 5-minute period of no-flow ischemia. When hypoperfusion was initiated, pH_i quickly increased to 6.73±0.05 and remained constant until the end of low-flow ischemia. No splitting of the P_i peak was observed [figure 2(b), peak 2]. During reperfusion pH_i recovered to 7.06±0.03 within 10 minutes.

In group (a) and (b), PCr levels at the end of low-flow ischemia amounted to 13±8% and 26±6% of pre-ischemic levels, respectively. During reperfusion, PCr recovery was better in group b: 67±12% vs 23±11%. In group (a) and (b), ATP levels at the end of low-flow ischemia were 5±10% and 19±9%, respectively. During reperfusion no significant changes in ATP were observed (figure 2).

At present little information is available about the mechanisms by which an initial short period of severe ischemia can trigger the development of a state with preserved viability during a subsequent period of sustained hypoperfusion. At first sight, the decrease of pH_i from 7.08 to 6.55 during the 5-minute period of no-flow ischemia [figure 3(a)] does not seem to be dramatic. It should be noted, however, that the actual pH_i at the end of no-flow ischemia may have been well below 6.55, since pH_i values were average values of 5-minute periods. Although a rapid decrease in pH_i will initiate a rapid decrease in contractile function and will decrease the imbalance between energy supply and energy demand, the role of a low pH_i in triggering the development of short-term hibernation is unclear at present.

Recently, it has been reported that short-term hibernation in isolated rat hearts (8 minutes of no-flow ischemia, followed by 292 minutes of low-flow ischemia) was linked to an increase of heat shock protein 72 (hsp72), while low-flow ischemia alone failed to induce hsp72 [22]. It has been shown that hsp72 is involved in the "second window" (after 24 hours) of preconditioning-mediated myocardial protection [23]. Finally, it has been reported that a short period of no-flow ischemia in isolated rat hearts induces a translocation of the glucose transporter GLUT-4 from intracellular locations to the plasma membrane, associated with an increased myocardial glucose uptake [24]. The possible relevance of this observation to short-term hibernation will be discussed in the next section.

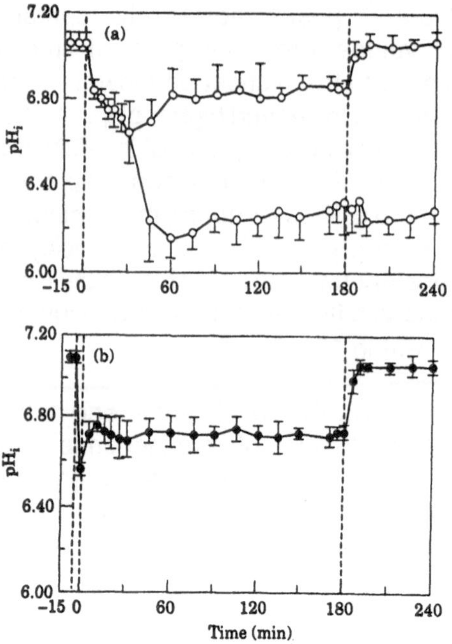

Figure 3. *Intracellular pH (pH_i) of isolated rat hearts, calculated from the chemical shift of the intracellular inorganic phosphate (P_i) peak, relative to the PCr peak of ^{31}P NMR spectra. Perfusion sequences: see legend to figure 1. In group* ***(a)*** *splitting of the P_i peak occurred after approximately 30 minutes of low-flow ischemia. From this point of time two pH_i values are given, corresponding with the highest and lowest chemical shift values of the P_i peaks present. Reproduced with permission from ref. 21.*

Glucose uptake and glycolysis in hibernation

The main conclusion from the in situ pig heart study by Schulz et al. [16] was that the beneficial effect on infarct size of an episode of no-flow ischemia prior to low-flow ischemia, was related to preconditioning rather than to hibernation because of the involvement of ATP-dependent potassium channels. Their experimental protocol cannot be considered a classic ischemic preconditioning protocol because the brief period of no-flow ischemia was not followed by full reperfusion but by low-flow ischemia. Ischemic preconditioning without intermittent reperfusion is a controversial issue. In anesthetized pigs, infarct size after 60 minutes of coronary artery occlusion was reduced by a preceding 30-minute period of partial coronary stenosis, enough to decrease coronary blood flow by 70%, when compared with pigs undergoing only 60 minutes of coronary artery occlusion [25]. Likewise, in isolated perfused rabbit hearts, 10 minutes of global hypoxia decreased infarct size after a subsequent 30-minute period of regional no-flow ischemia, demonstrating that intermittent reoxygenation is not required for ischemic preconditioning [26]. However, in anesthetized dogs, 15 minutes of partial coronary stenosis, sufficient to reduce coronary blood flow by 50%, did not reduce infarct size after subsequent total coronary artery occlusion for 60 minutes without intermittent reperfusion [27]. It was suggested that the reduction of coronary blood flow during the initial ischemic period in the latter study may have been insufficient to increase the resistance to lethal myocyte injury during the subsequent more prolonged period of ischemia [16].

The protocol Janier et al. [28] used was similar to our protocol [20,21] but was more closely related to ischemic preconditioning, as an episode of no-flow ischemia was followed by reperfusion before sustained low-flow ischemia was imposed. The protective effect of this intervention on the functional and metabolic status of the heart during low-flow ischemia and reperfusion was similar to that reported by us [20,21]. Furthermore, these authors reported an enhanced glucose uptake and an increased lactate production during low-flow ischemia [28]. They concluded that the cycle of total ischemia followed by reperfusion prior to sustained low-flow ischemia stimulated anaerobic glycolysis and thereby improved the functional and metabolic condition of the heart. By increasing glucose and insulin concentrations in the perfusate, Eberli et al. [29] showed a similar protection of the functional and metabolic state of the heart during sustained low-flow ischemia, as was observed by Janier et al. [28]. The change in perfusate composition resulted in enhanced glucose uptake with an increased glycolytic flux, a better preserved diastolic function during low-flow ischemia, and an increased recovery of developed pressure upon reperfusion. The data from the latter two studies suggest that an enhanced glucose uptake and increased anaerobic glycolysis are key factors in the protection of the myocardium during sustained low-flow ischemia.

Evidence has been provided that glycolysis plays a critical role in maintaining Ca^{2+} homeostasis and diastolic function [30-32]. It has been reported that glycolytically generated ATP may play an important role in cellular Ca^{2+} handling by driving the Ca^{2+} pump of the sarcoplasmic reticulum [33]. Furthermore, Cross et al. proposed that sustained glycolysis during low-flow ischemia provides the energy to maintain sufficient Na^+/K^+ ATPase activity to prevent a deleterious increase of intracellular Na^+ [34].

The observation that diastolic function was better preserved in the hearts of group (b) [figure 1(b)] strongly suggests that glycolytic flux was increased when low-flow ischemia was preceded by no-flow ischemia. The onset of ischemic contracture has been associated with a cessation of glycolytic flux[35]. Therefore, a critically reduced or halted glycolysis in certain areas of the heart may have caused contracture in the hearts of group (a) [figure 1(a)], resulting in a relative hypoperfusion in these areas and a further decrease of pH_i due to an attenuated lactate washout and continuing depletion of ATP [figure 3(a)].

Whether ischemic preconditioning leads to a higher (or longer) glycolytic activity during ischemia is a highly controversial issue. In most studies on preconditioning a decreased lactate accumulation was observed during ischemia [36,37]. However, as mentioned before, Janier et al. [28] measured an increased lactate release during low-flow ischemia in preconditioned rat hearts, and recently, a higher lactate accumulation during total ischemia was observed in preconditioned rat hearts than in hearts that were not preconditioned [38]. It has also been reported that in hypothermic rabbit hearts ischemic preconditioning has no effect on tissue lactate content [39]. Interestingly, Ferrari et al. [20] observed a lower lactate release during the last hour of low-flow ischemia in the hearts that had a preceding period of no-flow ischemia, compared with the hearts that were subjected to only low-flow ischemia. This observation would be in line with the finding that in short-term hibernation lactate production is attenuated [7,9] and myocardial PCr content recovers to near control values [8,9,40,41], pointing to recovery of aerobic metabolism. The relation between glucose uptake, as demonstrated with FDG PET, and glycogen accumulation [42-44] in chronically hibernating myocardium has recently been discussed by Borgers [45]. The author speculated that storage of glycogen may be the consequence of impaired catabolism of glycogen [46], an increase of glycogen synthase activity [47], or a translocation of the glucose transporter GLUT-4 to the plasma membrane and an associated increase of glucose uptake as mentioned in the previous section [24].

Conclusion

Much more investigation is needed on animal models of short-term hibernation. The results may be relevant to the clinical situation because it is reasonable to assume that short-term hibernation is the precursor of long-term hibernation. Long-term hibernation, however, will remain a controversial issue until animal models become available in which the various aspects of long-term hibernation can be reproduced. The question whether chronic dysfunction in patients reflects true long-term hibernation, or repetitive episodes of ischemia and reperfusion (repetitive stunning) remains unresolved at present. In the context of this chapter it is interesting to note that it has recently been reported [48] that in chronically instrumented pigs, repetitive stunning of the circumflex region resulted in an increased glucose uptake, measured with FDG PET, and an increased tissue glycogen content.

Acknowledgment

This study was supported by The Netherlands Heart Foundation (Grant 94.103) and performed within the framework of the EEC Biomed Concerted Action CT 95-838. The assistance of I.E. Mercalina is gratefully acknowledged.

References

1. Rahimtoola SH. Coronary bypass surgery for chronic angina - 1981. A perspective. Circulation 1982;65:225-41.
2. Rahimtoola SH. A perspective on the three large multicenter randomized clinical trials of coronary bypass surgery for chronic stable angina. Circulation 1985;72:V123-35.
3. Vanoverschelde JL, Wijns W, Borgers M, et al. Chronic myocardial hibernation in humans. From bedside to bench. Circulation 1997;95:1961-71.
4. Wijns W, Melin JA. Clinical imaging of chronic myocardial dysfunction. In: Heyndrickx GR, Vatner SF, Wijns W, editors. Stunning, hibernation, and preconditioning: clinical pathophysiology of myocardial ischemia. Philadelphia: Lippincott-Raven, 1997: 307-29.
5. Ferrari R, Cargnoni A, Curello S, Ceconi C, Volpini M, Visioli O. Metabolic adaptation of underperfused isolated rabbit heart: an insight into molecular mechanisms underlying hibernation [abstract]. Circulation 1993; 88 (4 suppl): I188.
6. Ross J. Myocardial perfusion-contraction matching: Implications for coronary heart disease and hibernation. Circulation 1991;83:1076-83.
7. Fedele FA, Gewirtz H, Capone RJ, Sharaf B, Most AS. Metabolic response to prolonged reduction of myocardial blood flow distal to a severe coronary artery stenosis. Circulation 1988;78:729-35.
8. Pantely GA, Malone SA, Rhen WS et al. Regeneration of myocardial phosphocreatine in pigs despite continued moderate ischemia. Circ Res 1990;67:1481-93.
9. Schulz R, Guth BD, Pieper K, Martin C, Heusch G. Recruitment of an inotropic reserve in moderately ischemic myocardium at the expense of metabolic recovery. A model of short-term hibernation. Circ Res 1992;70:1282-95.
10. Mills I, Fallon JT, Wrenn D, et al. Adaptive responses of coronary circulation and myocardium to chronic reduction in perfusion pressure and flow. Am J Physiol 1994;266:H447-H57.
11. Liedtke AJ, Renstrom B, Nellis SH, Hall JL, Stanley WC. Mechanical and metabolic functions in pig hearts after 4 days of chronic coronary stenosis. J Am Coll Cardiol 1995;26:815-25.
12. Canty JM Jr, Klocke FJ. Reductions in regional myocardial function at rest in conscious dogs with chronically reduced regional coronary artery pressure. Circ Res 1987;61:II107-16.
13. Shen Y-T, Vatner SF. Mechanism of impaired myocardial function during progressive coronary stenosis in conscious pigs. Hibernation versus stunning? Circ Res 1995;76:479-88.
14. Fallavollita JA, Perry BJ, Canty JM. ^{18}F-2-deoxyglucose deposition and regional flow in pigs with chronically dysfunctional myocardium: Evidence for transmural variations in chronic hibernating myocardium. Circulation 1997;95:1900-9.
15. Heusch G, Ferrari R, Hearse DJ, Ruigrok TJC, Schulz R. 'Myocardial hibernation' - questions and controversies. Cardiovasc Res. In press 1997.
16. Schulz R, Post H, Sakka S, Wallbridge DR, Heusch G. Intraischemic preconditioning. Increased tolerance to sustained low-flow ischemia by a brief episode of no-flow ischemia without intermittent reperfusion. Circ Res 1995;76:942-50.

17. Schulz R, Rose J, Heusch G. Involvement of activation of ATP-dependent potassium channels in ischemic preconditioning in swine. Am J Physiol 1994;267:H1341-52.
18. Schulz R, Rose J, Post H, Heusch G. Regional short-term myocardial hibernation in swine does not involve endogenous adenosine or KATP channels. Am J Physiol 1995;268:H2294-301.
19. Murry CE, Jennings RB, Reimer KA. Preconditioning with ischemia. A delay of lethal cell injury in ischemic myocardium. Circulation 1986;74:1124-36.
20. Ferrari R, Cargnoni A, Bernocchi P, et al. Metabolic adaptation during a sequence of no-flow and low-flow ischemia. A possible trigger for hibernation. Circulation 1996;94:2587-96.
21. Van Binsbergen XA, Van Emous JG, Ferrari R, Van Echteld CJ, Ruigrok TJ. Metabolic and functional consequences of successive no-flow and sustained low-flow ischaemia; A ^{31}P MRS study in rat hearts. J Mol Cell Cardiol 1996;28:2373-81.
22. Ferrari R, Bongrazio M, Cargnoni A, et al. Heat shock protein changes in hibernation: a similarity with heart failure? J Mol Cell Cardiol 1996;28:2383-95.
23. Marber MS, Latchman DS, Walker JM, Yellon DM. Cardiac stress protein elevation 24 hours after brief ischemia or heat stress is associated with resistance to myocardial infarction. Circulation 1993;88:1264-72.
24. Sun D, Nguyen N, DeGrado TR, Schwaiger M, Brosius FC 3rd. Ischemia induces translocation of the insulin-responsive glucose transporter GLUT4 to the plasma membrane of cardiac myocytes. Circulation 1994;89:793-8.
25. Koning MM, Simonis LA, DeZeeuw S, Nieukoop S, Post S, Verdouw PD. Ischaemic preconditioning by partial occlusion without intermittent reperfusion [published erratum in Cardiovasc Res 1994;28:1736]. Cardiovasc Res 1-994;28:1146-51.
26. Walsh RS, Borges M, Thornton JD, Cohen MV, Downey JM. Hypoxia preconditions rabbit myocardium by an adenosine receptor-mediated mechanism. Can J Cardiol 1995;11:141-6.
27. Ovize M, Przyklenk K, Kloner RA. Partial coronary stenosis is sufficient and complete reperfusion is mandatory for preconditioning the canine heart. Circ Res 1992;71:1165-73.
28. Janier MF, Vanoverschelde JL, Bergmann SR. Ischemic preconditioning stimulates anaerobic glycolysis in the isolated rabbit heart. Am J Physiol 1994;267:H1353-60.
29. Eberli FR, Weinberg EO, Grice WN, Horowitz GL, Apstein CS. Protective effect of increased glycolytic substrate against systolic and diastolic dysfunction and increased coronary resistance from prolonged global underperfusion and reperfusion in isolated rabbit hearts perfused with erythrocyte suspensions. Circ Res 1991;68:466-81.
30. Steenbergen C, Murphy E, Watts JA, London RE. Correlation between cytosolic free calcium, contracture, ATP, and irreversible ischemic injury in perfused rat heart. Circ Res 1990;66:135-46.
31. Jeremy RW, Koretsune Y, Marban E, Becker LC. Relation between glycolysis and calcium homeostasis in postischemic myocardium. Circ Res 1992;70:1180-90.
32. Nakamura K, Kusuoka H, Ambrosio G, Becker LC. Glycolysis is necessary to preserve myocardial Ca^{2+} homeostasis during beta-adrenergic stimulation. Am J Physiol 1993;264:H670-8.

33. Xu KY, Zweier JL, Becker LC. Functional coupling between glycolysis and sarcoplasmic reticulum Ca^{2+} transport. Circ Res 1995;77:88-97.
34. Cross HR, Radda GK, Clarke K. The role of Na^{+}/K^{+} ATPase activity during low flow ischemia in preventing myocardial injury: a ^{31}P, ^{23}Na and ^{87}Rb NMR spectroscopic study. Magn Reson Med 1995;34:673-85.
35. Kingsley PB, Sako EY, Yang MQ, et al. Ischemic contracture begins when anaerobic glycolysis stops: a ^{31}P-NMR study of isolated rat hearts. Am J Physiol 1991;261:H469-78.
36. Murry CE, Richard VJ, Reimer KA, Jennings RB. Ischemic preconditioning slows energy metabolism and delays ultrastructural damage during a sustained ischemic episode. Circ Res 1990;66:913-31.
37. Asimakis GK, Inners-McBride K, Medellin G, Conti VR. Ischemic preconditioning attenuates acidosis and postischemic dysfunction in isolated rat hearts. Am J Physiol 1992;263:H887-94.
38. Doenst T, Guthrie PH, Chemnitius J-M, Zech R, Taegtmeyer H. Fasting, lactate, and insulin improve ischemia tolerance in rat heart: a comparison with ischemic preconditioning. Am J Physiol 1996;270:H1607-15.
39. Illes RW, Wright JK, Inners-McBride K, Yang CJ, Tristan A. Ischemic preconditioning improves preservation with crystalloid cardioplegia. Ann Thorac Surg 1994;58:1481-5.
40. Downing SE, Chen V. Myocardial hibernation in the ischemic neonatal heart. Circ Res 1990;66:763-72.
41. Arai AE, Pantely GA, Anselone CG, Bristow J, Bristow JD. Active downregulation of myocardial energy requirements during prolonged moderate ischemia in swine. Circ Res 1991;69:1458-69.
42. Vanoverschelde JL, Wijns W, Depré C, et al. Mechanisms of chronic regional postischemic dysfunction in humans. New insights from the study of noninfarcted collateral-dependent myocardium. Circulation 1993;87:1513-23.
43. Maes A, Flameng W, Nuyts J et al. Histological alterations in chronically hypoperfused myocardium. Correlation with PET findings. Circulation 1994;90:735-45.
44. Depré C, Vanoverschelde JL, Melin JA, et al. Structural and metabolic correlates of the reversibility of chronic left ventricular ischemic dysfunction in humans. Am J Physiol 1995;268:H1265-75.
45. Borgers M. Pathologic findings in chronic hibernating myocardium. In: Heyndrickx GR, Vatner SF, Wijns W, editors. Stunning, hibernation, and preconditioning: clinical pathophysiology of myocardial ischemia. Philadelphia: Lippincott-Raven, 1997: 287-306.
46. Stull JT, Mayer SE. Biochemical mechanisms of adrenergic and cholinergic regulation of myocardial contractility. In: Berne RM,Sperelakis N, Geiger SR, editors. Handbook of physiology; Section 2, The Cardiovascular System. Volume I, The heart; Bethesda, Maryland: American Physiological Society, 1979: 741-74.
47. McNulty PH, Luba MC. Transient ischemia induces regional myocardial glycogen synthase activation and glycogen synthesis in vivo. Am J Physiol 1995;268:H364-70.
48. McFalls EO, Baldwin DR, Marx D, Jaimes D, Ward HB. The effects of repetitive stunning on regional myocardial glucose uptake in swine. [abstract]. Circulation 1997;96 (8 Suppl):I 537.

Chapter 12

MYOCARDIAL HIBERNATION: BLOOD FLOW AND METABOLISM

Jean-Louis J. Vanoverschelde, Bernhard L. Gerber and Jacques A. Melin

Introduction

The term "hibernation" was employed for the first time by Diamond et al. in 1978 [1] to describe the chronic wall motion abnormalities of patients with coronary artery disease but no previous myocardial infarction and their reversibility upon revascularization. The overall concept of myocardial hibernation was subsequently developed by Rahimtoola[2,3] and popularized by Braunwald and Rutherford.[4] In his 1989 description of the syndrome, Rahimtoola postulated that myocardial hibernation resulted from the "relatively uncommon response to reduced myocardial blood flow at rest whereby the heart downgrades its myocardial function to the extent that blood flow and function are once again in equilibrium, and as a result, neither myocardial necrosis or ischemic symptoms are present."[2]

The definition of myocardial hibernation, as formulated by Rahimtoola, raises several questions, many of which still lack experimental demonstration. These include:

1) can the heart spontaneously adapt to chronic underperfusion?
2) can a new steady state between perfusion and contraction be reached?
3) can this new equilibrium be maintained for a prolonged period of time?
4) does chronic left ventricular ischemic dysfunction in humans represent an adaptive response to a chronic reduction of resting myocardial blood flow?

Van der Wall et al. (eds.),
Advanced Imaging in Coronary Artery Disease, 199-214.

It is the purpose of this chapter to review available data on flow - function relationships during various ischemic conditions [5] and to examine how these concepts can be applied to improve our understanding of the pathophysiology of chronic myocardial hibernation in humans.

Myocardial blood flow in experimental models of regional ischemic dysfunction

Flow-function relations during partial coronary occlusion

The tight coupling between coronary flow, myocardial oxygen consumption and contractile performance of the heart is a fundamental principle of cardiac physiology. Because of the small extraction reserve of oxygen, decreases in coronary blood flow rapidly translate into decreases in contractile performance.[6] Several studies have examined the relation between regional myocardial blood flow (radioactive microspheres) and function (sonomicrometry) in both open-chest [7] and conscious dogs [8,9] undergoing graded reductions in coronary flow. These studies have demonstrated the existence of a close coupling between the supply of myocardial substrates, including oxygen, of which the measurement of regional perfusion provides a rough estimate,[10] and myocardial energy demand, as reflected by the steady state level of regional contraction. The proportional decrease in regional myocardial flow and function in this setting has been termed "acute perfusion-contraction matching" and is typical of acute myocardial ischemia. Reperfusion after very short periods of low coronary flow (less than 10 minutes) usually results in rapid and complete restoration of cardiac performance. There is no necrosis, and myocardial ultrastructure is normal. More prolonged periods of coronary flow reduction, up to 15-20 minutes, do not usually cause tissue necrosis, but, with reperfusion, are associated with a prolonged, albeit reversible, dysfunction which has been termed myocardial stunning.[11] Further increases in the duration of ischemia usually result in variable degree of irreversible cell damage.[12]

Adaptive responses to sustained nonlethal reductions of resting myocardial blood flow

The observation that, under acute conditions, myocardial contraction decreases to a level matched to the available blood supply, has prone investigators to examine whether sustained perfusion-contraction matching could be achieved without inducing necrosis. Studies in open-chest anesthetized animals undergoing 1 to 5 hours partial coronary occlusion have shown that the heart can indeed adapt to a sustained reduction of resting myocardial blood flow.[13-18] Several investigators have reported on the successful development of sustained low-flow perfusion-contraction matching (also called short-term hibernation) in both the dog [13] and the pig heart.[14-18] Ischemia was produced by incomplete coronary occlusion leading to a 20-70% reduction of transmural myocardial blood flow. Despite continuing low-flow and dysfunction, intriguing phenomena were observed, including the spontaneous resolution of some of the metabolic markers of ischemia (mainly lactate production)[13,14] and the regeneration of phosphocreatine back to nearly normal levels.[15-18] Short-term hibernation is a fragile and unstable condition, however, as superimposition of a chronotropic or inotropic stress invariably results in increased lactate production, decreased phosphocreatine and eventually myocardial necrosis.[17,18]

Very few data are presently available to indicate that such a perfusion-contraction matching can persist for more than 5 hours in chronic animals. To date, the only indication in favor of this possibility as been provided by Chen et al.[19] These authors studied pigs with a severe left anterior descending coronary artery stenosis resulting in a sustained reduction of resting coronary flow (to $\pm$ 60% of baseline) and myocardial contraction (to $\pm$ 30% of baseline) during 24 hours. The reduction of regional coronary flow initially produced acute myocardial ischemia, as evidenced by regional lactate production and a decrease in regional coronary venous pH. At 24 hours, however, the markers of ischemia had almost completely disappeared. Morphologically, 6 of the 11 pigs studied were free of myocardial infarction; and 5 others had patchy necrosis. The morphological changes also included a partial loss of myofibrils, an increase in mitochondria and glycogen deposition, [19] and evidence of myocyte apoptosis.[20] These studies thus support the contention that sustained perfusion-contraction matching can be maintained in pigs with coronary stenoses for at least 24 hours and perhaps longer without inducing (too much) necrosis. There is, however, a possible caveat to the studies of Chen et al.,[19,20] i.e. the absence of data on tissue perfusion. The authors indeed relied solely on electromagnetic flow measurements to estimate flow in the left anterior descending coronary artery, assuming that, in the absence of preformed collaterals, flow in the left anterior descending coronary artery and tissue perfusion should be equal. Although this was probably true during the first 24 hours, collateral growth, which is known to occur in pigs and was not taken into account, could have confounded their late results. This view is supported by recent data from Mc Falls et al., who demonstrated, in a similar model, that flow does not significantly changes over time in the ischemic region, whereas it tended to increase in the non-ischemic region.[21]

Adaptation to chronic coronary artery disease

Despite considerable interest, the development of animal models of chronic but reversible left ventricular ischemic dysfunction mimicking human myocardial hibernation has proven to be tremendously difficult. So far, most investigators who have succeeded in reproducing chronic (>1 week) but reversible regional left ventricular ischemic dysfunction in the experimental lab have almost invariably ended up with models of perfusion-contraction mismatch. Canty and Klocke [22] examined the temporal response of regional function after ameroid implantation in conscious dogs. In their model, regional contraction was found to decrease progressively during the course of ameroid occlusion. Yet, at the time of ameroid occlusion (2 to 4 weeks), the measurements of regional endocardial blood flow showed a dissociation between flow and function. Bolukoglu et al.[23] and Liedtke et al.[24] achieved sustained reduction in segmental shortening without necrosis in swine undergoing a 50% reduction of the left anterior descending coronary artery flow velocity for 7 days. In these experiments too, the decrease in segmental function was progressive over time and was not associated with reduced subendocardial blood flow by day 4. More recently, Shen et al.[25] and Fallavollita et al.[26] in pigs as well as Gerber et al.[27] in dogs succeeded in producing regional contractile dysfunction over periods of 1, 3 and 6 months respectively. In each of these studies, the severity of regional dysfunction was found to be out of proportion to the reduction in myocardial blood flow, thus demonstrating perfusion-contraction mismatch. While the above studies do not dismiss the possibility that chronic perfusion-contraction matching could exist in intact animals over prolonged periods of time, they nevertheless suggest that chronic underperfusion is not a necessary prerequisite to the development of chronic dysfunction in the presence of chronic coronary artery stenoses.

Chronic reduction in myocardial blood flow as a consequence rather than the cause of chronic hibernation

The fact that chronic contractile dysfunction in the presence of severe coronary artery disease likely results from repeated episodes of ischemia followed by a state of chronic stunning, does not exclude the possibility that myocardial blood flow may eventually become reduced in the affected segments. There is indeed increasing evidence to suggest that myocardial blood flow progressively downgrades in response to reduced contractile function. Back in 1975, Heyndrickx et al.[11] already indicated that myocardial blood flow, measured 4 to 6 hours after reperfusion, was often decreased by 20 - 25% in acutely stunned myocardium. Canty and Klocke [22] made very similar observations in their dog model of chronic ameroid occlusion. In their experiments, subendocardial blood flow, which had remained normal up to the time of ameroid occlusion and peak contractile dysfunction, gradually decreased after ameroid occlusion. Interestingly, this occurred in face of a progressive increase in coronary perfusion pressure and a slow normalization of regional contractile function. Recently, Berman et al.[28] studied the effects of sustained demand-induced ischemia in a pig model of short-term hibernation. They made the intriguing observation that, despite no changes in myocardial blood flow during stress, transmural blood flow decreased after cessation of the stress and remained depressed for a prolonged period of time. Although it is possible that the above observations are related to some form of microvascular stunning, it is tempting to hypothesize that the progressive reduction in myocardial blood flow seen under these conditions is somehow secondary to the reduction in resting contractile function,[29] and serves a means to increase residual myocardial perfusion reserve.[30]

Myocardial blood flow in the human hibernating myocardium

Assessment of perfusion-contraction matching in patients with hibernating myocardium requires the ability to measure blood flow and function simultaneously.[5] Direct assessment of resting myocardial blood flow in patients is complicated by two factors: the difficulty of measuring myocardial blood flow in absolute terms in the clinical setting and the known tissue heterogeneity of ischemically injured myocardium. The contention that flow is decreased in human hibernating myocardium is based on the results of clinical studies of the relative distribution of radiolabeled flow tracers such as ^{201}Thallium [31-33], ^{82}Rubidium [34] or ^{99m}Tc-MIBI.[35] The interpretation of these scintigrams usually assumes that the segments with maximum tracer uptake have normal flow and that any region with an apparent reduction of tracer uptake is underperfused. As perfusion scintigraphy only provides estimates of relative differences in tracer distribution, a seemingly decreased perfusion to a dysfunctional segment may result in part from an absolute increase in flow to the remote hyperfunctioning tissue.[36] The accuracy of relative perfusion scintigraphy is further affected by the limited spatial resolution of the current single photon emission computed tomography (SPECT) devices. This results in significant underestimation of true regional activity concentrations, a phenomenon known as "partial volume effect," which describes how counts measured from a myocardial region with reduced wall thickness will always be fewer than those measured from a region with a normal wall thickness.[37] The partial volume effect is particularly relevant to the situation of the hibernating myocardium as the sole loss of systolic wall thickening is expected to result in a 20 to

25% underestimation of regional counts.[38] The degree of underestimation can even be larger in the presence of significant wall thinning. Taken together, these limitations make it difficult to determine whether a dysfunctional myocardial segment which exhibits reduced radiolabeled flow tracer uptake at rest with SPECT is truly underperfused or not. Recent refinements in myocardial perfusion imaging, and particularly the advent of positron emission tomography (PET), have greatly enhanced our ability to measure flow directly in patients with coronary artery disease.[39-41] PET is a truly quantitative method. It has a much better spatial resolution than SPECT; it allows for accurate correction of photon attenuation and, to some extent, of partial volume effects; finally, when mathematically and physiologically appropriate models are used to describe the biological behavior of the radiotracers in blood and myocardium, it allows for computation of quantitative estimates of regional myocardial perfusion. Several investigators have attempted to assess the level of resting myocardial blood flow in patients with hibernating myocardium using PET. Initial studies in patients with previous myocardial infarction indicated that reversibly dysfunctional segments corresponded to areas with qualitatively reduced perfusion but preserved metabolism.[42-44] However, quantitative studies using ^{13}N-ammonia found that reversibly dysfunctional segments after revascularization had normal or only mildly reduced baseline flow compared with remote normally contracting areas in the same patients, while myocardial segments with persistent dysfunction had even lower values (Table 1).[41-43]

	Remote	Viable	Nonviable
^{13}N-ammonia			
Grandin et al.	90 ± 18	77 ± 20*	51 ± 9 ‡
Depré et al.	100 ± 18	88 ± 23	61 ± 12‡
Gerber et al.	81 ± 20	84 ± 27	60 ± 26†
Sun et al.	70 ± 18	53 ± 33	28 ± 9‡
Gerber et al.	75 ± 8	84 ± 16	46 ± 12†
Depré et al.	-	90 ± 29	63 ± 20‡
^{15}O-water			
De Silva et al.	97 ± 22	73 ± 18	73 ± 18
Marhino et al.	92 ± 25	87 ± 31	82 ± 40
Gerber et al.	83 ± 12	74 ± 12	82 ± 18

Myocardial blood flow is in ml.(min.100g)$^{-1}$
† $p<0.01$ versus remote and viable; ‡ $p<0.001$ versus remote and viable; * $p<0.05$ versus remote

Table 1. *Myocardial blood flow in remote, viable and nonviable myocardium of patients with previous myocardial infarction*

On the basis of these studies, one could inadvertently conclude that the hibernating myocardium is indeed characterized by a mildly reduced perfusion. Two important aspects must nonetheless be considered. First, the level of flow reduction in most studies is not sufficient to justify ischemic dysfunction.[8] Second, many, if not all the above studies have included a variable proportion of patients with previous myocardial infarction, which greatly complicates the interpretation of the flow data. Flow estimates with PET are indeed critically dependent on the mass of tissue that actively participates in tracer exchange within the region of interest. In the presence of marked spatial tissue heterogeneity, such as occurs in previously infarcted myocardium, flow estimates represent the transmural average between several values from very low in micro-infarcted areas to almost normal in the non-infarcted epicardial zones and may thus not reflect the actual level of flow seen by the viable part of the wall. One approach to circumvent this problem is to study carefully selected patients with hibernating myocardium in whom any evidence of previous myocardial infarction is lacking. Vanoverschelde et al.[36] studied 26 patients whose clinical and angiographic characteristics were quite similar to those initially described by Rahimtoola. All had symptomatic coronary artery disease, no previous myocardial infarction and complete chronic occlusion of a major coronary artery. In patients with normal resting wall motion, no difference in myocardial blood flow measured with ^{13}N-ammonia and PET was found between normal and collateral-dependent myocardium. In patients with abnormal resting wall motion, myocardial blood flow was higher in remote compared to collateral dependent segments (95 ± 27 vs. 77 ± 25 ml.(min.100g)$^{-1}$, $p < 0.001$). Yet, no difference was found among collateral dependent segments of patients with and without wall motion abnormalities (77 ± 25 versus 85 ± 14 ml.(min.100g)$^{-1}$, p=ns) . To corroborate their surprising results, these authors also investigated regional myocardial oxygen consumption using ^{11}C-acetate and PET. In patients with normal resting wall motion, oxygen consumption was comparable between remote and collateralized segments. In patients with resting wall motion abnormalities, myocardial oxygen consumption was higher in remote compared with collateral dependent segments. It did not differ significantly, however, among collateral dependent segments of patients with and without regional wall motion abnormalities. Similar findings were also reported by Sambuceti et al.[48] and by Knuuti et al.[49,50] Another approach to circumvent the problems of tissue heterogeneity is to use $H_2{}^{15}O$ and PET to measure myocardial blood flow.[51,52] Quantitation of myocardial blood flow using $H_2{}^{15}O$ indeed allows to incorporate into the kinetic model an estimate of the fraction of tissue in the region of interest that is exchanging the freely diffusible water.[51,52] This approach provides values of flow per gram of perfusable tissue as opposed to gram of region of interest. Since, for any practical purposes, the exchange of water by scar tissue can be regarded as negligible, this technique thus predominantly measures flow in the non necrotic part of the wall. Using $H_2^{15}O$, De Silva et al.,[53] Marinho et al.,[54] Conversano et al.,[55] and Gerber et al.[56] found baseline flow values that are within the range of resting flow values measured in normal regions in the majority of hibernating segments (Table 2).

	Patients with hibernating myocardium	
	Remote	Dysfunctional
Vanoverschelde et al.	95 ± 27	77 ± 25 *
Sambucetti et al.	77 ± 26	66 ± 19*
Maki et al.	101 ± 23	81 ± 27*
Maki et al.	81 ± 14	76 ± 17

Myocardial blood flow is in $ml.(min.100g)^{-1}$
* $p<0.05$ versus remote

Table 2. *Myocardial blood flow in remote and dysfunctional myocardium of patients in the absence of a previous myocardial infarction*

Repeated stunning as a plausible mechanism for chronic myocardial hibernation

If resting flow is not reduced, which can then be the trigger for the chronic reduction in mechanical function? Even if resting perfusion is nearly normal, perfusion reserve is highly abnormal in hibernating segments. Vanoverschelde et al. [36] investigated the regional flow reserve of collateral dependent myocardium using dipyridamole as the hyperemic agent. They found a wide range of hyperemic transmural flow values, from a 4-fold increase to a 20% decrease in basal flow. Importantly, the collateral flow reserve of the dysfunctional segments was markedly blunted and correlated with the severity of chronic regional wall motion abnormalities. Accordingly these authors suggested that repetitive intermittent episodes of ischemia (either exercise-induced or related to primary reductions in coronary blood flow [plaque events, vasoconstriction, platelet aggregation, etc.]) followed by stunning could be the mechanism leading to chronic regional ischemic dysfunction. It is worth mentioning that Braunwald and Kloner had already proposed such mechanism back in 1982.[57] Although, because of the study design, no single episode of stunning could be demonstrated in the study of Vanoverschelde et al.,[32] subsequent observations by Shen and Vatner[25] have provided evidence that chronic dysfunction in collateral-dependent myocardium can result from repeated episodes of ischemia followed by a perpetuated state of chronic stunning. These authors examined the time course of regional dysfunction after ameroid implantation in chronically instrumented pigs and found that the onset of dysfunction was not associated with permanently reduced subendocardial blood flow but was always preceded by repeated episodes of acute dysfunction induced by transient increases in regional demand. Altogether, these data suggest that repetitive stunning is a plausible mechanism that can account for the sustained prolonged contractile dysfunction of the hibernating myocardium. Alternatively, chronic dysfunction could result from a chronic decrease in coronary perfusion pressure in the post-stenotic bed.[58,59] Coronary pressure has been shown to regulate contractile performance acutely, even in the absence of changes in coronary flow.[60] Whether a decrease in coronary perfusion pressure can be involved in long-term regulation of contractile function in the hibernating myocardium is unknown and requires further investigation.

Metabolic alterations in the hibernating myocardium

Several investigators have indeed reported that, under fasting conditions, the hibernating myocardium was taking up glucose more avidly than remote normal myocardium,[44,49,61] a feature that has been utilized to predict the reversibility of regional dysfunction after revascularization.[40] The comparison of morphological data with the findings on metabolic imaging (which demonstrates increased rate of FDG transport and phosphorylation) has risen intriguing questions about the biochemical fate of exogenous glucose in "hibernating" cells.[62,63] Although it was originally suggested that the increased glucose uptake in the hibernating myocardium resulted from stimulation of anaerobic metabolism by chronic ischemia,[64] this explanation now appears unlikely in view of the normal or nearly normal levels of absolute myocardial blood flow[36,45-50,53-56] and oxygen consumption[36,65] measured in these segments. It would also hardly explain the accumulation of glycogen, a quite unusual finding in the setting of ongoing ischemia, rather expected to result in the opposite.[66] Even if ongoing ischemia is not implicated, it remains possible that a change in the pattern of myocardial substrate utilization, from fatty acid to glucose, contributes to the metabolic alterations of the hibernating myocardium. In this regard, it is worth mentioning that Liedtke et al.[24] recently presented strong evidence that such a metabolic switch occurred in pigs with chronic coronary stenosis. Chronic activation of glycogen synthase by ischemia has also been proposed to account for the metabolic alterations seen in the hibernating myocardium. McNulty and Luba [67] have recently shown that transient ischemia induced a sustained activation of the glucose-6-phosphate independent form of glycogen synthase, allowing for a rapid replenishment of the glycogen stores during reperfusion. Similar observations were also reported by Bolukoglu et al.[68] Altogether, these data thus suggest that the alterations of glucose metabolism seen in experimental myocardial ischemia and hibernation could result from a concerted deregulation of glycolysis and glycogen synthesis. Further studies are nonetheless required to verify this hypothesis in the clinical setting. Finally, because the uptake of glucose by dysfunctional but metabolically active myocardium was shown to be relatively independent of the hormonal milieu and dietary conditions,[49,61] some investigators have postulated that a change in the activity or in the expression of the 2 major cardiac glucose transporters, GLUT-1 and GLUT-4, could be involved in this phenomenon. So far, only 2 preliminary studies have attempted to measure the messenger RNA of these 2 glucose transporters by quantitative PCR in dysfunctional segments of patients with hibernating myocardium, and came up with opposite results.[69,70]

Conclusions

The recent refinements in myocardial perfusion imaging and the results of morphological studies of biopsy specimens from human hibernating myocardium have shed a new light on our understanding of chronic myocardial hibernation. The pathophysiology of this peculiar condition now appears to be much more complex than previously anticipated. It likely involves a combination of repetitive post-ischemic dysfunction, which is perpetuated because of renewed episodes of ischemia, and from ischemia/reperfusion-induced changes in cell phenotype, which eventually culminate into the dramatic morphological alterations which have been described. In the end, however, this adaptation may not be as successful as initially anticipated. Evidence is indeed accumulating that the hibernating myocardium represents an unstable and precarious condition that requires, if nor urgent, at least rapid revascularization. Failure to revascularize hibernating segments has been associated with an increased rate of adverse events and a poor prognosis.[71-73] Much is still to be learnt about the pathophysiology of myocardial hibernation and particularly how the hibernating phenotype develops. Future progress in this field will require the development of relevant animal models of chronic hibernation and a better understanding of how ischemia, reperfusion and their various metabolic and mechanical consequences eventually interfere with myocardial gene expression. Identification of the various steps leading to the final picture is mandatory to develop new and better therapeutic strategies and to hasten functional recovery after revascularization.

References

1. Diamond GA, Forrester JS, DeLuz PL, Wyatt HL, Swan HJ. Post-extrasystolic potentiation of ischemic myocardium by atrial stimulation. Am Heart J 1978;95:204-9.
2. Rahimtoola SH. The hibernating myocardium. Am Heart J 1989; 117:211-21.
3. Rahimtoola SH. A perspective on the three large multicenter randomized clinical trial of coronary bypass surgery for chronic stable angina. Circulation 1985; 72:V123-35.
4. Braunwald E, Rutherford JD. Reversible ischemic left ventricular dysfunction: evidence for "hibernating myocardium". J Am Coll Cardiol 1986;8:1467-70.
5. Ross J Jr. Myocardial perfusion-contraction matching. Implications for coronary heart disease and hibernation. Circulation 1991;83:1076-83.
6. Tennant R, Wiggers CJ. The effect of coronary occlusion on myocardial contraction. Am J Physiol 1935;112:351-61.
7. Gallagher KP, Kumada T, Koziol JA, McKown MD, Kemper WS, Ross J Jr. Significance of regional wall thickening abnormalities relative to transmural myocardial perfusion in anesthetized dogs. Circulation 1980;62:1266-74.
8. Gallagher KP, Matsuzaki M, Koziol JA, Kemper WS, Ross J Jr. Regional myocardial perfusion and wall thickening during ischemia in conscious dogs. Am J Physiol 1984;247:H727-38.
9. Vatner SF. Correlation between acute reductions in myocardial blood flow and function in conscious dogs. Circ Res 1980;47:201-7.
10. Eckenhoff JE, Hafkenschiel JH, Landmesser CM, Harmel M. Cardiac oxygen metabolism and control of the coronary circulation. Am J Physiol 1947;149:634-49.
11. Heyndrickx GR, Millard RW, McRitchie RJ, Maroko PR, Vatner SF. Regional myocardial functional and electrophysiological alterations after brief coronary artery occlusion in conscious dogs. J Clin Invest 1975;56:978-85.
12. Jennings RB, Sommers HM, Smyth GA, Flack HA, Linn H. Myocardial necrosis induced by temporary occlusion of a coronary artery in the dog. AMA Arch Pathol 1960;70:68-78.
13. Matsuzaki M, Gallagher KP, Kemper WS, White F, Ross J Jr. Sustained regional dysfunction produced by prolonged coronary stenosis: gradual recovery after reperfusion. Circulation 1983;68:170-82.
14. Fedele FA, Gewirtz H, Capone RJ, Sharaf B, Most AA. Metabolic response to prolonged reduction of myocardial blood flow distal to a severe coronary artery stenosis. Circulation 1988;78:729-35.
15. Pantely GA, Malone SA, Rhen WS, et al. Regeneration of myocardial phosphocreatine in pigs despite continued moderate ischemia. Circ Res 1990;67:1481-93.
16. Arai AE, Pantely GA, Anselone CG, Brislow J, Brislow JD. Active downregulation of myocardial energy requirements during prolonged moderate ischemia in swine. Circ Res 1991;69:1458-69.
17. Schulz R, Guth BD, Pieper K, Martin C, Heusch G. Recruitment of an inotropic reserve in moderately ischemic myocardium at the expense of metabolic recovery. A model of short- term hibernation. Circ Res 1992;70:1282-95.
18. Schulz R, Rose J, Martin C, Brodde OE, Heusch G. Development of short-term myocardial hibernation. Its limitation by the severity of ischemia and inotropic stimulation. Circulation 1993;88:684-95.

19. Chen C, Chen L, Fallon JT, et al. Functional and structural alterations with 24-hour myocardial hibernation and recovery after reperfusion. A pig model of myocardial hibernation. Circulation 1996;94:507-16.
20. Chen C, Ma L, Linfert DR, et al. Myocardial cell death and apoptosis in hibernating myocardium. J Am Coll Cardiol 1997;30:1407-12.
21. McFalls EO, Baldwin D, Palmer B, Marx D, Jaimes D, Ward HB. Regional glucose uptake within hypoperfused swine myocardium as measured by positron emission tomography. Am J Physiol 1997;H272:H343-9.
22. Canty JM Jr, Klocke FJ. Reductions in regional myocardial function at rest in conscious dogs with chronically reduced regional coronary artery pressure. Circ Res 1987;61:II107-16.
23. Bolukoglu H, Liedtke AJ, Nellis SH, Eggleston AM, Subramanian R, Renstrom B. An animal model of chronic coronary stenosis resulting in hibernating myocardium. Am J Physiol 1992;263:H20-9.
24. Liedtke AJ, Renstrom B, Nellis SH, Hall JL, Stanley WC. Mechanical and metabolic functions in pig hearts after 4 days of chronic coronary stenosis. J Am Coll Cardiol 1995;26:815-25.
25. Shen YT, Vatner SF. Mechanism of impaired myocardial function during progressive coronary stenosis in conscious pigs. Hibernation versus stunning? Circ Res 1995;76:479-88.
26. Fallavollita JA, Perry BJ, Canty JM Jr. Transmural variations in 18F-2-deoxyglucose (FDG) deposition in pigs with collateral-dependent myocardium and chronic hibernation [abstract]. Circulation 1995;92(Suppl I):I386.
27. Gerber B, Laycock SK, Melin JA, Flameng W, Vanoverschelde JL. Perfusion-contraction matching, inotropic reserve and vasodilatory capacity in a canine model of dysfunctional collateral-dependent myocardium [abstract]. Circulation 1995;92(Suppl I):I314.
28. Berman M, Fischman AJ, Southern J, et al. Myocardial adaptation during and after sustained, demand-induced ischemia. Observations in closed-chest, domestic swine. Circulation 1996;94:755-62.
29. Sherman AJ, Harris KR, Hedjbeli S, et al. Proportionate reversible decreases in systolic function and myocardial oxygen consumption after modest reductions in coronary flow: hibernation versus stunning. J Am Coll Cardiol 1997;29:1623-31.
30. Mills I, Fallon JT, Wrenn D, et al. Adaptive responses of coronary circulation and myocardium to chronic reduction in perfusion pressure and flow. Am J Physiol 1994;266:H447-57.
31. Berger BC, Watson DD, Burwell LR, et al. Redistribution of thallium at rest in patients with stable and unstable angina and the effects of coronary artery bypass graft surgery. Circulation 1979;60:1114-25.
32. Iskandrian AS, Hakki AH, Kane SA, et al. Rest and redistribution thallium-201 myocardial scintigraphy to predict improvement in left ventricular function after coronary arterial bypass grafting. Am J Cardiol 1983;51:1312-6.
33. Ragosta M, Beller GA, Watson DD, Kaul S, Gimple LW. Quantitative planar rest-redistribution 201Tl imaging in detection of myocardial viability and prediction of improvement in left ventricular function after coronary bypass surgery in patients with severely depressed left ventricular function. Circulation 1993;87:1630-41.

34. Marwick TH, MacIntyre WJ, Lafont A, Nemec JJ, Salcedo EE. Metabolic responses of hibernating and infarcted myocardium to revascularization. A follow-up study of regional perfusion, function and metabolism. Circulation. 1992;85:1347-53.
35. Udelson JE, Coleman PS, Metherall J, et al. Predicting recovery of severe regional ventricular dysfunction. Comparison of resting scintigraphy with 201Tl and 99mTc-sestamibi. Circulation 1994;89:2552-61.
36. Vanoverschelde JL, Wijns W, Depré C, et al. Mechanisms of chronic regional postischemic dysfunction in humans. New insights from the study of noninfarcted collateral- dependent myocardium. Circulation 1993; 87:1513-23.
37. Hoffman EJ, Huang SC, Phelps ME. Quantitation in positron emission computed tomography: 1. Effect of object size. J Comput Assist Tomogr 1979;3:299-308.
38. Parodi O, Schelbert HR, Schwaiger M, Hansen H, Selin C, Hoffman EJ. Cardiac emission computed tomography: underestimation of regional tracer concentrations due to wall motion abnormalities. J Comput Assist Tomogr 1984;8:1083-92.
39. Schelbert HR, Phelps ME, Hoffman EJ, Huang SC, Selin CE, Kuhl DE. Regional myocardial perfusion assessed with N-13 labeled ammonia and positron emission computerized axial tomography. Am J Cardiol 1979; 43:209-18.
40. Bergmann SR, Herrero P, Markham J, Weinmheimer CJ, Walsh MN. Noninvasive quantitation of myocardial blood flow in human subjects with oxygen-15-labeled water and positron emission tomography. J Am Coll Cardiol 1989; 14:639-52.
41. Bol A, Melin JA, Vanoverschelde JL, et al. Direct comparison of [13N] ammonia and [15O] water estimates of perfusion for quantification of regional myocardial blood flow by microspheres. Circulation 1993;87:512-25.
42. Marshall RC, Tillisch JH, Phelps ME, et al. Identification and differentiation of resting myocardial ischemia and infarction in man with positron computed tomography, 18F-labeled fluorodeoxyglucose and N-13 ammonia. Circulation 1983;67:766-78.
43. Tillisch J, Brunken R, Marshall R, et al. Reversibility of cardiac wall motion abnormalities predicted by positron tomography. N Engl J Med 1986;314:884-8.
44. Tamaki N, Yonekura Y, Yamashita K, et al. Positron emission tomography using fluorine-18 deoxyglucose in evaluation of coronary artery bypass grafting. Am J Cardiol 1989;64:860-5.
45. Grandin C, Wijns W, Melin JA, et al. Delineation of myocardial viability with PET. J Nucl Med 1995;36:1543-52.
46. Gerber BL, Vanoverschelde JL, Bol A, et al. Myocardial blood flow, glucose uptake, and recruitment of inotropic reserve in chronic left ventricular ischemic dysfunction. Implications for the pathophysiology of chronic myocardial hibernation. Circulation 1996;94:651-9.
47. Sun KT, Czernin J, Krivokapich J, et al. Effects of dobutamine stimulation on myocardial blood flow, glucose metabolism, and wall motion in normal and dysfunctional myocardium. Circulation 1996;94:3146-54.
48. Sambuceti G, Parodi O, Marzullo P, et al. Regional myocardial blood flow in stable angina pectoris associated with isolated significant narrowing of either the left anterior descending or left circumflex coronary artery. Am J Cardiol 1993;72:990-4.

49. Maki M, Luotolahti M, Nuutila P, et al. Glucose uptake in the chronically dysfunctional but viable myocardium. Circulation 1996;93:1658-66.
50. Maki MT, Haaparanta MT, Luotolahti MS, et al. Fatty acid uptake is preserved in chronically dysfunctional but viable myocardium. Am J Physiol 1997;273:H2473-80.
51. Iida H, Rhodes CG, De Silva R, et al. Myocardial tissue fraction - correction for partial volume effects and measure of tissue viability. J Nucl Med 1991;32:2169-75.
52. Herrero P, Staudenherz A, Walsh JF, Gropler RJ, Bergmann SR. Heterogeneity of myocardial perfusion provides the physiological basis of perfusable tissue index. J Nucl Med 1995;36:320-7.
53. De Silva R, Yamomoto Y, Rhodes CG, et al. Preoperative prediction of the outcome of coronary revascularization using positron emission tomography. Circulation 1992;86:1738-42.
54. Marinho NV, Keogh BE, Costa DC, Lammertsma AA, Ell PJ, Camici PG. Pathophysiology of chronic left ventricular dysfunction. New insights from the measurement of absolute myocardial blood flow and glucose utilization. Circulation 1996;93:737-44.
55. Conversano A, Walsh JF, Geltman EM, Perez JE, Bergmann SR, Gropler RJ. Delineation of myocardial stunning from hibernation by positron emission tomography in advanced coronary artery disease. Am Heart J 1996;131:440-50.
56. Gerber BL, Melin JA, Bol A, et al. Differences in 13N-ammonia and 15O-water estimates of absolute myocardial perfusion in patients with chronic left ventricular ischemic dysfunction. J Nucl Med. In press 1998.
57. Braunwald E, Kloner RA. The stunned myocardium: prolonged, postischemic ventricular dysfunction. Circulation 1982;66:1146-9.
58. Kitakaze M, Marban E. Cellular mechanism of the modulation of contractile function by coronary perfusion pressure in ferret hearts. J Physiol (Lond) 1989;414:455-72.
59. Bache RJ, Schwartz JS. Effect of perfusion pressure distal to a coronary stenosis on transmural myocardial blood flow. Circulation 1982;65:928-35.
60. Weisfeldt ML, Shock NW. Effect of perfusion pressure on coronary flow and oxygen usage of nonworking heart. Am J Physiol 1970;218:95-101.
61. Gerber B, Melin JA, Bol A, Vanoverschelde JL. Attenuated response of myocardial glucose utilization to insulin stimulation in hibernating myocardium [abstract]. Circulation 1995;92 (suppl 1):I313.
62. Depré C, Vanoverschelde JL, Melin JA, et al. Structural and metabolic correlates of the reversibility of chronic left ventricular ischemic dysfunction in humans. Am J Physiol 1995;268:H1265-75.
63. Depré C, Vanoverschelde JL, Gerber B, Borgers M, Melin JA, Dion R. Correlation of functional recovery with myocardial blood flow, glucose uptake, and morphologic features in patients with chronic left ventricular ischemic dysfunction undergoing coronary artery bypass grafting. J Thorac Cardiovasc Surg 1997;113:371-8.
64. Schelbert HR, Buxton D. Insights into coronary artery disease gained from metabolic imaging. Circulation 1988; 78:496-505.
65. Gropler RJ, Geltman EM, Sampathkumaran K, et al. Functional recovery after coronary revascularization for chronic coronary artery disease is dependent on maintenance of oxidative metabolism. J Am Coll Cardiol 1992;20:569-77.

66. Vanoverschelde JL, Janier MF, Bakke JE, Marshall DR, Bergmann SR. Rate of glycolysis during ischemia determines extent of ischemic injury and functional recovery after reperfusion. Am J Physiol 1994;267:H1785-94.
67. McNulty PH, Luba MC. Transient ischemia induces regional myocardial glycogen synthase activation and glycogen synthesis in vivo. Am J Physiol 1995;268:H364-70.
68. Bolukoglu H, Goodwin GW, Guthrie PH, Carmical SG, Chen TM, Taegtmeyer H. Metabolic fate of glucose in reversible low-flow ischemia of the isolated working rat heart. Am J Physiol 1996;270:H817-26.
69. Brosius FC 3rd, Sun DQ, England R, Nguyen N, Schwaiger M. Altered glucose transporter mRNA levels in cardiac ischemia [abstract]. Circulation 1993;88(Suppl I):I542.
70. Depré C, Vanoverschelde JL, Grillenberger K, et al. Correlation of glucose transporter messenger RNA expression with morphological pattern and glucose uptake in chronically dysfunctional myocardium [abstract]. Circulation 1995;92(Suppl 1):I651.
71. Lee KS, Marwick TH, Cook SA, et al. Prognosis of patients with left ventricular dysfunction, with and without viable myocardium after myocardial infarction. Relative efficacy of medical therapy and revascularization. Circulation 1994;90:2687-94.
72. Di Carli MF, Davidson M, Little R, et al. Value of metabolic imaging with positron emission tomography for evaluating prognosis in patients with coronary artery disease and left ventricular dysfunction. Am J Cardiol 1994;73:527-33.
73. Pasquet A, Gerber B, D'Hondt AM, De Kock M, Melin JA, Vanoverschelde JL. Value of dobutamine echocardiography and FDC-PET in evaluating prognosis in patients with chronic left ventricular ischemic dysfunction [abstract]. Circulation 1995;92 (Suppl 1):I268.

Chapter 13

IMAGING TECHNIQUES IN DETERMINING MYOCARDIAL VIABILITY AND HIBERNATION

Mark Gunning and Richard Underwood

Introduction

Coronary artery disease is the leading cause of heart failure in the Western world. Left ventricular function is an important determinant of prognosis and parameters which reflect function such as left ventricular ejection fraction (LVEF), end-diastolic volume, end diastolic pressure, and exercise capacity can all be used to help predict outcome [1,2]. The advent of drugs such as ACE inhibitors[3], angiotensin II inhibitors[4], and more recently beta-blocking agents such as carvedilol [5] have provided means of improving prognosis in heart failure, but nevertheless overall outcome on medical treatment remains poor . Data from the CASS registry showed that in patients with left ventricular dysfunction on medical therapy, mortality increased in a curvilinear fashion in relation to reduction in LVEF [6]. Furthermore it was shown that a survival benefit was conferred by surgical revascularization even in patients where LVEF was less than 25%, with a 1 year mortality of 15% in the surgical group and 24% in the medical group. Surgical and anesthetic techniques have improved since this data was published and most recent reports suggest an advantage of revascularization over medical therapy in patients with ischemic left ventricular dysfunction.[7,8]

However peri-operative mortality in patients with impaired left ventricular function is relatively high. Differentiation of viable myocardium with potential for recovery from scar is useful in determining the suitability of patients for

Van der Wall et al. (eds.),
Advanced Imaging in Coronary Artery Disease, 215-235.

this high risk coronary intervention, as it is they who benefit most from revascularization. Imaging techniques which identify these regions of viable tissue play a valuable role.

Hibernating Myocardium - History and Definition

Several studies carried out in the 1970's challenged the contemporary concept that chronic regional myocardial dysfunction was synonymous with infarction [9,10]. Rees and colleagues reported improvement in regional left ventricular wall motion following coronary artery bypass surgery with an associated improvement in global function [11]. This implied that regional abnormalities could represent areas of viable myocardium, and that correction of impaired perfusion could restore contractile function. Bodenheimer and colleagues [12] assessed the relationship between the epicardial ECG, histology and nitroglycerine induced improvement in contractility, and showed that regions which improved function with nitrates contained more viable myocytes than those which did not improve.

Early methods used to identify viability in areas of impaired function included nitroglycerine induced contractile reserve [13], post extra-systolic potentiation of function [14], and the absence of Q waves in patients with previous myocardial infarction[15]. With the advent of myocardial perfusion scintigraphy, a new perspective emerged. In 1979, Berger and colleagues showed that a resting injection of thallium-201 was useful for identifying viable myocardium in hypokinetic regions, although this study did not assess the potential to predict recovery of function after revascularization[16]. Since then imaging techniques such as positron emission tomography (PET) conventional radionuclide perfusion imaging, and stress echocardiography or magnetic resonance imaging (MRI) have all been assessed.

In 1982, Rahimtoola first proposed that resting dysfunction might be the result of persistent painless hypoperfusion which could be reversed by revascularization[17]. In spite of the supportive results of studies in the preceding decade, the concept did not initially attain widespread acceptance. He used the term "hibernating myocardium" to suggest that regional myocardial contractile function was down-regulated in order to redress imbalance of oxygen supply and demand in this setting. When Braunwald and Rutherford stressed the potential clinical importance of the phenomenon in 1986 [18], general support for the concept was achieved. Despite many recent studies the pathophysiology of hibernating myocardium remains unclear, and controversy persists whether reduced resting perfusion or repetitive episodes of stunning are responsible. It is likely that hibernating myocardium is not ischemic at rest [19], but that coronary flow reserve is reduced making it susceptible to repeated episodes of stunning [20].

In current literature the terms "viability" and "hibernation" are often used synonymously, but this approach is not ideal. "Viable myocardium" is relatively non-specific and might include anything from normal tissue to partial thickness infarction. Ischemia may or may not be superimposed. A simple definition for "hibernation" is viable, hypocontractile myocardium, supplied by a coronary vessel with a flow limiting stenosis, which improves function following revascularization. The final point, recovery of function, is the defining criterion. Therefore, the identification of viability must be followed by further steps to ensure that it is hibernating.

Imaging

Over almost two decades imaging techniques which identify hibernating myocardium have been refined and improved. The choice is rather diverse as no single technique simultaneously assesses all of the features of hibernation. Therefore while conventional radionuclide imaging provides information on perfusion together with cell viability, and PET assesses perfusion and metabolism, functional techniques such as echocardiography or MRI evaluate the functional reserve of poorly contractile regions unveiled when stimulated with inotropic agents. In this chapter we focus on the basis and relative merits of these methods.

Positron Emission Tomography

Positron emission tomography will be covered in more detail elsewhere in this book, but it bears mention in this chapter as it is perhaps the most accurate method of identifying viable and hibernating myocardium, and can predict both segmental and global recovery of function following revascularization.[21,22] Positron emitting radionuclides can be used to assess both perfusion and myocardial metabolism. Perfusion tracers include ^{82}Rb, ^{13}N ammonia, and ^{15}O labeled water. ^{82}Rb is a potassium analogue which is generator produced. It has a short half life (76s) and thus it allows repeated measurements of flow [23]. Myocardial extraction at high flow rates is reduced, and therefore the uptake/flow relationship becomes non-linear.

^{13}N ammonia is a widely used agent which yields excellent image quality and has a longer half life(10 min)[24]. Although flow is also underestimated at high rates, this effect is less pronounced. ^{15}O water has a short half life (20s) and because uptake and flow rates are linearly related, accurate assessment of perfusion can be performed [25].

The most widely used metabolic tracer is ^{18}F fluoro-deoxyglucose (FDG). This is a glucose analogue and regional uptake reflects myocardial glucose utilization [26]. In the fasting state free fatty acids are the preferred substrate but with ischemia or following a glucose load this preference switches to glucose [27]. Therefore normal or increased uptake of FDG is indicates the presence of viable myocardium. Most institutions use a glucose clamp in order to control serum glucose during FDG injection. The basis of the perfusion/metabolism PET protocol in identifying myocardial hibernation centres around the identification of regions of "mismatch", where hibernating territory displays impaired perfusion but normal or increased uptake of FDG, and myocardial scar shows impaired uptake of both the perfusion and metabolic tracers. This technique has been widely used, and studies report positive and negative predictive accuracy for the recovery of regional left ventricular dysfunction ranging from 72% to 95% and 75% to 100% respectively [28,29,30].

In addition the presence of FDG/perfusion mismatch predicts improvement in global left ventricular function after revascularization [28,31]. Besozzi and colleagues[32] assessing 56 patients found that the mean LVEF of patients with mismatch increased from 29 to 41% following coronary artery bypass surgery (CABG) whereas in patients without mismatch it fell from 43 to 39%. Moreover Di Carli and colleagues found that PET mismatch predicted improvement in patient symptoms and functional capacity following revascularization. The same study and that of Eitzmann and colleagues also suggested that patients with ischemic LV dysfunction and hibernation, identified by FDG/PET pre-operatively, had reduced mortality if treated surgically compared with those who remained on medical therapy alone.

Fatty acids are an important substrate for myocytes, and therefore analogues such as 1-^{11}C-palmitate have been developed [33]. Clearance of fatty acid tracers is related to beta-oxidation and diminished magnitude and rate of this clearance is consistent with myocardial ischemia. Difficulties arise however with variables such as serum free fatty acids, changes in substrate metabolism during and following ischemia, and back-diffusion of unaltered tracer into ischemic regions. 1-^{11}C-acetate is a marker of oxidative metabolism and uptake is not affected by the substrate environment[34]. As a metabolic tracer it has compared favorably with FDG and recent reports suggest that if it is also used as a marker of myocardial blood flow, the need for two separate tracers can be avoided[35].

Thallium-201

The use of thallium-201 for identifying myocardial viability and hibernation has been widely reported[36-38] and it was the first tracer technique to be used for this purpose. However it is disadvantaged by a number of properties such as a low energy X-ray emission and a long half life leading to appreciable radiation exposure to patients[39]. The tracer behaves as a potassium analogue and myocardial uptake depends upon regional flow and upon an intact sarcolemmal membrane to facilitate transport[40]. Therefore thallium provides information on both flow and cell viability. A simple rest/redistribution protocol underestimates the amount of viable myocardium present and therefore alternative protocols have been developed.

These include late imaging from 8 to 72 hours (after stress injection)[41,42] reinjection of tracer on the same day[43], a resting injection on a separate day or the adjunctive use of agents such as ribose[44] or nitrates[45]. Late imaging shows redistribution in up to 54%[46] of defects that are fixed 4 hours after stress injection. Reinjection identifies increased uptake in 49% of segments and nine studies using this technique had positive and negative predictive accuracies of 69% and 89% respectively for improvement of function after revascularization[47].

There are several different features of thallium scintigraphy which have been put forward as criteria for hibernation. The identification of stress induced perfusion abnormalities has not been predictive of functional recovery per se, therefore most recent studies have concentrated on resting image characteristics. The most widely reported criterion is simply the extent of regional thallium uptake. On quantitative analysis activity of more than 50% of maximum in hypokinetic segments has been used as a criterion but this threshold has been arbitrarily defined. A higher tracer uptake reflects higher proportion of muscle versus fibrous tissue, so thallium activity should be seen as part of a spectrum rather than a dichotomy in the identification of viability. Perroni-Fillardi and colleagues found a linear relationship between thallium uptake and the likelihood of functional recovery[48]. Receiver operating characteristic (ROC) curves have been used and the ideal uptake has ranged between 55 and 60%.[49,50,51]

Other aspects of thallium imaging have also been evaluated. Redistribution following resting injection has been reported as a marker of hibernation although several studies combine this criterion with resting uptake greater than 50%.[52] Ragosta and colleagues identified rest-redistribution in 58 of 141 severely asynergic segments, 34 of which improved function after CABG. Gunning and colleagues identified this phenomenon in only 26 of 145 severely impaired segments, and this criterion in isolation was found to have a specificity of 83% but sensitivity of 18%. Therefore rest-redistribution was a relatively uncommon observation but was highly predictive of improvement in function. Authors who compared regions with reverse-redistribution of thallium after stress injection with FDG uptake suggest that this too may be marker of hibernation.[53] However we identified this phenomenon in only 7 of 145 severely impaired segments, 5 of which improved function. Therefore this criterion, like rest redistribution, appears to be a specific but insensitive predictor of hibernation.

Using these criteria separately or in combination, studies have shown that thallium imaging can accurately predict both regional and global functional recovery. Reports on resting uptake with or without rest-redistribution show positive predictive accuracies for regional improvement ranging from 57 to 92% and negative predictive accuracies from 62 to 100%[54]. One study demonstrated that redistribution after resting injection of thallium was an adverse prognostic marker for patients with left ventricular dysfunction who remained on medical therapy alone[55]. The full prognostic importance of these and other imaging features has not yet been clarified by controlled studies. Therefore notwithstanding some of the disadvantages of this tracer, described above, thallium remains a valuable imaging tool for hibernation. Many potential substitutes have been assessed.

Technetium labeled tracers

Technetium-99m labeled tracers have advantages such as a shorter half-life with lower radiation load to the patient, a higher energy gamma emission which diminishes soft tissue attenuation, and the potential for ECG gated acquisition. The comparison between these agents and thallium has fuelled considerable debate. Of the technetium labeled agents the most widely reported is Tc-99m-sestamibi (MIBI) and head to head comparative studies have been performed. Some authors have found thallium to be superior to MIBI[56,57,58] in the identification of viability, while others have found the two tracers to be comparable[59]. Most studies have assessed viability rather than hibernation, some comparing the results with those of PET techniques or histology, and others comparing the relative uptake of MIBI and thallium after quantitative analysis. Kaufmann and colleagues using quantitative analysis of tracer activity found MIBI uptake to be comparable to thallium after a resting injection, even in severe perfusion defects. This contradicts the findings of others such as Maurea and colleagues who reported significantly lower MIBI uptake (67%) than thallium (72%) in regions with severely impaired regional ventricular function. It has been suggested that uptake of technetium labeled radionuclides is flow dependent and is therefore likely to be diminished in regions of low flow, whereas transport of thallium into myocytes relies upon both flow and the integrity of the sarcolemmal membrane. Thallium exhibits a greater degree of redistribution than MIBI although it has recently been suggested that the extent of MIBI redistribution has been underestimated[60]. The controversy regarding which is the superior marker for hibernation is likely to continue but the current balance of favor supports thallium. Notwithstanding this the sensitivity and specificity of MIBI for predicting functional recovery have been reported as high as 83% and 71% respectively so it is undeniably a useful radionuclide. As discussed in more detail below, concurrent use of nitrates to increase myocardial uptake improves it's value.

Tetrofosmin is a cationic diphosphine which has been recently developed. It is a retention agent and displays little redistribution. There is less experience using this agent in the identification of hibernation. Matsunari and colleagues found that it underestimated the amount of viable muscle when compared to thallium[61]. Another study showed that it was less sensitive than thallium (66% vs 76% respectively), and specificity was similarly low (49% vs 44%) in identifying hibernation. As the results of further investigations emerge it is expected that results for tetrofosmin will be similar to those reported for MIBI.

Nitrates and Other Adjuncts

As mentioned previously, a simple stress/redistribution thallium protocol underestimates the amount of viable myocardium and resting injection has improved the sensitivity of this technique. However both thallium and the technetium agents are still less sensitive that PET on resting injection alone and therefore additional agents have been used together with the tracers in order to augment myocardial uptake.

In regions of reduced tracer counts both thallium and MIBI activity have been improved using sublingual or intravenous nitrates.[62,63] Nitrate administration improves regional coronary blood flow. It is likely that coronary vasodilation leads to better tracer delivery to areas where perfusion is reduced, thereby enhancing uptake. Sciagra and colleagues showed that defect severity calculated from polar plots was lower using nitrate enhanced MIBI single photon emission computed tomography (SPECT) when compared with standard imaging and the identification of hibernating segments was improved[64]. Moreover Bisi and colleagues showed that the identification of nitrate induced perfusion changes per se predicted improvement in function after revascularization. It is likely these effects would also be applicable to tetrofosmin imaging.

Some believe that food intake following thallium injection reduces the degree of tracer redistribution as the rate of washout from the myocytes is increased. Wilson and colleagues demonstrated that glucose-insulin-potassium infusion given after thallium delivery resulted in a net decrease in regional myocardial activity [65]. However more recent studies contradict this finding. Tartagni and colleagues carried out simultaneous infusion of thallium, glucose and insulin and found that regional counts were increased when compared to thallium injection alone [66]. Similarly intravenous loading with glucose solution prior to rest thallium imaging improved thallium uptake in regions of previous myocardial infarction [67]. The use of glucose and insulin has not been applied to predicting functional recovery but it is probable that the sensitivity of standard tracer techniques would be improved.

An infusion of D-ribose increases stores of high energy phosphates such as 5-phosphoribosyl-1-pyrophosphate. Hegewald and Perlmutter [68] together with colleagues showed that an infusion of D-ribose after stress thallium imaging improved redistribution in up to 50% of segments. A more recent study showed that a bolus injection of D-ribose conferred little benefit on the identification of thallium redistribution. At present D-ribose is not widely used in clinical imaging and no data exists on the effects of an infusion on redistribution [69] after resting injection of thallium.

Therefore additional agents can be used to optimize identification of hibernation. At present the results seem best using nitrates which are easy to administer and readily available, and they should now become routinely incorporated into resting imaging protocols in clinical practice.

Recent Developments

The ideal imaging modality for myocardial hibernation should be able to accurately and simultaneously assess tissue viability, wall motion and regional perfusion. At present no technique fulfils this "gold standard" requirement. However gated tomography using radionuclide tracers adds another dimension to scintigraphic imaging techniques. Thallium is not ideally suited to gated tomography due to its low energy X-ray emission, whereas the Tc-99m labeled tracers have better physical characteristics for this purpose. Gated SPECT using both MIBI and tetrofosmin has been evaluated for measurement of left ventricular volumes and ejection fraction and results have been promising.[70,71] In addition studies have compared regional wall motion assessment by gated SPECT with more conventional techniques such as echocardiography or MRI.[72,73] In patients with normal left ventricular function and well maintained resting tracer uptake gated SPECT has agreed closely with MRI. However the assessment of regional wall motion and thickening is more difficult in territories which have previously suffered myocardial infarction, where counts are poor. As a consequence results for gated SPECT in patients with ischemic left ventricular dysfunction are not as good.

However, in identifying areas of myocardium with preserved viability and impaired wall motion, an inability to comment on regions of full thickness infarction should not prove a major limitation as these areas are unlikely to recover function. Therefore, in theory at least, gated SPECT should be suitable for detecting hibernation. In a recent study gated tetrofosmin SPECT using tetrofosmin was as sensitive as standard tetrofosmin SPECT coupled with MRI (62% vs 58%) [74]. These relatively low sensitivities could have been improved with the concurrent use of nitrates. Larger studies may well reveal the full potential of gated tomography.

PET has certain advantages over conventional radionuclide tomography (SPECT). Spatial resolution is higher (4-8mm vs 10mm) and the technique routinely corrects for soft tissue attenuation of counts. In addition radiation dosimetry is lower and studies may be repeated over short time intervals. The principal disadvantage is the low availability of PET in clinical centres and the expense of each study. A cyclotron is required for production of most of the tracers and this should be on-site or nearby as the agents have a relatively short half life. These limitations have stimulated the development of alternative ways of imaging radionuclides such as FDG. Standard imaging equipment can be modified with collimators designed for 511 keV SPECT, and early studies show that the correlation between SPECT and

PET using FDG to identify viable but hypokinetic myocardium is good.[75,76,77] On the whole the image quality with PET remains better. As this field develops SPECT protocols combining FDG with perfusion tracers such as MIBI or thallium are likely to provide a fairly comprehensive assessment of hibernating tissue providing information on viability, metabolism, in addition to stress and resting perfusion.

Other metabolic tracers suitable for conventional nuclear medicine facilities have also been developed. ^{123}I-iodopentadecanoic acid (IPPA) is a radiolabeled fatty acid fatty acid, and like ^{11}C-palmitate which is used in PET, clearance from the myocardium is dependent on beta-oxidation and is therefore a marker of intact metabolism[78]. It has compared favorably with FDG PET and thallium in identifying viability although more data on hibernation is awaited.[79,80] It is possible that the clearance rates might be influenced by variables such as serum free fatty acid levels. ^{123}I-methyl-IPPA(BMIPP) is a modified free fatty acid which is retained longer in the myocardium that other free fatty acid analogues and this makes it more suitable for SPECT. The full application of these tracers in hibernation assessment needs to be further assessed.

Inotropic Reserve and Myocardial Contractility

In hypokinetic areas of the left ventricle the improvement in regional contractility with inotropic stimulation descriminates between reversible and fixed functional impairment. Early methods of unveiling this functional reserve included administration of nitroglycerin, epinephrine [81], isopropterenol[82] or dipyridamole[83]. In addition the identification of improved wall motion following an extrasystole was also used. However dobutamine is currently the most widely used inotrope for this purpose. It is a synthetic cathecholamine which is positively inotropic at low doses (4-8 μ/kg/min) but this is mainifest as an increment in rate-pressure product only after infusion rates exceed about 10 μg/kg/min[84].

Studies have compared response to dobutamine with other techniques such as PET[85], both as a marker of viability and in predicting functional recovery[86,87]. The infusion of dobutamine has been combined with a number of imaging modalities including 2D transthoracic echocardiography (TTE), transesophageal echocardiography (TOE)[88] and cine MRI [89]. TTE is the most widely available technique and has the advantages of being inexpensive and relatively easy to perform. However in some patients the acoustic window is poor and the image quality suboptimal. Better spatial resolution is achieved with the other two techniques and MRI is particularly versatile because imaging may be carried out in any plane. This allows views to be aligned with the intrinsic axes of the left ventricle and it has the added advantage of providing better images of the apex than TTE or TOE.

The reported accuracy of dobutamine stress imaging in identifying myocardial viability and hibernation varies considerably. Infusion protocols vary. Some authors report the use of low doses (5-10 µg/kg/min) whereas others increment infusion rates starting with low doses and reaching 40 µg/kg/min[90]. The hemodynamic response stimulated when these higher doses are used can render ischemic regions of myocardium with reduced coronary reserve. The consequence of this is a reduction in contractility in that area and this is the principle behind diagnostic stress imaging for myocardial ischemia. Such changes may be evoked even at infusion rates as low as 10 µg/kg/min. However this may be used to good effect. The observation of functional improvement followed by deterioration in function has been referred to as the "biphasic response". It has been suggested that this increases the predictive power of dobutamine stress imaging in identifying hibernation[90].

A comparison of dobutamine TTE and FDG-PET demonstrated agreement in 76% of segments for myocardial viability[91]. Vanoverschelde and colleagues found that dobutamine TTE had a similar sensitivity to reinjection thallium SPECT in predicting functional recovery (75% vs 77%) but displayed higher specificity (86% vs 56%)[92]. It is difficult to combine all the data from different studies as the protocols vary. Nevertheless Bonow's cumulative analysis of information from available studies shows a positive predictive accuracy of 83% and a negative predictive accuracy of 81% for identifying hibernation. Baer and colleagues compared dobutamine cine MRI with FDG-PET with the results of PET being regarded as the frame of reference for viability. On this basis MRI had a sensitivity of 81% and a specificity of 95%. When the same group compared TOE with PET similar figures where obtained. These results suggest that dobutamine stress techniques have a broad predictive accuracy.

However a more recent comparison between MRI, thallium and tetrofosmin showed that in patients with severe left ventricular impairment, inotropic response to dobutamine was relatively insensitive but highly specific for hibernation. The converse applied to thallium which was sensitive but not specific. Gerber and colleagues showed that hibernating myocardium did not respond to inotropic stimulation in up to 25% of segments[93]. These findings showing reduced sensitivity of dobutamine techniques in severely impaired regions of myocardium may be a reflection of a delicate balance between reduced perfusion and function, where the supply-demand balance is breached even at low doses and the segment becomes ischemic. Recent studies indicate a discordance between the finding of rest thallium imaging and dobutamine stress techniques. Arnese and colleagues identified myocardial viability in 49 of 112 akinetic segments which showed no response to dobutamine[94]. Similarly Panza and colleagues demonstrated that 84% of 311 dysfunctional segments were deemed viable by thallium criteria but only 56% exhibited inotropic response[95]. If there is appreciable discordance between dobutamine and radionuclide imaging techniques for identifying hibernation, consideration has to be given to a suitable algorithm for clinical use where the two techniques can be combined in order to improve the diagnostic yield.

Hibernation Imaging and the Clinician

Despite much attention focused on various imaging techniques for identifying myocardial hibernation in medical literature, the place of this in a clinical strategy has not been as clearly defined as might be expected. Detection of hibernation is most important in patients where left ventricular performance is markedly reduced. Perhaps one reason for underutilization of imaging in this context is that the reported global ejection fraction changes following revascularization are often small,[96,97] and if this is regarded by clinicians as the only measure of successful intervention they are less likely to be influenced by hibernation studies. More importantly no randomised clinical trial has yet been carried out which compares medical and surgical treatment of patients with or without hibernation present. The only information available comes from non randomizd studies.

Di Carli and colleagues assessed the survival of 93 patients investigated with FDG-PET. The mean ejection fraction was 25%. Fifty patients remained on medical treatment alone and 43 underwent surgery. Follow-up was carried out over 14 months and the results showed that the highest mortality of 41% was identified in patients with PET mismatch (a marker for hibernation) on medical treatment only. The subgroup with hibernation who were revascularized had a much lower mortality of 12% and all deaths in this group occurred in the immediate post-operative period. This is in keeping with the expected high peri-operative mortality in patients with poor left ventricular function. Patients with no mismatch had lower overall mortality whether treated medically (9%) or surgically (6%). These findings are very similar to those reported by Eitzmann and colleagues in a similar study of 82 patients. Again the highest mortality was reported in the hibernation subgroup on medical therapy (33%) while in this report the lowest was in the hibernation subgroup who underwent surgery. These findings indicate the importance of detecting hibernation as a prognostic marker and reveal a need for early revascularization when it is found.

An improvement in regional and global left ventricular systolic function may not be the only worthwhile objective in revascularizing hibernating myocardium. Lee and colleagues found a reduction in non-fatal ischemic events if patients with hibernation underwent angioplasty or bypass grafting[98]. Gunning and colleagues showed that surgery in similar patients significantly improved symptoms whereas medical treatment did not.[96] Again no controlled study has assessed the place of these different treatment strategies but the evidence to date favours intervention where hibernating myocardium is identified.

Practical issues dictate the choice of imaging technique employed clinically. The availability of PET, MRI, radionuclide imaging and echocardiography varies between centres and the cost of investigations plays an increasingly important role. This applies particularly to PET which, although widely acclaimed as an accurate technique, is not widely available and is expensive. Echocardiography on the other hand is widely available, convenient and less expensive. There are many comparative studies which have attempted to identify the most accurate technique. In the clinical context the more specific techniques such as dobutamine stress imaging will identify the patient with a high likelihood of functional recovery, but have the disadvantage of a lower sensitivity. Therefore using this approach alone, a proportion of patients with potential for improvement in systolic function may not be put forward for revascularization. The converse may apply to the radionuclide techniques which are sensitive but relatively non-specific. If patients are revascularized on the basis of these images alone a proportion will fail to improve. Therefore the best strategy may involve a combination of these two techniques if PET is not available.

This approach is based on the currently available reports, most of which assess imaging techniques in predicting functional recovery. However if prospectively conducted studies in the future show that the identifying and revascularizing hibernating myocardium lowers the risk of future cardiac events and improves mortality even in the absence of an increment in systolic function, then the relative insensitivity of techniques such as thallium tomography may prove less limiting. In the current management of patients with coronary disease and left ventricular dysfunction, the evaluation of myocardial hibernation should play a pivotal role in determining medical or interventional treatment. There is a very real need for large controlled studies in this field to more clearly delineate correct clinical practice.

References

1. Cohn JN, Johnson GR, Shabeti R. et al. Ejection fraction, peak exercise oxygen consumption, cardiothoracic ratio, ventricular arrhythmias and plasma norepinephrine as determinants of prognosis in heart failure. The V-Heft VA Cooperative Studies Group. Circulation 1993;87: (6 Suppl):V5-16.
2. Parameshwar J, Keegan J, Sparrow J, Sutton GC, Poole-Wilson PA. Predictors of prognosis in severe chronic heart failure. Am Heaff J 1992;123:421-6.
3. Effects of enalapril on mortality in severe congestive heart failure. Results of the Cooperative North Scandinavian Enalapril Survival Study (CONSENSUS). The CONSENSUS Trial Study Group. N Eng J Med 1987;316:1429-35.
4. Pitt B, Segal R, Martinez FA, et al. Randomised trial of losartan versus captopril in patients over 65 with heart failure. (Evaluation of Losartan in the Elderly Study, ELITE). Lancet 1997;349;747-52.
5. Packer M, Bristow MR, Cohn JN, et al. The effect of carvedilol on morbidity and mortality in patients with chronic heart failure. U.S. Carved. Heart Failure Study Group. N Engl J Med 1996;334:1349-55.
6. Mock MB, Ringqvist I, Fisher LD, et al. Survival of medically treated patients in the coronary artery surgery study (CASS) registry. Circulation 1982;66:562-8.
7. Mickleborough LL, Maruyama H, Takagi Y, Mohamed S, Sun Z, Ebisuzaki L. Results of revascularisation in patients with severe leftventriculardysfunction. Circulation 1995;92 (9 Suppl):II73-9.
8. Luciani GB, Faggian G, Razzolini R, Livi U, Bortolotti U, Mazzucco A. Severe ischemic left ventricular failure: coronary operation or heart transplantation? Ann Thorac Surg 1993;55:719-23.
9. Chatterjee K, Swan HJ, Parmley, Sustaita H, Marcus HS, Matloff I. Influence of direct myocardial revascularization on left ventricular asynergy and function in patients with coronary artery disease. With and without previous myocardial infarction. Circulation 1973;47:276-86.
10. Bonchek LI, Rahimtoola SH, Chaitman BR, Rosch I, Anderson RP, Starr A. Vein graft occlusion. Immediate and late consequences and therapeutic implications. Circulation 1974;50(2 Suppl):II84-97.
11. Rees G, Bristow JD, Kremkau EL, et al. Influence of aortocoronary bypass surgery on left ventricular performance. N En.ql J Med 1971;284:1116-20.
12. Bodenheimer MM, Banka VS, Hermann GA, Trout RG, Pasdan H, Helfant RH. Reversible asynergy. Histopathologic and electrocardiographic correlations in patients with coronary artery disease. Circulation 1976;53:792-6.
13. McAnulty JH, Hattenhauer MT, Rosch J, Kloster FE, Rahimtoola SH. Improvement in left ventricular wall motion abnormalities after nitroglycerin. Circulation 1975:51:140-5.
14. Popio KA, Gorlin R, Bechtel D, Levine JA. Postextrasystolic potentiation as a predictor of potential myocardial viability: preoperative analyses compared with studies after coronary bypass surgery. Am J Cardiol 1977;39:944-53.
15. Banka VS, Bodenheimer MM, Helfant RH. Determinants of reversible asynergy. Effect of pathological Q waves, coronary collaterals, and anatomic location. Circulation 1974;50:714-9.
16. Berger BC, Watson DD, Burwell LR, et al. Redistribution of thallium at rest in patients with stable and unstable angina and the effect of coronary bypass surgery. Circulation 1979;60:1114-25.
17. Rahimtoola SH. Coronary bypass surgery for chronic angina - 1981. A perspective. Circulation 1982;65:225-41.

18. Braunwald E, Rutherford JD. Reversible ischemic left ventricular dysfunction evidence for the "hibernating myocardium". J Am Coll Cardiol 1986;8:1467-70.
19. Fedele FA, Gerwitz H, Capone RJ, Sharaf B, Most AS. Metabolic response to prolonged reduction of myocardial blood flow distal to a severe coronary artery stenosis. Circulation 1988;78:729-35.
20. Vanoverschelde J-LJ, Wijns W, Depre C, et al. Mechanisms of chronic regional postischemic dysfunction in humans: new insights from the study of non-infarcted collateral dependent myocardium. Circulation 1993;87: 1513-23.
21. Di Carli MF, Davidson M, Little R, et al. Value of metabolic imaging with positron emission tomography for evaluating prognosis in patients with coronary artery disease and left ventricular dysfunction. Am J Cardiol 1994;73:527-33.
22. Eitzman D, Al-Aouar Z, Kanter HL, et al. Clinical outcome of patients with advanced coronary artery disease after viability studies with positron emission tomography. J Am Coll Cardiol 1992;20:559-65.
23. Vom Dahl J, Muzik O, Wolfe ER Jr, Allman C, Hutchins G, Schwaiger M. Myocardial rubidium-82 tissue kinetics assessed by dynamic positron emission tomography as a marker of myocardial cell membrane integrity and viability. Circulation 1996;93:238-45.
24. Schwaiger M, Muzik O. Assessment of myocardial perfusion by positron emission tomography. Am J Cardiol 1991 ;67:35D-43D.
25. Lida H, Kanno I, Takahashi A, et al. Measurement of absolute myocardial blood flow with $H_2{}^{15}O$ and dynamic positron-emission tomography. Strategy for quantification in relation to the partial-volume effect. [published erratum appears in Circulation 1988;78:1078.] Circulation 1988;78:104-15.
26. Choi Y, Brunken RC, Hawkins RA, et al. Factors affecting myocardial 2-[F-18]fluoro-2-deoxy-D-glucose uptake in positron emission tomography studies of normal humans. Eur J Nucl Med 1993;20:308-18.
27. Camici P, Araujo LI, Spinks T, et al. Increased uptake of '5F-fluorodeoxyglucose in postischemic myocardium of patients with exercise-induced angina. Circulation 1986;74:81-8.
28. Lucignani G, Paolini G, Landoni C, et al. Presurgical identification of hibernating myocardium by combined use of technetium-99m hexakis 2-methoxyisobutylisonitrile single photon emission tomography and fluorine-18 fluoro-2-deoxy-D-glucose positron emission tomography in patients with coronary artery disease Eur J Nucl Med 1992; 19:874-81.
29. Gropler RJ, Geltman EM, Sampathkumaran K, et al. Comparison of carbon-11-acetate with fluorine-18-fluorodeoxyglucose for delineating viable myocardium by positron emission tomography. J Am Coll Cardiol 1993;22:1587-97.
30. Tamaki N, Ohtani H, Yamashita K, et al. Metabolic activity in the areas of new fill-in after thallium-201 reinjection: comparison with positron emission tomography using fluorine-18-deoxyglucose. J Nucl Med 1991;32:673-8.
31. Tillisch J, Brunken R, Marshall R, et al. Reversibility of cardiac wall-motion abnormalities predicted by positron tomography. N Engl J Med 1986;314:884-8.
32. Bessozi MC, Brown MD, Hubner KF, et al. Retrospective posttherapy evaluation of cardiac function in 208 coronary artery disease patients evaluated by positron emission tomography [abstract] J Nucl Med 1992;33:(5 Suppl):885.

33. Schelbert HR, Henze E, Sochor H, et al. Effects of substrate availability on myocardial C-11 palmitate kinetics by positron emission tomography in normal subjects and patients with ventricular dysfunction. Am Heart J 1986; 111:1055-64.
34. Brown MA, Myears DW, Bergmann SR. Validity of estimates of myocardial oxidative metabolism with carbon-11 acetate and positron emission tomography despite altered patterns of substrate utilization. J Nucl Med 1989;30:187-93.
35. Wolpers HG, Burchert W, van den Hoff J, et al. Assessment of myocardial viability by use of ^{11}C-acetate and positron emission tomography. Treshold criteria of reversible dysfunction. Circulation 1997;95:1417-24.
36. Mori T, Minamiji K, Kurogane H, Ogawa K, Yoshida Y. Rest injected thallium-201 imaging for assessing viability of severe asynergic regions. J Nucl Med 1991 ;32: 1718-24.
37. Ragosta M, Beller GA, Watson DD, Kaul S, Gimple LW. Quantitative planar rest-redistribution 201-Tl imaging in detection of myocardial viability and prediction of improvement in left ventricular function after coronary bypass surgery in patients with severely depressed left ventricular function. Circulation 1993;87:1630-41.
38. Ohtani H, Tamaki N, Yonekura Y, et al. Value of thallium-201 reinjection after delayed SPECT imaging for predicting reversible ischemia after coronary artery bypass grafting. Am J Cardiol 1990;66:394-9.
39. Kiat H, Maddahi J, Roy LT, et al. Comparison of technetium 99m methoxy isobutyl isonitrile with thallium 201 for evaluation of coronary artery disease by planar and tourographic methods. Am Heart J 1989; 117:1-11.
40. Pohost GM, Alpert NS, Ingwall JS, Strauss HW. Thallium redistribution: mechanisms and clinical utility. Semin Nucl Med 1980;10:70-93.
41. Kiat H, Berman DS, Maddahi J, et al. Late reversibility of tomographic myocardial thallium-201 defects: an accurate marker of myocardial viability. J Am Coll Cardiol 1988; 12:1456-63.
42. Kayden DS, Sigal S, Soufer R, Mattera I, Zaret BL, Wackers FJ. Thallium-201 for assessment of myocardial viability: quantitative comparison of 24 hour redistribution imaging with imaging after reinjection at rest. [published erratum appears in J Am Coll Cardiol 1991;19-1121] J Am Coll Cardiol 1991;18:1480-6.
43. Dilsizian V, Rocco TP, Freedman NM, Leon MB, Bonow RO. Enhanced detection of ischemic but viable myocardium by the reinjection of thallium after stress-redistribution imaging. N Engl J Med 1990;323:141-6.
44. Hegewald MG, Palac RT, Angello DA, Perlmutter NS, Wilson RA. Ribose infusion accelerates thallium redistribution with early imaging compared with late 24-hour imaging without ribose. J Am Coll Cardiol 1991;18:1671-81.
45. He ZX, Darcourt J, Guignier A, et al. Nitrates improve detection of ischemic but viable myocardium by thallium-201 reinjection SPECT. [published erratum appears in J Nucl Med 1993;34:1909]. J Nucl Med 1993;34:1472-7.
46. Bonow RO. The hibernating myocardium: implications for management of congestive heart failure. Am J Cardiol 1995;75:17A-25A.
47. Bonow RO. Identification of viable myocardium. Circulation 1996;94:2674-80.
48. Perrone-Filardi P, Pace L, Prastaro M, et al. Assessment of myocardial viability in patients with chronic coronary artery disease. Rest-4-hour-24-hour ^{201}Tl tomography versus dobutamine echocardiography Circulation 1996;94:2712-9.

49. Vanoverschelde JL, D'Hondt AM, Marwick T, et al. Head-to-head comparison of exercise-redistribution-reinjection thallium single-photon emission computed tomography and low dose dobutamine echocardiography for prediction of reversibility of chronic left ventricular ischemic dysfunction. J Am Coll Cardiol 1996;28:432-42.
50. Gunning MG, Knight CJ, Anagnostopoulos C, et al. Identification of hibernating myocardium: a comparison of Tl-201, Tc-99m tetrofosmin, and dobutamine cine. Magnetic resonance imaging [abstract] Heart 1996;75(Suppl 1):p.72.
51. Udelson JE, Coleman PS, Metherall J, et al. Predicting recovery of severe regional ventricular dysfunction. Comparison of resting scintigraphy with ^{201}Tl and ^{99m}Tc-sestamibi. Circulation 1994;89:2552-61.
52. Lomboy CT, Schulman DS, Grill HP, Flores HR, Orie JE, Granato JE. Rest-redistribution thallium-201 scintigraphy to determine myocardial viability early after myocardial infarction. J Am Coll Cardiol 1995;25:210-7.
53. Marin Neto JA, Dilsizian V, Arrighi JA, et al. Thallium reinjection demonstrates viable myocardium in regions with reverse redistribution. Circulation 1993;88:1736-45.
54. Maddahi J, Schelbert H, Brunken R, Di Carli M. Role of thallium-201 and PET imaging in evaluation of myocardial viability and management of patients with coronary artery disease and left ventricular dysfunction. J Nucl Med 1994;35:707-15.
55. Gioia G, Milan E, Giubbini R, De Pace N, Heo J, Iskandrian AS. Prognostic value of tomographic rest-redistribution thallium 201 imaging in medically treated patients with coronary artery disease and left ventricular dysfunction. J Nuc/ Cardiol 1996;3:150-6.
56. Cuocolo A, Pace L, Ricciardelli B, Chiariello M, Salvatore M. Identification of viable myocardium in patients with chronic coronary artery artery disease: comparison of thallium-201 scintigraphy with reinjection and technetium-99m methoxyisobutyl isonitrile. J Nucl Med 1992;33:505-11.
57. Maurea S, Cuocolo A, Pace L, et al. Rest injected thallium-201 redistribution and resting technetium-99m methoxyisobutylisonitrile uptake in coronary artery disease: relation to the severity or coronary artery stenosis. Eur J Nucl Med 1993;20:502-10.
58. Dilsizian V, Arrighi JA, Diodati JG, et al. Myocardial viability in patients with chronic coronary artery disease. Comparison of ^{99m}Tc-sestamibi with thallium reinjection and [^{18}F-] fluorodeoxyglucose. [published erratum appears in Circulation 1995;91:3026] Circulation 1994;89:578-87.
59. Kauffman GJ, Boyne TS, Watson DD, Smith WH, Beller GA. Comparison of rest thallium-201 imaging and rest technetium-99m sestamibi imaging for assesment of myocardial viability in patients with coronary artery disease and severe left ventricular dysfunction. J Am Coll Cardiol 1996;27:1592-7.
60. Maurea S, Cuocolo A, Soricelli A, et al. Myocardial viability index in chronic coronary artery disease: technetium-99m-methoxy isobutyl isonitrile redistribution. J Nucl Med 1995;36:1953-60.
61. Matsunari I, Fujino S, Taki J, et al. Myocardial viability assessment with technetium-99m-tetrofosmin and thallium-201 reinjection in coronary artery disease. J Nucl Med 1995;36:1961-7.
62. Bisi G, Sciagra R, Santoro GM, Rossi V, Fazzini PF. Technetium-99m-sestamibi imaging wiht nitrate infusion to detect viable hibernating myocardium and predict postrevascularization recovery. J Nucl Med 1995; 36:1994-2000.

63. Maurea S, Cuocolo A, Soricelli A, et al. Enhanced detection of viable myocardium by technetium-99m-MIBI imaging after nitrate administration in chronic coronary artery disease. J Nucl Med 1995;36:1945-52.
64. Sciagra R, Bisi G, Santoro GM, Agnolucci M, Zoccarato O, Fazzini PF. Influence of the assessment of defect severity and intravenous nitrate administration during tracer injection on the detection of viable hibernating myocardium with data-based quantitative technetium 99m-labeled sestamibi single photon emission computed tomography. J Nucl Cardiol 1996;3:221-30.
65. Wilson RA, Okada RD, Strauss HW, Pohost MG. Effect of glucose-insulin-potassium infusion on thallium myocardial clearance. Circulation 1983;68:203-9.
66. Tartagni F, Fallani F, Corbelli C, et al. Detecting hibernated myocardium with SPECT and thallium-glucose-insulin infusion. J Nucl Med 1995;36:1377-83.
67. Chiba H, Kusuoka H, Ohno J, Nishimura T. Glucose-loading thallium-201 myocardial SPECT. J Nucl Med 1997;38:573-7.
68. Perlmutter NS, Wilson RA, Angello DA, Palac RT, Lin J, Brown BG. Ribose facilitates thallium-201 redistribution in patients with coronary artery disease. J Nucl Med 1991;32: 193-200.
69. Gunning MG, Clunie G, Bradley J, Gupta NK, Bomanji JB, Ell PJ. Slow bolus injection of ribose in the identification of thallium-201 redistribution following combined adenosine/dynamic exercise stress. Eur Heart J 1996;17:1438-43.
70. DePuey EG, Nichols K, Dobrinsky C. Left ventricular ejection fraction assessed from gated technetium-99m-sestamibi SPECT. J Nucl Med 1993;34: 1871-6.
71. Mochizuki T, Murase K, Tanaka H, Kondoh T, Hamamoto K, Tanxe WN. Assessment of left ventricular volume using ECG-gated SPECT with technetium-99m-MIBI and technetium-99m-tetrofosmin. J Nucl Med 1997;38:53-7.
72. Gunning MG, Anagnostopoulos C, Davies G, Forbat SM, Ell PJ, Underwood SR. Gated technetium-99m-tetrofosmin SPECT and cine MRI to assess left ventricular contraction. J Nucl Med 1997;38:438-42.
73. Chua T, Kiat H, Germano G, et al. Gated technetium-99m sestamibi for simultaneous assessment of stress myocardial perfusion, postexercise regional ventricular function and myocardial viability. Correlation with echocardiography and rest thalliu-201 scintigraphy. J Am Coll Cardiol 1994;23:1107-14.
74. Gunning MG, Anagnostopoulos C, Davies G, et al. Gated Tc-99m tetrofosmin SPECT in the identification of myocardial hibernation: comparison with thallium-201 SPECT and cine magnetic resonance imaging. [abstract] Eur Heart J 1996:17(Abstract suppl):220.
75. Bax JJ, Cornel JH, Visser FC, et al. Prediction of recovery of myocardial dysfunction after revascularization. Comparison of fluorine-18 fluorodeoxyglucose/thallium-201 SPECT, thallium-201 stress-reinjection SPECT and dobutamine echocardiography. J Am Coll Cardiol 1996;28:558-64.
76. Bax JJ, Visser FC, Blanksma PK, et al. Comparison of myocardial uptake of fluorine-18-fluorodeoxyglucose imaged with PET and SPECT in dyssynergic myocardium. J Nucl Med 1996;37:1631-6.
77. Chen EQ, Macintyre WJ, Go RT, et al. Myocardial viability studies using fluorine-18-FDG SPECT: a comparison with fluorine-18-FDG PET. J Nucl Med 1997;38:582-6.
78. Reske SN. ^{123}I-phenylpentadecanoic acid as a tracer of cardiac free fatty acid metabolism. Experimental and clinical results. Eur Heart J 1985;6(suppl B):39-47.

79. Murray GL, Schad NC, Magill HL, Van der Zwaag R. Myocardial viability assessment with dynamic low-dose iodine-123-iodophenylpentadecanoic acid metabolic imaging: comparison with myocardial biopsy and reinjection SPECT thallium after myocardial infarction. J Nucl Med 1994;35(4 suppl):43S-48S.
80. Hansen CL. Preliminary report of an ongoing phase I/II dose range, safety and efficacy study of iodine-123-phenylpentadecanoic acid for the identification of viable myocardium. J Nucl Med 1994;35(4 suppl):38S-42S.
81. Horn HR, Teicholz LE, Cohn PF, Herman MV, Gorlin R. Augmentation of left ventricular contraction pattern in coronary artery disease by an inotropic catecholamine: the epinephrine ventriculogram. Circulation 1974;49:1063-71.
82. Hinnen ML, Kremkau EL, Kloster FE, Rosch J. Influence of isoproterenol on left ventricular function in coronary artery disease [abstract]. Circulation 1972;46(suppl 11):11-22.
83. Picano E, Marzuilo P, Gigli G. Identification of viable myocardium by dipyridamole-induced improvement in regional left ventricular function assessed by echocardiography in myocardial infarction and comparison with thallium scintigraphy at rest. Am J Cardiol 1992;70:703-10.
84. Tuttle RR, Pollock D, Todd G, MacDonald B, Tust R. Dusenberry W. The effect of dobutamine on cardiac oxygen balance, regional blood flow and infarction severity after coronary artery narrowings in dogs . Circ Res 1977;41:357-64.
85. Chan RK, Lee KJ, Calafiore P, Berlangieri SU, McKay WJ, Tonkin AM. Comparison of dobutamine echocardiography and positron emission tomography in patients with chronic ischemic left ventricular dysfunction. J Am Coll Cardiol 1996;27:1601-7.
86. La Canna G, Alfieri O, Giubbini R, Gargano M, Ferrari R, Visioli O. Echocardiography during infusion of dobutamine for identification of reversibly dysfunction in patients with chronic coronary artery disease. J Am Coll Cardiol 1994;23:617-26.
87. Cigarroa CG, deFilippi CR, Brickner E, Alvarez LG, Wait MA, Grayburn PA. Dobutamine stress echocardiography identifies hibernating myocardium and predicts recovery of left ventricular function after revascularization. Circulation 1993;88:430-6.
88. Baer FM, Voth E, Deutsch HJ, Schneider CA, Schicha H, Sechtem U. Assessment of viable myocardium by dobutamine transesophageal echocardiography and comparison with fluorine-18 fluorodeoxyglucose positron emission tomography. J Am Coll Cardiol 1994;24:343-53.
89. Baer FM, Voth E, Schneider CA, Theissen P, Schicha H, Sechtem U. Comparison of low-dose dobutamine-gradient echo magnetic resonance imaging and positron emission tomography with [^{18}F]fluorodeoxyglucose in patients with chronic coronary artery disease. A functional and morphological approach to the detection of residual myocardial viability. Circulation 1995;91:1006-15.
90. Afridi I, Kleinman NS, Raizner AE, Zoghbi WA. Dobutamine echocardiography in myocardial hibernation. Optimal dose and accuracy in predicting recovery of ventricular function after coronary angioplasty. Circulation 1995;91:663-70.
91. Sawada S, Elsner G, Segar DS, et al. Evaluation of patterns of perfusion and metabolism in dobutamine responsive myocardium. J Am Coll Cardiol 1997;29:55-61.

92. Gerber BL, Vanoverschelde JL, Bol A, et al. Myocardial blood flow, glucose uptake, and recruitment of inotropic reserve in chronic left ventricular ischemic dysfunction. Implications for the pathophysiology of chronic myocardial hibernation. Circulation 1996;94:651-9.
93. Arnese M, Cornel JH, Salustri A, et al. Prediction of improvement of regional left ventricular function after surgical revascularization. A comparison of low dose dobutamine echocardiography with 201Tl single-photon emission computed tomography. Circulation 1995;91:2748-52.
94. Panza JA, Dilsizian V, Laurienzo JM, Curici RV, Katsiyiannis PT. Relation between thallium uptake and contractile response to dobutamine. Implications regarding myocardial viability in patients with chronic coronary artery disease and left ventricular dysfunction. Circulation 1995;91:990-8.
95. Gunning MG, Chua TP, Harrington D, et al. Hibernating myocardium: clinical and functional response to revascularisation. Eur J Cardiothorac Surg 1997; 11:1105-12.
96. Nagueh SF, Vaduganathan P, Ali N, et al. Identification of hibernating myocardium: comparative accuracy of myocardial contrast echocardiography, rest-redistribution thallium-201 tomography and dobutamine echocardiography. J Am Coll Cardiol 1997;29:985-93.
97. Lee KS, Marwick TH, Cook SA, et al. Prognosis of patients with left ventricular dysfunction, with and without viable myocardium after myocardial inf arction. Relative efficacy of medical therapy and revascularization. Circulation 1994:90:2687-94.

Chapter 14

IMPROVEMENT OF LV FUNCTION BY A PET BASED REVASCULARIZATION STRATEGY: A PROSPECTIVE RANDOMIZED COMPARISON WITH SPECT

Hans-Marc J. Siebelink, Ad J. van Boven and Paul K. Blanksma

Introduction

Treatment of patients with coronary artery disease (CAD) and evidence of ischemia is an important clinical issue. Patients benefit from revascularization if viable or jeopardized myocardium is present. Various myocardial perfusion imaging techniques with different radioisotopes [thallium-201, ^{99m}Tc (technetium-99m)-sestamibi, ^{13}N (nitrogen-13)-ammonia, ^{18}F-fluoro-deoxyglucose (FDG)] have been proven to delineate myocardium that shows functional recovery after revascularization [1-9]. Dobutamine stress echocardiography is also used to detect myocardium that could benefit from revascularization [10]. However, for all these techniques varying numbers for sensitivity and specificity for recovery of left ventricular function are reported. This has also been demonstrated in a recent meta-analysis [11]. Stress/rest sestamibi single photon emission computed tomography (SPECT) imaging is a widely used technique to detect myocardial perfusion abnormalities. In revascularization strategies, sestamibi SPECT results are frequently used to demonstrate whether viable myocardium with stress induced ischemia is present. For prediction of recovery of left ventricular function good sensitivity and specificity have been reported [11]. Nitrogen-ammonia/FDG positron emission tomography (PET) myocardial perfusion imaging is used for detection of hibernating

Van der Wall et al. (eds.),
Advanced Imaging in Coronary Artery Disease, 237-247.

myocardium and/or stress induced ischemia. Since FDG imaging represents myocardial glucose metabolism, PET is thought to detect viability better than sestamibi SPECT. Moreover PET imaging has a higher resolution and higher energy emission voltage resulting in better image quality. However PET imaging is more expensive and is less widely available. Since both imaging modalities can predict recovery of left ventricular function the question remains whether in clinical practice revascularization strategies involving viability questions should be based on sestamibi SPECT or on nitrogen-ammonia/FDG PET imaging? Bax et al. showed in a meta-analysis that FDG PET imaging has a slightly better sensitivity and specificity than sestamibi SPECT [11]. Therefore, we hypothesized that a revascularization strategy based on PET improves left ventricular function and clinical outcome compared to sestamibi SPECT. To test this hypothesis we compared revascularization strategies based on nitrogen-ammonia/FDG PET to sestamibi SPECT imaging in a prospective randomized study. In addition we also hypothesized that revascularization decision based on PET is more cost effective than revascularization based on SPECT.

Methods

Patients

Patients with anginal complaints and/or objective evidence of myocardial ischemia underwent coronary angiography and ventriculography in our hospital for evaluation of CAD. Patients were asked to participate in our study if left ventricular wall motion abnormalities were present in the area supplied by a stenosed coronary artery. Furthermore a team consisting of cardiologists and thoracic surgeons had to be non-conclusive about viability in this particular area and because patients had no contraindications for revascularization, the amount of viable myocardium in the area with wall motion abnormalities determined the revascularization strategy [percutaneous transluminal coronary angioplasty (PTCA), coronary artery bypass surgery (CABG) or medical treatment]. Patients younger than 20 and older than 80 years, patients with unstable angina, and patients with recent (<4 weeks) myocardial infarction were excluded from the study. Patients hypersensitive to dipyridamole, patients on aminophylline medication and women with child-bearing potential were not included. Patients with non-cardiovascular life-threatening disease were also excluded. After written informed consent was obtained patients underwent history taking, physical examination and routine laboratory investigation.

Exercise Tolerance Test

A symptom-limited exercise tolerance test (ETT) was done on a bicycle ergometer using a 20 or 10 Watt increase per minute depending on the estimated pretest exercise capacity. Endpoints for bicycle exercise were either severe chest pain, severe fatigue, more than 0.3 mV ST-segment depression, significant hypotension, severe arrhythmias or the attainment of 85% of age predicted maximal heart rate.

Echocardiography

Two dimensional echocardiography was performed to assess wall motion score index (WMSI) for regional wall motion. Single or biplane images were obtained and stored on erasable optical disc. Then wall motion was scored by an independent observer using a 16-segment model and scoring: 1= hyper and normokinesis, 2 = hypokinesis, 3 = dyskinesis, 4 = akinesis [12]. WMSI was calculated as the summed score of at least 12 segments divided by the number of segments assessed. Using this method a number of 1 reflects normal wall motion and a number greater than 1 reflects some degree of wall motion abnormality.

SPECT imaging protocol

Patients were referred to the Nuclear Medicine Department for stress/rest sestamibi SPECT myocardial imaging using a 2 day protocol. For stress imaging infusion of dipyridamole (0.56 mg/kg body weight in 4 minutes) was done and 600 MBq of sestamibi was injected 8 minutes after start of dipyridamole infusion. After 60 minutes imaging was started. Rest imaging was done 60 minutes after 600 MBq of sestamibi was injected at rest. Imaging was performed using a single head gamma camera (Siemens Orbiter) equipped with a low energy high resolution collimator. A 15% window was set over the 140 KeV photon peak. Sixty-four projection images were obtained in supine position in a 180-degree arc imaging 20 seconds per view. All images were acquired on computer in a 64x64 matrix (word mode) and stored on optical disk. Images were reconstructed and corrected for uniformity and center-of-rotation offset. No attenuation or scatter correction was applied. Images were prefiltered with a two-dimensional Butterworth filter, with order equal to 6. The cut-off frequency was 0.5. After ramp-filtered back projection, slices of 2 pixels were generated. Slices were reorientated according to the anatomic axis of the heart. Reconstructed slices were displayed as short-axis slices and horizontal and vertical long-axis slices. Analysis was done using the ICON software. Unprocessed planar images were processed in cine format for evidence of significant patient motion or breast or diaphragmatic attenuation. None of the SPECT studies had defects that could potentially be explained as artifacts.

Displayed short-axis slices and horizontal and vertical long-axis slices were normalized to the hottest pixel and shown in colour scale for semiquantitative analysis. From short-axis slices a polar map for rest and stress was reconstructed. Images were analyzed by the consensus of two experienced readers and classified as having either a reversible defect (ischemia), a partially reversible defect (ischemia and scar) or a fixed defect (scar). A fixed defect was assumed when the lowest activity in the defect was smaller than 50% of maximum activity and did not recover more than 10%.

PET imaging protocol

Patients underwent dynamic nitrogen-ammonia rest, nitrogen-ammonia dipyridamole and FDG PET imaging using a one-day protocol. Imaging was done in supine position with a Siemens ECAT 951 positron camera measuring 31 planes simultaneously over 10.8 cm. Measured resolution of the system is 6 mm full width at half maximum. Data were automatically corrected for accidental coincidence and dead time. Patients were positioned with the help of a rectilinear scan. Photon attenuation was measured using a retractable external ring source filled with 68GE/68GA. Dynamic rest imaging was started at the time of injection of 370 MBq nitrogen-ammonia and was continued for 15 minutes (frames: 12x10 sec, 1x2 min, 1x4 min, 1x7 min). Dipyridamole stress testing (DST) was performed infusing dipyridamole (0.56 mg/kg body weight in 4 minutes). Stress imaging was started injecting 370 MBq nitrogen-ammonia 6 minutes after start of dipyridamole and imaging was continued for 15 minutes (frames: 12x10 sec, 1x2 min, 1x4 min, 1x7 min). Then myocardial glucose uptake was studied using FDG using the method of Krivokapic [13] and Ratib[14]. To stimulate FDG uptake patients were given 50 gram of glucose orally before the scanning procedure and in diabetic patients FDG imaging was done with hyperinsulinemic euglycemic glucose clamp technique [15]. FDG imaging was performed after injection 185 MBq of FDG and continued for 55 minutes (frames: 8x15 sec 4x30 sec, 1x1 min, 1x5 min, 1x10 min, 1x15 min, 1x20 min).

During PET imaging a 12 lead electrocardiogram, heart rate and blood pressure were continously monitored. The data of dipyridamole nitrogen-ammonia study and the FDG study were corrected for remaining activity by subtracting the last frame of the preceding study. Data processing and analysis for flow, metabolism, stress induced ischemia and nonviable myocardium were performed as described previously using a quantitative parametric polar map method [16]. Parametric polar maps of nitrogen-ammonia imaging were constructed using the perfusion model [17] and for

FDG using the Patlak analysis [13,14]. To assess stress induced ischemia (mismatch defect) and nonviable myocardium (match defect) ratio maps were calculated of the FDG study and the stress nitrogen-ammonia study. The calculated values in these polar maps were compared with the 95% confidence interval of a normal database consisting of normal volunteers. This resulted in mismatch and match polar maps where the amount of myocardium with stress induced ischemia and nonviable myocardium could be detected with 95% certainty.

Randomization and revascularization strategy

After PET and SPECT imaging were performed patients were randomized to use either PET or SPECT results for determination of revascularization strategy. Randomization was done independently by the trial coordination center on basis of sex, age and one-vessel or multivessel disease. For determination of revascularization strategy a blinded polar map was designed to display PET and SPECT results (figure 1).

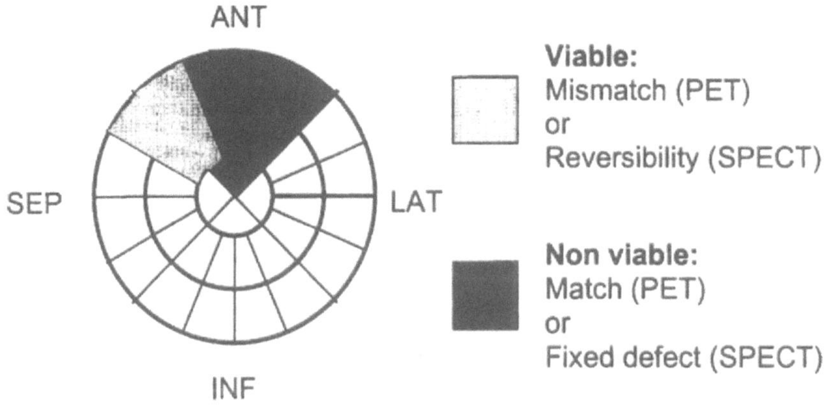

Figure 1. *Blinded PET result or SPECT result for revascularization strategy discussion*

Physicians from the Department of Nuclear Medicine displayed the areas with reversibility (complete reversibility or partial reversibility) and fixed defect detected with SPECT in the blinded polar map. The physicians from the PET center did the same for de PET results depicting mismatch and match defect in the blinded polar map. Then the polar map of the technique to which the patient was randomized was given to a team consisting of cardiologists and thoracic surgeons. The team discussed the results of the polar map together with the results obtained from coronary angiography and ventriculography to determine revascularization strategy. The team could decide to perform PTCA, CABG or to treat patient medically depending on the amount of viable myocardium present in the area with regional myocardial dysfunction.

Six months follow up
CABG and PTCA were performed as soon as possible in the regular schedule. Follow up visit was performed 6 months after patients received the selected treatment. Patients were seen at the outpatient clinic for history taking, recording adverse events, assessing physical situation and routine laboratory investigation. A symptom limited ETT and echocardiography for assessment of WMSI were again performed both using the same protocol as before treatment.

Two years follow up
Two years after receiving treatment follow up of all patients was performed. Information on cardiac events (death, myocardial infarction, re-intervention) was obtained by consulting the patients cardiologist and/or general practitioner. A flow chart of the study is shown in figure 2.

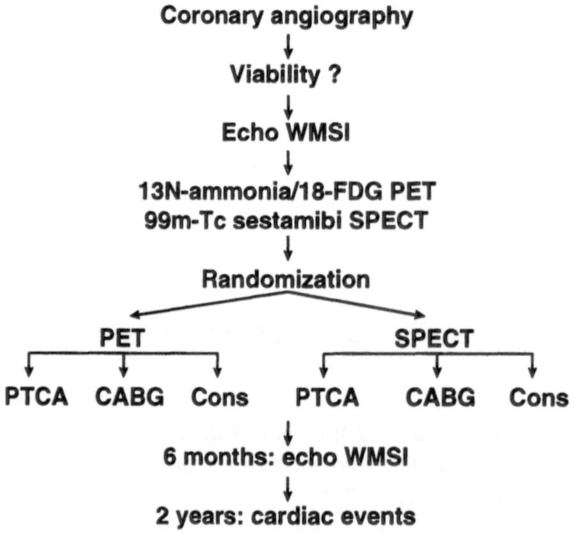

Figure 2. *Flow chart of the PET-SPECT study*

Statistics

Comparison of groups was done with a Student *t*-test, a paired Student *t*-test and Wilcoxon two sample test. For statistical analysis, a statistical package (SAS, version 6.12) was used.

Results

During a period of two and a half years 110 patients were included in the study. Baseline characteristics of the total population and of patients randomized to PET or SPECT for revascularization strategy are shown in table 1. There were no differences in baseline characteristics and medical history between the PET and SPECT group.

	Total population	PET	SPECT
Number of patients	110	54	56
Age	61.8	61.0 ± 1.5	62.6 ± 1.3
Sex	95 male	45 male	50 male
NYHA class	2.4	2.4 ± 0.1	2.5 ± 0.1
One Vessel Disease	29	15	14
Multi Vessel Disease	81	39	42
Previous myocardial infarction	97	47	50

Values are displayed as mean + SD or numbers.
NYHA: New York Heart Association class.
p=NS for comparison PET vs SPECT.

Table 1. *Baseline characteristics of total study population and subgroups*

An interim analysis of echocardiographic results of 40 patients was performed. Twenty patients were randomized to use PET for revascularization decision and 20 other patients to use SPECT. As for the 110 patients, in this subpopulation there were no significant differences in baseline characteristics and medical history. Both groups contained 18 male patients, mean age was 58±10 and 60±11 and there were 12 and 14 multivessel disease patients in the PET and SPECT group respectively. In the PET group 6 patients received PTCA, 4 patients CABG and 10 patients were treated medically. In the SPECT group 7 patients received PTCA, 4 patients CABG and 9 patients were treated medically. Baseline WMSI in the PET group was 1.66±0.45 and 1.54±0.36 in the SPECT group (p=NS). After 6 months WMSI in the PET group changed to 1.43±0.38 ($p<0.004$ compared to baseline) and in the SPECT group WMSI changed to 1.49±0.31 (p=NS compared to baseline). The change in WMSI in the PET group was significantly different from the SPECT group (p=0.04) (figure 3).

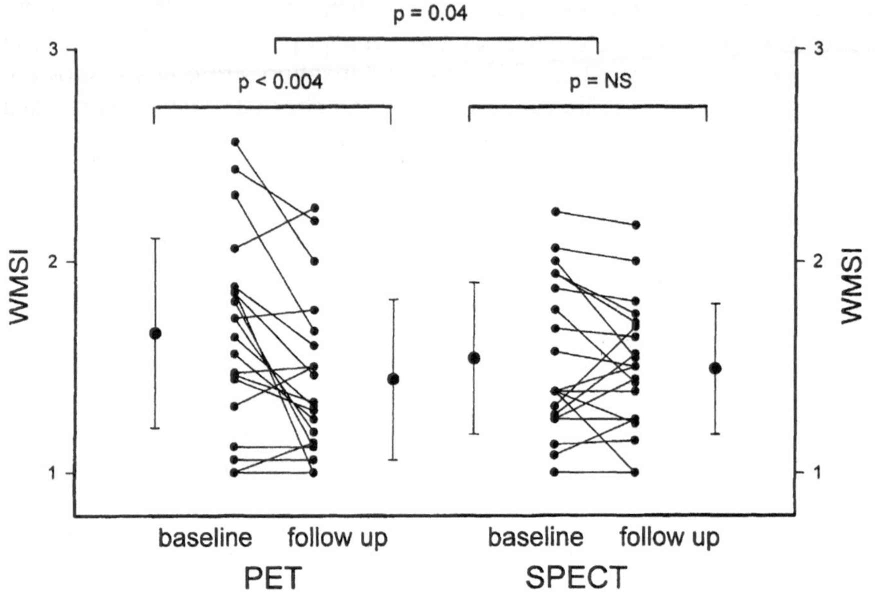

Figure 3. *Change in Wall Motion Score Index (WMSI) after 6 months in patients with revascularization strategy based on PET or SPECT*

Discussion

In CAD patients with left ventricular wall motion abnormalities and questionable viability the interim results of 40 patients show that the improvement in WMSI is more pronounced when the revascularization decision is based on PET results, as compared to the decision based on SPECT results. This suggests that for determination of revascularization strategy in patients with questionable viability nitrogen-ammonia/FDG PET is a better imaging modality than stress/rest sestamibi SPECT.

Both PET and SPECT imaging have been proven to predict recovery of left ventricular function after revascularization. However in a recent meta-analysis [11] different numbers for sensitivity and specificity are reported. Since PET imaging with FDG represents myocardial glucose metabolism, detection of myocardial viability is likely to be more accurate than with stress/rest sestamibi imaging. Moreover higher energy emission voltage, higher spatial resolution and attenuation correction of PET imaging result in favorable imaging properties compared to SPECT imaging. Soufer et al. compared sestamibi SPECT with ammonia/FDG PET and found that PET was more accurate in delineating viability in the inferior wall region[5]. The advantage of SPECT imaging above PET imaging is the wide availability and the considerably less costs. For determination of revascularization strategy, the advantages of PET imaging above SPECT imaging have not been proven to make a difference in the clinical situation since PET and SPECT imaging have not been compared in a randomized fashion for revascularization strategy. Tamaki et al. compared the use of rest-redistribution thallium-201 SPECT and FDG PET imaging for prediction of recovery of LV function. They concluded that FDG PET was a better predictor for future cardiac events than rest-redistribution Thallium-201 [1]. The reason we did not compare nitrogen-ammonia/FDG PET imaging to thallium-201 SPECT is that thallium-201 SPECT has lower overall accuracy than sestamibi.

The present study was designed to assess the value of PET imaging for determination of revascularization strategy in a prospective randomized clinical situation compared to conventional viability assessment with sestamibi SPECT imaging. The interim results suggest that in a selected population where strategy depends on presence or absence of viability a decision based on PET imaging results in a better recovery of left ventricular wall motion. However if this enhanced recovery of left ventricular wall motion is correlated with an improved clinical outcome for patients and if PET imaging is a cost-effective imaging modality needs further investigation. The results from the two years follow up will address these questions.

References

1. Tamaki N, Kawamoto M, Takahashi N, et al. Prognostic value of an increase in fuorine-18 deoxyglucose uptake in patients with myocardial infarction: comparison with stress thallium imaging. J Am Coll Cardiol 1993;22:1621-7
2. Knuuti MJ, Sarraste M, Nuutila P, et al. Myocardial viability: fluorine-18-deoxyglucose positron emission tomography in prediction of wall motion recovery after revascularization. Am Heart J 1994;127:785-96
3. Beller GA, Ragosta M, Watson DD, Gimple LW. Myocardial thallium-201 scintigraphy for assessment of viability in patients with severe left ventricular dysfunction. Am J Cardiol 1992;70:18E-22E.
4. Tillisch J, Brunken R, Marshall R, et al. Reversibility of cardiac wall motion abnormalities predicted by positron tomography. N Engl J Med 1986;314:884-8.
5. Soufer R, Dey HM, Ng CK, Zaret BL. Comparison of sestamibi single photon emission computed tomography with positron emission tomography for estimating left ventricular myocardial viability. Am J Cardiol 1995;75:1214-9.
6. Bax JJ, Cornel JH, Visser FC, et al. Prediction of improvement of contractile function in patients with ischemic ventricular dysfunction after revascularization by fluorine-18 fluorodeoxyglucose single photon emission Computed Tomography. J Am Coll Cardiol 1997;30:377-83.
7. Tamaki N, Ohanti H, Yamashita K, et al. Metabolic activity in the areas of new fill-in after thallium-201 reinjection: comparison with positron emission tomography using fluorine -18-deoxyglucose. J Nucl Med 1991;32:673-8.
8. Tamaki N, Kawamoto M, Tadamura E, et al. Prediction of reversible ischemia after revascularization. Perfusion and metabolic studies with positron emission tomography. Circulation 1995;91:1697-705.
9. Vom Dahl J, Eitzman DT, Al-Aouar ZR, et al. Relation of regional function, perfusion and metabolism in patients with advanced coronary artery disease undergoing surgical revascularization. Circulation 1994;90:2356-66.
10. Afridi I, Kleiman NS, Raizner AE, Zoghbi WA. Dobutamine echocardiography in myocardial hibernation. Optimal dose and accuracy in predicting recovery of ventricular function after coronary angioplasty. Circulation 1995;91:663-70.
11. Bax JJ, Wijns W, Cornel JH, Visser FC, Boersma E, Fioretti PM. Accuracy of currently available techniques for prediction of functional recovery after revascularization in patients with left ventricular dysfunction due to chronic coronary artery disease : comparison of pooled data. J Am Coll Cardiol 1997;30:1451-60.
12. Breekland A, Blanksma PK, Kengen RA, Pieper EG, Crijns HJ, Visser CA. Categorization of abnormal left ventricular function: comparison between radionuclide angiographic and echocardiographic technique in postinfarction patients. Am J Cardiol 1997;79:108-11.
13. Huang SC, Phelps ME, Hoffman EJ, Sideris K, Selin CJ, Kuhl DE. Noninvasive determination of local cerebral metabolic rate of glucose in man. Am J Physiol 1980;238:E69-82.
14. Ratib O, Phelps ME, Huang SC, Henze E, Selin CE, Schelbert HR. Positron tomography with deoxyglucose for estimating local myocardial glucose metabolism. J Nucl Med 1982;23:577-86.
15. Knuuti MJ, Nuutila P, Ruotsalainen U, et al. Euglycemic hyperinsulinemic clamp and oral glucose load in stimulating myocardial glucose utilization during positron emission tomography. J Nucl Med 1992;33:1255-62.

16. Blanksma PK, Willemsen AT, Meeder JG, et al. Quantitative myocardial mapping of perfusion and metabolism using parametric polar map displays in cardiac PET. J Nucl Med 1995;36:153-8.
17. Shelbert HR, Phelps ME, Huang SC, et al. N-13 ammonia as an indicator of myocardial blood flow. Circulation 1981;63:1259-72.

Chapter 15

FDG SPECT TO ASSESS MYOCARDIAL VIABILITY

Jeroen J. Bax, Frans C. Visser, Jan H. Cornel, Paolo M. Fioretti, Arthur van Lingen and Cees A. Visser

Introduction

Coronary revascularization may lead to improved regional and global LV function in patients with coronary artery disease and left ventricular (LV) dysfunction [1,2]. Rahimtoola introduced the concept of hibernation to explain reversal of contractile function after revascularization [3]. The asynergic but viable segments are likely to improve in contractile function, whereas the scarred segments will not improve. Reversibility of regional dyssynergy after revascularization can be predicted with positron emission tomography (PET) in combination with F18-fluorodeoxyglucose (FDG) [4-10]. In addition, FDG uptake has been imaged successfully with single photon emission computed tomography (SPECT) [11-13] and, more recently, we have demonstrated that FDG SPECT can also predict improvement of ventricular function after revascularization [14]. In the FDG PET studies and in the reports on FDG SPECT, the hallmark of viability was increased FDG uptake in areas of hypoperfusion (FDG-perfusion mismatch) [4-10,14,15].

Moreover, the finding of a FDG-perfusion mismatch was highly predictive of functional recovery after revascularization [4-10,14,15]. In addition, it has recently been shown that many segments with normal perfusion demonstrate improvement of function after revascularization [11]. The presence of concordantly reduced perfusion and FDG uptake (FDG-perfusion match) was highly predictive of absence of recovery [4-10,14,15]. In many other FDG

Van der Wall et al. (eds.),
Advanced Imaging in Coronary Artery Disease, 249-260.

PET studies a mild reduction in both perfusion and/or FDG uptake (mild match) was also considered as viable tissue [16-19]. In these studies however, functional outcome after revascularization was not studied. Recently, vom Dahl et al. [10] reported low predictive accuracy for functional recovery in segments with a mild match. The present study was designed to compare the predictive values for functional recovery of these different patterns of viability, including normal perfusion, FDG-perfusion mismatch, mild match and FDG-perfusion match.

Methods

Patients and Study Protocol

Twenty-one consecutive patients with regional dyssynergy on two-dimensional echocardiography, scheduled for revascularization, were included. Eight patients underwent a percutaneous transluminal coronary angioplasty (PTCA) and 13 patients underwent coronary artery bypass grafting (CABG). All patients had coronary angiography within 3 months before the SPECT study. Functional outcome data of 10 of these patients have been published previously [14]. Each patient underwent resting Tl-201 SPECT to evaluate regional perfusion, followed by FDG SPECT during hyperinsulinemic glucose clamping. Regional wall motion was evaluated with two-dimensional echocardiography before revascularization and repeated 3 months after revascularization. All patients gave informed consent to the study protocol that was approved by the Ethical Committees of The Free University Hospital Amsterdam and the Thorax Center Rotterdam.

SPECT Studies

The SPECT studies were performed with a dual head rotating gamma camera system (ADAC Laboratories, Milpitas, CA, USA). The method has been previously described in detail [11]. Briefly, resting perfusion was evaluated with thallium-201 chloride (111 MBq). Imaging was performed <15 min after tracer injection. Imaging was performed over 360°, with a total imaging time of 16 min. Data were stored in a 64x64, 16-bit matrix. For FDG SPECT the camera system was equipped with 511 keV-collimators (van Mullekom, Nuclear Fields, Boxmeer, The Netherlands) to detect 511 keV photons [20]. The FDG study was performed during hyperinsulinemic euglycemic glucose clamping, to optimize and standardize metabolic conditions [21]. Separate venous infusions of glucose and insulin were given; insulin infusion rate was 100 mU/kg/h and remained constant during the study. Normoglycemia was maintained by adapting the glucose infusion rate every 10 min, guided by the determination of the plasma glucose concentration. After 60 min of clamping, 185 MBq FDG was injected; 45 min later the SPECT images were obtained [22].

Reconstruction and Analysis of SPECT Images

Transaxial slices were reconstructed by filtered back projection using a Hanning filter (fc = 0.63 cycle/cm). Slices were not corrected for attenuation. Further reconstruction yielded long- and short-axis projections perpendicular to the heart-axis. Corresponding series of Tl-201 and FDG images (long and short-axis) were displayed side by side on a videoscreen. In addition, the Tl-201 and FDG short-axis images were presented in a polar map display with a quantitative color scale. The LV myocardium was divided into 9 segments: apical, 4 distal and 4 basal segments (anterior, lateral, inferior and septal). Two experienced observers visually interpreted the uptake of Tl-201 and FDG in each of the segments using a semi-quantitative scoring scale: 1=normal uptake, 2=mildly reduced uptake, 3=severely reduced uptake, 4=absent uptake, comparable to background activity.

Definition of Viability on FDG SPECT

Myocardial viability was assessed by comparing perfusion (assessed by resting Tl-201 SPECT) with FDG uptake (table 1).

Viability Classification	Perfusion Score	FDG Uptake Score
Normal	1	-*
Mild Match	2	2
Viable With Mismatch	2	1
	3	1,2
	4	1,2
Necrosis	3	3,4
	4	3,4

* in the segments with normal perfusion, the FDG score was considered irrelevant. FDG: F18-fluorodeoxyglucose.

Table 1. *Definition of viable myocardium according to the different patterns of perfusion and FDG uptake*

Pre-interventional wall motion was not considered in the assessment of viable myocardium. Normal myocardium was defined as normal Tl-201 uptake (normal perfusion) regardless of the FDG uptake. Viable myocardium was defined as described previously by Vom Dahl et al. [10]. Mildly reduced Tl-201 uptake (score 2) and mildly reduced FDG uptake (score 2) was considered viable myocardium without a mismatch pattern (mild match). Mildly or severely reduced or absent Tl-201 uptake (scores 2,3,4) with normal or mildly reduced FDG uptake (scores 1,2) was considered viable myocardium with a mismatch pattern. Severely reduced or absent Tl-201 uptake (scores 3,4) and severely reduced or absent FDG uptake (scores 3,4) was considered as necrotic tissue.

Regional Wall Motion Analysis

Two-dimensional echocardiograms were recorded in 4 standard views of the left ventricle (parasternal long- and short-axis, apical 2- and 4-chamber views) using standard equipment. Off-line analysis was performed by digitizing the videotaped images in a computer system (Prevue III, Nova-Microsonics, USA) using an ECG R-wave triggered mechanism. The stored images were displayed side-by-side in a cine-loop format on a quad-screen; thus, the baseline and follow-up images were displayed simultaneously in either one of 4 standard views. The left ventricle was divided into 9 segments, matching the SPECT segments. Wall motion was scored semi-quantitatively by 2 combined experienced observers who were blinded to the SPECT data. Each segment was scored as 0) normal (normal endocardial excursion and systolic wall thickening), 1) hypokinetic (reduced excursion and wall thickening), 2) akinetic (absence of excursion and wall thickening) or 3) dyskinetic (paradoxic outward movement in systole). A segment was considered improved if systolic thickening (either hypokinetic or normokinetic) became apparent in a segment that was a- or dyskinetic before revascularization, or if a hypokinetic segment returned to normal contraction after the intervention. Postoperative paradoxical wall motion has been described in the septal region [23]; for this reason special attention was paid to the endocardial thickening in these regions to study improvement after the revascularization.

Cardiac Catheterization

All patients had coronary arteriography and left ventriculography. Lesions >50% reduction in luminal cross-section diameter in 1 or more of the major coronary arteries were considered significant. The LV ejection fraction was calculated from the right anterior oblique view of the LV angiogram.

Statistical Analysis

All results are expressed as mean±SD. Patient data were compared using the Student's t-test for paired data. Comparison of proportions was performed using chi-square analysis. A p-value <0.05 was considered significant.

Results

Clinical Data

There were 19 men and 2 women with a mean age of 63±8 years (range 48-76). Eighteen patients had a previous myocardial infarction. Q waves were present on the ECG in 11 patients. Three patients were studied within one month after infarction, 15 had an infarction more than 1 month ago. They had a mean number of stenosed vessels of 2.3±0.8. The mean LV ejection fraction was 46±15% (range 13-67%). All were receiving cardiac medication, that was continued during the SPECT study. Three patients had diabetes mellitus type II, which was well-regulated on oral hypoglycemics; furthermore, using the clamping technique good image quality of cardiac FDG SPECT studies can be obtained in this subset of patients [24]. The mean time interval of the SPECT study to revascularization was 2.3±2.3 month (range 1 week - 9 months, 90% of patients ≤5 months).

Baseline Data

Of 189 segments that were analyzed initially, 10 (5%) segments that were not revascularized adequately, were excluded from further analysis. In these 10 segments, regional wall motion remained unchanged after revascularization. The baseline characteristics of the remaining 179 segments are presented in Table 2. Ninety-seven (54%) segments were classified as normal myocardium. The Tl-201 score was 1 and the FDG score was 1.08±0.27. Eighty-five (88%) of the segments classified by SPECT as normal myocardium had normal wall motion; the mean segmental WMS was 0.16±0.47. Sixty (34%) segments were classified as viable; 31 had a mismatch pattern (Tl-201 score 2.48±0.50, FDG score 1.42±0.49), whereas 29 segments did not have a mismatch pattern (Tl-201 score 2, FDG score 2). In the segments classified as viable without a mismatch, 12 segments had normal wall motion, and 17 had wall motion abnormalities. In the segments classified as viable with a mismatch, 10 were normokinetic and 21 had wall motion abnormalities. The segmental WMS was not significantly different between both groups with viable myocardium: 0.90±0.88 vs 1.06±0.84 (NS). Twenty-two (12%) segments were classified as non-viable (Tl-201 score 2.91±0.73, FDG score 3.27±0.45). Twenty (91%) of the non-viable segments had wall motion abnormalities; the segmental WMS was 1.55±0.72 (P<0.01 vs viable or normal myocardium).

	Perfusion	FDG uptake	WMS
Normal perfusion (n=97 segments)	1.0±0.0	1.08±0.27	016±0.47*
Mild match (n=29 segments)	2.0±0.0	2.0±0.0	0.90±0.88
Viable myocardium with mismatch (n=31 segments)	2.48±0.50	1.42±0.49	1.06±0.84
Necrotic myocardium (n=22 segments)	2.91±0.73	3.27±0.45	1.55±0.72*

* P<0.01 vs all other groups.
FDG: F18-fluorodeoxyglucose; WMS: wall motion score

Table 2. *Characteristics of all analyzed segments (n=179) at baseline*

SPECT Data Versus Functional Outcome

The mean change in segmental wall motion after revascularization of the different groups of segments (grouped according to their SPECT findings) is demonstrated in figure 1. In the segments with normal perfusion, the WMS decreased from 0.16±0.47 to 0.05±0.22 (P<0.01) after revascularization. In the mild match segments the WMS did not change significantly: 0.90±0.88 before vs 0.79±0.80 (NS) after the procedure, whereas in the viable segments with a mismatch pattern the WMS decreased significantly from 1.06±0.84 to 0.52±0.56 (P<0.05). In the non-viable segments the WMS remained unchanged: 1.55±0.72 vs 1.64±0.77 (NS). The outcome of dyssynergic segments (grouped according to their SPECT classification) is demonstrated in table 3 and figure 2. The pattern of normal perfusion on SPECT had a predictive value of 92% for improvement in regional wall motion after revascularization. The predictive values for improvement of viable segments with a mismatch pattern was 71% and for the mild match segments 23%. The pattern of necrotic myocardium showed a predictive value of 95% for absence of improvement after revascularization.

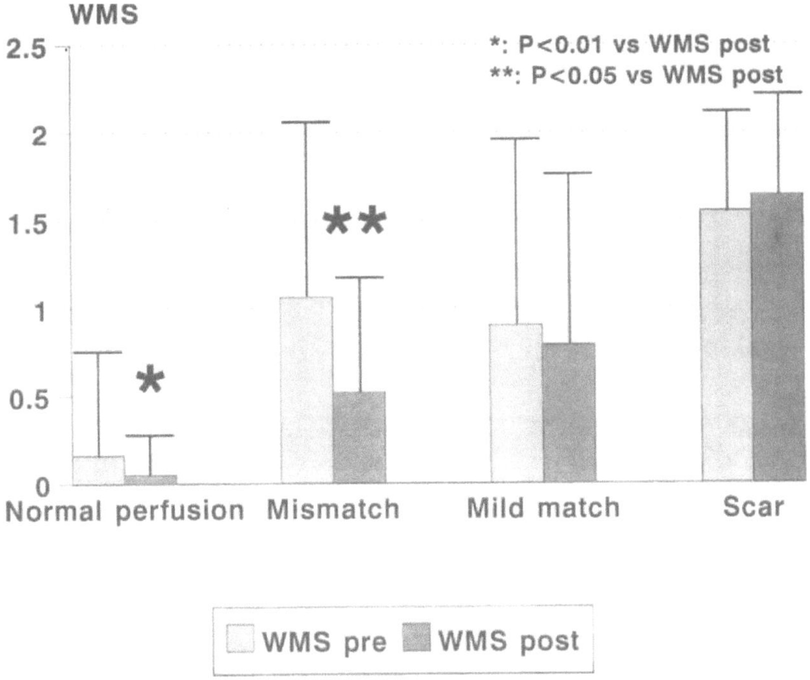

Figure 1. *The pre- and post-revascularization mean segmental wall motion scores according to tissue characterization on FDG SPECT*

Tissue characterization on SPECT	Improvement post-revasc	No improvement post-revasc
Normal perfusion (n=12 segments)	11 (92%)	1 (8%)
Mild match (n=17 segments)	4 (24%)	13 (76%)
Viable myocardium with mismatch (n=21 segments)	15 (71%)	6 (29%)
Necrotic myocardium (n=20 segments)	1 (5%)	19 (95%)

Post-revasc: post-revascularization

Table 3. *Outcome of dyssynergic segments (grouped according to tissue characterization on SPECT) after revascularization*

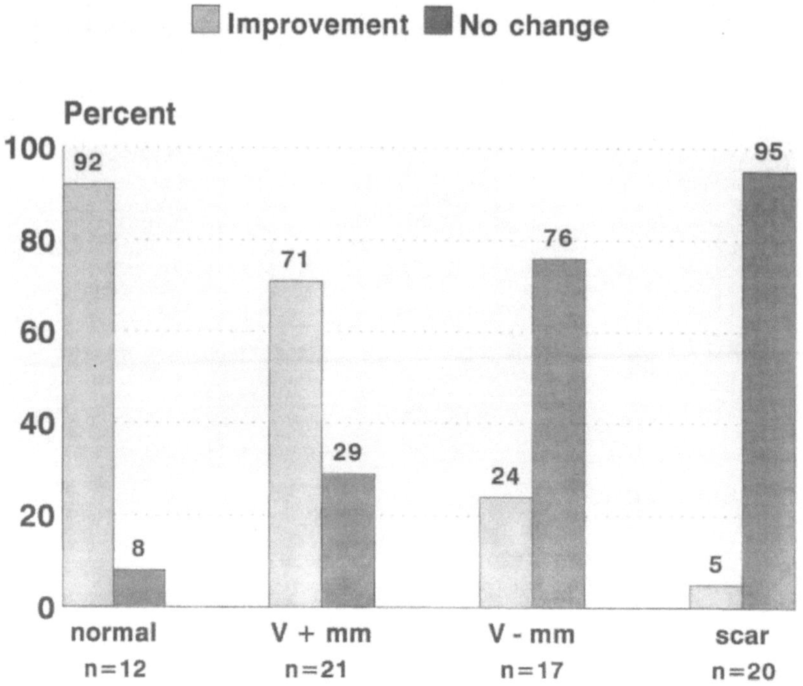

Figure 2. Number of segments with and without improvement after revascularization in the different subsets of segments. V+mm = mismatch segments; V-mm = mild match segments

Discussion

This study evaluated the use of FDG SPECT imaging to predict functional recovery in dyssynergic segments after revascularization using different criteria of viability. The presence of a FDG-perfusion mismatch pattern or normal perfusion had a high predictive value for functional recovery after revascularization, whereas segments with severely reduced perfusion and FDG uptake (consistent with necrotic tissue) had a high predictive value for absence of recovery. These findings confirmed earlier findings with FDG PET [4-10,15] and SPECT [14] in patients undergoing revascularization. In contrast to the viable myocardium with a mismatch, myocardium with a mild match showed a low predictive value for functional recovery.

Predictive Value of Different SPECT Patterns

It has been pointed out previously, that different conditions may lead to regional dyssynergy, including (repetitive) stunning, hibernation or scar formation due to infarction [25]. In transmural infarction the scar formation involves the entire myocardial wall, whereas in non-transmural infarction the scar formation is restricted the subendocardium or to localized parts of the myocardial wall. Improvement of contractile function after revascularization is unlikely in the situation of either transmural or non-transmural infarction. In transmural infarction, both perfusion and FDG uptake will be reduced throughout the entire myocardial wall, leading to severe perfusion defects associated with severely decreased FDG uptake on SPECT and consistent with absence of recovery in contractile function after revascularization, as demonstrated previously [4-10,14,15] and in the present study. In non-transmural infarction, with a mixture of scar and viable tissue, the reduction in perfusion and FDG uptake will be localized to certain parts of the myocardial wall. The spatial resolution of SPECT however, does not allow detection of these regions, resulting in a mild reduction of both perfusion and FDG uptake throughout the entire myocardial wall. Thus, the pattern of mild match may represent a situation after non-transmural infarction with a mixture of necrotic and viable myocytes. Revascularization of these regions will not lead to improvement of contractile function, as supported by the findings in the present study. Similar findings were reported by Vom Dahl et al[10] using FDG PET, showing poor predictive value for recovery of segments with a mild reduction in both perfusion and FDG uptake.

These findings have important clinical implications as the areas with a mild reduction in perfusion and FDG uptake are not likely to recover in function after revascularization, although they contain viable myocytes. Moreover, according to the severity of the reduction in perfusion and FDG uptake, Maddahi et al [15] suggested to divide "matched" defects into transmural and non-transmural matches. In previous studies using FDG [4-10,14,15] and in the present study, the presence of a mismatch pattern was predictive of recovery of contractile function after revascularization. The FDG-perfusion mismatch pattern is thought to indicate hibernating myocardium, which is defined as chronically reduced perfusion at rest, associated with regional dyssynergy, that can be improved after successful revascularization [1]. Although most of the patients in the present study had a myocardial infarction more than 1 month before the SPECT study, 3 patients were studied after a recent infarction. In these patients stunning (defined as reversibly impaired contractile function after ischemic events, in the absence of perfusion defects) may have been the cause of regional dyssynergy. [25] Moreover, 92% of segments without a perfusion defect, showed recovery of contractile function. Although the majority of segments with a mismatch pattern improved in function after revascularization, some segments did not improve. In this study vessel or graft patency was not determined after the procedure. Reocclusion may partly account for the failure of some mismatches to recover. In addition, although no patient suffered a peri-operative infarction, myocardial ischemia may have occurred during surgery, thereby affecting recovery after revascularization. Finally, Marwick et al [7] suggested that despite the increased FDG uptake, some segments may contain cells that are too severely injured to recover in function after revascularization.

Limitations

One limitation of the present study is the visual analysis of the images, using a semi-quantitative scoring system. Another limitation of this study is that we examined a selected population of patients referred for revascularization instead of an unselected group of patients. Finally, no quantitative data on improvement of LV ejection fraction as a measure of global ventricular function were obtained in this study. It was therefore not possible to correlate viability measured with FDG SPECT and improvement of global ventricular function.

Conclusions

The different patterns observed on FDG-perfusion imaging provide important information regarding outcome of regional myocardial dyssynergy after revascularization. A segment with severe reduction in both perfusion and FDG uptake represents necrotic tissue, which is not expected to recover in function. Conversely, a segment with a perfusion defect and increased FDG uptake represents compromised but viable myocardium, which is likely to improve in contractile function after revascularization. A mild perfusion defect with mildly decreased FDG uptake represents a mixture of viable and nonviable tissue, which has little chance to improve in contractile function after revascularization.

References

1. Brundage BH, Massie BM, Botvinick EH. Improved regional ventricular function after successful surgical revascularization. J Am Coll Cardiol 1984;3:902-8.
2. Dilsizian V, Bonow RO, Cannon RO 3rd, et al. The effect of coronary artery bypass grafting on left ventricular systolic function at rest: evidence for preoperative subclinical myocardial ischemia. Am J Cardiol 1988;61:1248-54.
3. Rahimtoola SH. The hibernating myocardium. Am Heart J 1989;117:211-3.
4. Tillisch J, Brunken R, Marshall R, et al. Reversibility of cardiac wall motion abnormalities predicted by positron tomography. N Engl J Med 1986; 314:884-8.
5. Tamaki N, Yonekura Y, Yamashita K, et al. Positron emission tomography using fluorine-18 deoxyglucose in evaluation of coronory artery bypass grafting. Am J Cardiol 1989;64:860-5.
6. Vanoverschelde JL, Wijns W, Depre C et al. Mechanisms of chronic regional postischemic dysfunction in humans. New insights from the study of noninfarcted collateral-dependent myocardium. Circulation 1993;87:1513-23.
7. Marwick TH, MacIntyre WJ, Lafont A, Nemec JJ, Salcedo EE. Metabolic responses of hibernating and infarcted myocardium to revascularization. A follow-up study of regional perfusion, and metabolism. Circulation 1992;85:1347-53.
8. Knuuti MJ, Nuutila P, Ruotsalainen U, et al. The value of quantitative analysis of glucose utilization in detection of myocardial viability by PET. J Nucl Med 1993;34:2068-75.
9. Maes A, Flameng W, Nuyts J, et al. Histological alterations in chronically hypoperfused myocardium. Correlation with PET findings. Circulation 1994;90:735-45.
10. Vom Dahl J, Eitzman DT, Al-Aouar ZR, et al. Relation of regional function, perfusion and metabolism in patients with advanced coronary artery disease undergoing surgical revascularization. Circulation 1994;90:2356-66.
11. Martin WH, Delbeke D, Patton JA, et al. FDG-SPECT: correlation with FDG-PET. J Nucl Med 1995;36:988-95.
12. Bax JJ, Visser FC, Blanksma PK et al. Comparison of myocardial uptake of fluorine 18-fluorodeoxyglucose imaged with PET and SPECT in dyssynergic myocardium. J Nucl Med 1996;37:1631-6.
13. Sandler MP, Videlefsky S, Delbeke D et al. Evaluation of myocardial ischemia using a rest metabolism/stress perfusion protocol with fluorine-18 deoxyglucose/technetium-99m MIBI and dual-isotope simultaneous-acquisition single-photon emission computed tomography. J Am Coll Cardiol 1995;26:870-8.
14. Bax JJ, Cornel JH, Visser FC et al. F18-fluorodeoxyglucose single-photon emission computed tomography predicts functional outcome of dyssynergic myocardium after surgical revascularization. J Nucl Cardiol 1997; 4: 302-8.
15. Maddahi J, Schelbert H, Brunken R, Di Carli M. Role of thallium-201 and PET imaging in evaluation of myocardial viability and management of patients with coronary artery disease and left ventricular function. J Nucl Med 1994;35:707-15.
16. Bonow RO, Dilsizian V, Cuocolo A, Bacharach SL. Identification of viable myocardium in patients with chronic coronary artery disease and left ventricular dysfunction. Comparison with thallium scintigraphy with reinjection and PET imaging with 18F-fluorodeoxyglucose. Circulation 1991;83:26-37.

17. Perrone-Filardi P, Bacharach SL, Dilsizian V, Maurea S, Frank JA, Bonow RO. Regional left ventricular wall thickening. Relation to regional uptake of 18-fluorodeoxyglucose and 201Tl in patients with chronic coronary artery disease and left ventricular dysfunction. Circulation 1992;86:1125-37.
18. Baer FM, Voth E, Deutsch HJ, Schneider CA, Schicha H, Sechtem U. Assessment of viable myocardium by dobutamine transesophageal echocardiography and comparison with fluorine-18 fluorodeoxyglucose positron emission tomography. J Am Coll Cardiol 1994;24:343-53.
19. Soufer R, Dey HM, Lawson AJ, Wackers FJ, Zaret BL. Relationship between reverse redistribution on planar thallium scintigraphy and regional myocardial viability: a correlative PET study. J Nucl Med 1995;36:180-7.
20. Van Lingen A, Huijgens PC, Visser FC, et al. Performance characteristics of a 511-keV collimator for imaging positron emitters with a standard gamma-camera. Eur J Nucl Med 1992;19:315-21.
21. Knuuti MJ, Nuutila P, Ruotsalainen U, et al. Euglycemic hyperinsulinemic clamp and oral glucose load in stimulating myocardial glucose utilization during positron emission tomography. J Nucl Med 1992;33:1255-62.
22. Phelps ME, Hoffman EJ, Selin C, et al. Investigation of [18F]2-fluoro-2-deoxyglucose for the measure of myocardial glucose metabolism. J Nucl Med 1978;19:1311-9.
23. Righetti A, Crawford MH, O'Rourke RA, Schelbert H, Daily PO, Ross J Jr. Interventricular septal motion and left ventricular function after coronary bypass surgery: evaluation with echocardiography and radionuclide angiography. Am J Cardiol 1977;39:372-7.
24. Bax JJ, Visser FC, van Lingen A, Raijmakers PG, Teule GJ, Visser CA. Image quality of F18-fluorodeoxyglucose SPECT studies in patients with coronary artery disease and diabetes mellitus type II [abstract]. Eur J Nucl Med 1994;21:824.
25. Bolli R. Myocardial "stunning" in man. Circulation 1992;86:1671-91.

Chapter 16

MYOCARDIAL ISCHEMIA IN HEART FAILURE: VALUE OF POSITRON EMISSION TOMOGRAPHY

Dirk J. van Veldhuisen, Ad F.M. van den Heuvel
and Maarten P. van den Berg

Introduction

Chronic heart failure (CHF) has become a major public health problem in the Western world and it constitutes one of the largest (cardiovascular) challenges for the next century [1]. In the majority of CHF patients, coronary artery disease is the underlying etiology, and in most of these patients, its progression leads to one or more myocardial infarctions, causing left ventricular (LV) dysfunction. In addition to irreversible myocardial damage, segmental (chronic) myocardial ischemia plays a role in this respect, as it may cause further ventricular dysfunction, often referred to as "myocardial hibernation" [2], which in turn may lead to another form of cell death or apoptosis [3].

Identification of these areas of non-contractile but viable myocardium is important, since they may recover after revascularization, leading to improved cardiac performance. Assessment of myocardial viability is possible with several techniques, including ^{201}Tl and ^{99m}Tc-sestamibi single photon emission computed tomography (SPECT), (dobutamine) stress echocardiography, and positron emission tomography (PET) [4], the latter being considered the gold standard [5]. There is thus convincing evidence that myocardial ischemia leads to impairment of myocardial relaxation and contraction.

Van der Wall et al. (eds.),
Advanced Imaging in Coronary Artery Disease, 261-271.

In recent years, evidence has accumulated, that a reverse relation may also be true, i.e. that LV dysfunction (and CHF) as such, may also lead to perfusion or flow impairment and ischemia, thus establishing a true reciprocal relation [6]. This is probably related to a number of changes, that take place in CHF, all leading to impairment of coronary blood flow and ischemia. First, endothelial function is impaired in several models of CHF and vascular disease [7,8], but also in patients with CHF due to idiopathic dilated cardiomyopathy [9]. Second, several plasma neurohormones, including norepinephrine, angiotensin II and endothelin, are increased in CHF, which cause vasoconstriction, including *coronary* vasoconstriction. Third, (compensatory) myocardial hypertrophy may occur in CHF which may lead to impairment of subendocardial perfusion during episodes of stress, such as exercise [10].

PET-imaging may be particularly suited to evaluate the presence of myocardial blood flow (MBF)- and MBF-reserve abnormalities and ischemia in patients with CHF. To examine this, we recently performed PET-imaging in a group of patients with CHF due to idiopathic dilated cardiomyopathy (IDC) [11], and in a group of patients with CHF due to coronary artery disease[12]; in addition, we examined the effect of cardiomyoplasty in patients with advanced CHF. In these patients, we related PET findings to parameters which reflect the severity of CHF, such as LV ejection fraction and peak oxygen consumption (Peak VO_2), and to LV stress [13].

In this paper we will discuss the various PET-techniques which may be used, and their potential value. In addition, the findings in the three patient groups discussed above will be reported.

Methods

Dynamic PET imaging permits noninvasive quantitation of MBF and metabolism, by using positron-emitting imaging tracers, taken up by the myocardium [14]. The technique we use in our institution has been described in detail recently [15,16]. MBF is estimated using nitrogen-ammonia as a perfusion tracer [17], both at rest and after infusion of a vasodilator such as adenosine or dipyridamole, to assess MBF-reserve.

Fluorine-18-fluorodeoxyglucose (FDG) is a positron-emitting metabolic imaging tracer, preferentially taken up by the myocardium which retains viability in the presence of severe ischemia. In these regions, metabolic function is maintained, even though myocardial blood flow is severely reduced. Simultaneous imaging with nitrogen-ammonia and FDG can demonstrate regions of "mismatch", where a reduced uptake of nitrogen-ammonia relative to maintained (or even increased) uptake of FDG is indicative of viable myocardium [18]. Indeed, in prospective studies, such mismatch patterns were found to be a good marker for the detection of myocardial ischemia [19].

In addition to these tracers, ^{11}C (Carbon-11)-acetate is used to quantitate myocardial oxidative metabolism. In normal myocardium, ^{11}C-acetate revealed monoexponential clearance of ^{11}C activity from myocardium after intravenous injection of ^{11}C-acetate [20]. Increased cardiac workload was associated with an increase in the ^{11}C clearance rate constant [21]. These characteristics make ^{11}C-acetate a useful tracer for clinical research to determine myocardial oxygen consumption.

Patient groups

A. Patients with chronic heart failure and idiopathic dilated cardiomyopathy[11].

We studied 19 patients with IDC, and they were compared to 19 age- and sex-matched healthy controls. All CHF patients had undergone left and right heart catheterization to assess the degree of coronary artery disease and to optimize the hemodynamic status. A diagnosis of IDC was made on the basis of clinical, laboratory and echocardiographic findings. In addition, coronary artery disease was excluded, and endomyocardial biopsy was performed in all patients to confirm the diagnosis. Patients were 32±4 years old, and all had mild to moderate CHF (New York Heart Association (NYHA) class II-III), mean LV ejection fraction by radionuclide ventriculography was 0.36±0.07 and mean peak VO_2 was 21±2 ml/min/kg.

At rest, MBF was similar between IDC patients and healthy volunteers (102±8 vs 102±6 ml/min/100g). In contrast, the increase in MBF after dipyridamole infusion was impaired in IDC patients (figure 1), with a consequent decrease in MBF-reserve (1.7±0.08 vs 2.7±0.04; $p<0.05$). This decrease in MBF-reserve correlated with the severity of heart failure, as assessed by LV ejection fraction ($r=+0.63$; $p=0.02$), and with peak VO_2 ($r=+0.5$, $p=0.04$). There was also a significant inverse correlation between MBF and wall stress, particularly after vasodilation ($p<0.01$). When perfusion and metabolism were related to each other, a mismatch pattern was observed in 80% of the IDC patients compared to none of the healthy volunteers ($p<0.05$). Further, the clearance rate of ^{11}C-acetate at rest and after dobutamine was not different from healthy volunteers, but in IDC, ^{11}C-acetate clearance (oxygen consumption) was significantly lower in regions with mismatch patterns ($r=-0.4$, $p<0.05$).

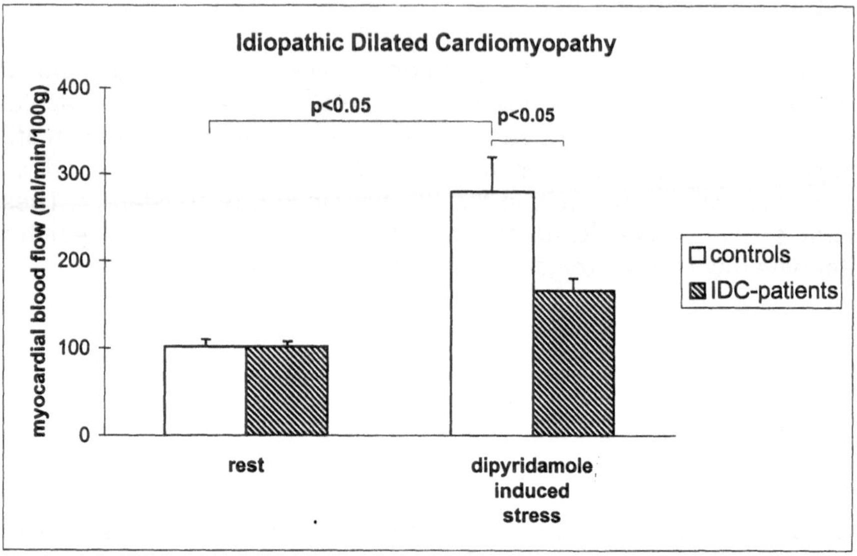

Figure 1. Myocardial blood flow at rest and after dipyridamole infusion (flow reserve) in patients with CHF and IDC and in controls (healthy volunteers)

It is concluded from this study in IDC patients, that MBF at rest is preserved, but that MBF-reserve is significantly impaired, and this impairment is related to the degree of LV-dysfunction and exercise impairment, and to ventricular wall-stress. When related to perfusion, both mismatch patterns and decreased oxygen consumption were found. These results suggest that, despite normal coronary artery anatomy, myocardial ischemia may play a role in IDC patients.

B. Patients with chronic heart failure and coronary artery disease [12].

In this protocol, 24 subjects were studied: 12 male patients with coronary artery disease and mild to moderate CHF, and 12 age-matched, male controls who had similar coronary disease but no CHF. Patients with CHF were 63±3 years old, and their mean LV ejection fraction was 0.34±0.02. Subjects in this protocol were therefore older than subjects in the IDC study.

MBF in *stenotic* (> 70%) arteries was normal at rest in both groups (normals and CHF), but MBF-reserve was significantly impaired in both groups (p= NS between the 2 groups). In *non-stenotic* (< 70%) coronary arteries, MBF was similar at rest in both groups. After dipyridamole, MBF increased in patients with normal LV function ("controls", although the increase was less pronounced than in healthy, and younger volunteers in the first protocol described above. The increase in MBF after dipyridamole infusion, however, was markedly impaired in patients with CHF (figure 2). MBF-reserve was therefore also markedly lower in patients with coronary artery disease and CHF (1.7 ± 0.06), as compared to those with coronary artery disease and normal LV function and no CHF (2.3 ± 0.05, p< 0.05). In CHF patients, MBF-reserve showed a significant relation (r=+0.6, p=0.03) with LVEF, but not with the severity of coronary narrowings. MBF-reserve impairment was also significantly related to ventricular wall stress in patients with CHF.

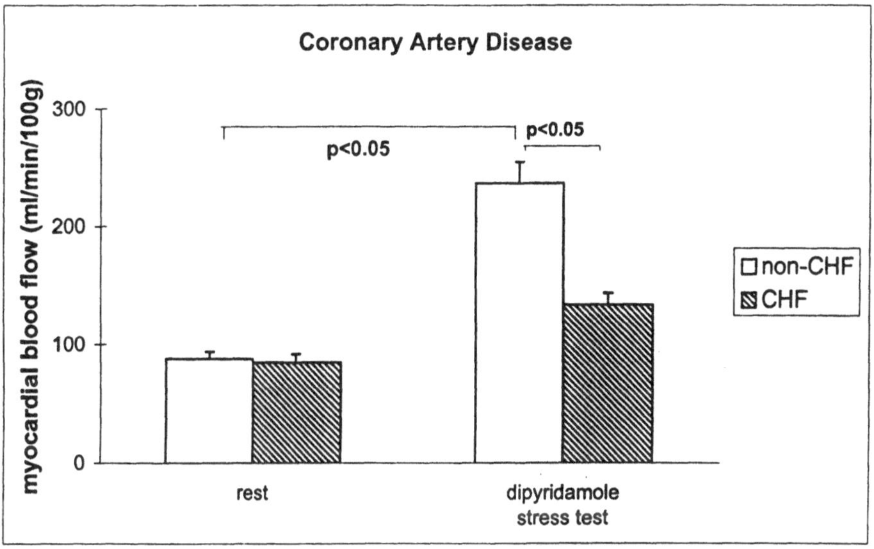

***Figure 2.** Myocardial blood flow at rest and after dipyridamole infusion in patients with coronary artery disease, measured in non-stenotic vessels and non-infarcted regions. A comparison in made between CHF patients, and patients with normal LV function (non-CHF)*

It was concluded from this study in patients with CHF and coronary artery disease, that MBF-reserve is impaired in the non-stenotic arteries, and that the degree of this impairment is related to the severity of the disease, but not to the severity of coronary stenosis. The findings regarding the relation ischemia and CHF of this study are thus comparable to the observations in patients with IDC.

C. Patients with advanced chronic heart failure, who underwent cardiomyoplasty.

Recently, we evaluated the effect of dynamic cardiomyoplasty on MBF and MBF-reserve as assessed by PET. Cardiomyoplasty was performed in our institution by using the technique of Carpentier et al [22], as previously reported [23]. We examined three patients with moderate to severe CHF, who were aged 54, 56, and 47 years old; their mean LV ejection fraction was 0.29, and their mean peak VO_2 was 14.0 ml/min/kg; all 3 were in NYHA functional class III-IV, despite optimal medication for CHF. At baseline, all three patients showed a markedly decreased MBF-reserve, which improved at 3 and 6 months after the procedure in two patients. Interestingly, the changes in PET parameters paralleled the clinical course of these patients.

Discussion

In most CHF patients, coronary artery disease is the underlying abnormality and besides *irreversible* myocardial damage, *reversible* damage caused by ischemia is an important factor in a large proportion of these patients [18,19]. It is now well established, that myocardial ischemia will lead to impairment of myocardial performance, but there is also increasing evidence that the reverse is true, and that LV dysfunction (and CHF) per se causes coronary perfusion abnormalities, and myocardial ischemia and hibernation, particularly after stress (such as pharmacologic interventions and exercise). In the present paper we reported three recent studies from our institution in which we examined MBF and its reserve (and myocardial metabolism) in patients with CHF. The data show that in patients with CHF, MBF-reserve is impaired and that this impairment is related to the severity of CHF and to left ventricular wall stress. Furthermore, improvement of cardiac function (by cardiomyoplasty) was found to partly reverse the abnormalities in MBF-reserve. Whether medical (drug) treatment will lead to a similar improvement in patients with LV dysfunction and CHF is currently unknown, but two such studies in which the effect of an ACE-inhibitor and a beta-blocker are examined, are currently ongoing in our institution.

In order to study abnormalities in MBF and its reserve, and to examine whether ischemia plays a role, IDC provides a "pure" model since the coronary arteries are by definition anatomically normal. In previous studies in patients with IDC, MBF abnormalities were also found, both at rest [24,25] and after administration of vasodilators [25,26]. In a similar study as the present, Neglia et al. [25] already showed MBF abnormalities in IDC patients who had no overt CHF, indicating that impairment of MBF occurs early in the disease. Further, one might speculate, that in combination with our findings, MBF abnormalities together with ischemia may be involved in the disease progression of CHF. In addition to this, we also showed that in patients with IDC, a substantial part of the myocardium showed a perfusion/metabolism mismatch, suggesting ischemia and/or hibernation. Since it has often been assumed that myocardial ischemia does not play a role in these patients, this latter finding is particularly interesting, and it supports earlier findings with ^{201}Tl scintigraphy in patients with IDC[27]. While IDC may present a "pure" model, patients with coronary artery disease and CHF obviously form a much larger population. The implications discussed above also hold for these patients, as long as non-infarct-related, non-stenotic vessels are studied, as is supported by our findings in such patients[12].

Potential explanations for impaired MBF reserve and ischemia in CHF

The regulation of MBF is complex, depending on coronary perfusion pressure, the presence of atherosclerotic narrowing, and/or vasomotor changes (including neurohumoral activation) in epicardial conduit vessels, the function of coronary microcirculation and extravascular forces, of which particularly intramyocardial pressure or wall stress plays an important role[10,28]. In CHF, several of these factors usually are involved. First, endothelial function is impaired in CHF, regardless of the underlying etiology of CHF in both patients with and without concomitant vascular disease [29].. Although the mechanism of this impairment is not completely understood, the balance between endothelium-derived relaxing and constricting factors is important in this respect.

Several explanations have been suggested, such as 1) alterations in endothelial cell surface receptors or abnormalities of postreceptor signal transduction; 2) abnormalities of endothelium-derived relaxing factor production or release; 3) rapid inactivation of endothelium-derived relaxing factor; 4) an increase in endothelium-derived contracting factor production and activity, as is observed in heart failure, and 5) other factors such as damaged endothelial cells due to exposure to viral infection, ethanol ingestion and/or oxygen-derived free radicals. A second important factor in CHF is the markedly increased (vasoconstrictive) plasma neurohormones, like (nor)epinephrine, angiotensin II, endothelin, and arginin-vasopressin etc. These neurohormones not only lead to (increased) coronary vasoconstriction, but they also have growth-promoting properties, leading to more structural vascular changes [30]. A third potential explanation for the occurrence of ischemia in CHF is the development of (compensatory) ventricular hypertrophy and elevated wall stress, which leads to an increased metabolic demand. Particularly in the subendocardium this may cause flow reserve impairment and ischemia [10].

Glucose metabolism (FDG) and oxygen consumption (^{11}C-acetate)

In areas where flow reserve (with nitrogen-ammonia) is impaired, a relative increase in FDG uptake (mismatch pattern) is generally considered to reflect myocardial ischemia [18,19]. This principle applies to patients with coronary artery disease, but we used it also in IDC patients. PET studies using FDG are mostly employed to assess myocardial viability, to predict recovery of regional contractility after coronary interventions, and it is also important in clinical decision making in such patients [31]. The impairment of MBF reserve in patients with IDC coincided with lower oxygen consumption (^{11}C-acetate washout) during dobutamine infusion. At rest, however, no abnormalities in MBF and oxygen consumption (^{11}C-acetate) were found. A decreased ^{11}C-acetate washout has been suggested to be of value in the differentiation between ischemic and non-ischemic myocardium [32], but studies on this issue are very scarse. Beanlands and Schwaiger [33] recently used this method in patients with IDC, in which they showed that myocardial oxygen consumption, as measured by ^{11}C-acetate washout (or kinetics), increased with dobutamine, while it decreased on nitroprusside. Given the importance of assessment of mycardial metabolism in patients with ischemia [34,35] and CHF, measurement of ^{11}C-acetate kinetics with PET will probably be of increasing value in CHF.

Clinical implications

Recently, there has been an increased awareness that both ischemia may play a role in patients who do not have (significant or obstructive) coronary artery disease [36], and that the condition of CHF per se may cause myocardial ischemia [6]. In this respect it is interesting to note, that a recent study in IDC, the beta-blocking agent metoprolol had a more favorable effect than the ACE-inhibitor captopril [37], which might indirectly also support the concept of the presence of ischemia in IDC. Further, it is tempting to speculate that the somewhat unexpected positive findings of both beta-blocking agents [38] and calcium antagonists [39] in patients with CHF due to IDC, as compared to those with coronary artery disease might also be related to their anti-ischemic effects.

References

1. Braunwald E. Shattuck lecture- Cardiovascular medicine at the turn of the millennium: triumphs, concerns, and opportunities. N Engl J Med 1997; 337: 1360-9.
2. Rahimtoola SH. The hibernating myocardium. Am Heart J 1989; 117: 211-21.
3. Chen C, Ma LJ, Linfert DR, et al. Myocardial cell death and apoptosis in hibernating myocardium. J Am Coll Cardiol 1997; 30: 1407-12.
4. Iskandrian AS, Heo J, Schelbert HR. Myocardial viability: methods of assessment and clinical relevance. Am Heart J 1996; 132: 1226-35.
5. Camici PG, Rosen SD. Does positron emission tomography contribute to the management of clinical cardiac problems? Eur Heart J 1996; 17: 174-81.
6. Van Veldhuisen DJ, Van den Heuvel AFM, Blanksma PK, Crijns HJGM. Ischemia and left ventricular dysfunction: a reciprocal relation? J Cardiovasc Pharmacol In press 1998.
7. Drexler H, Hayoz D, Munzel T, et al. Endothelial function in chronic congestive heart failure. Am J Cardiol 1992; 69: 1596-601.
8. Buikema H, Van Gilst WH, Van Veldhuisen DJ, et al. Endothelium dependent relaxation in two different models of chronic heart failure and the effect of ibopamine. Cardiovasc Res 1993; 27: 2118-24 .
9. Treasure CB, Vita JV, Cox DA, et al. Endothelium-dependent dilation of the coronary microvasculature is impaired in dilated cardiomyopathy. Circulation 1990; 83: 772-79.
10. Vatner SF, Shannon R, Hittinger L. Reduced subendocardial coronary reserve. A potential mechanism for impaired diastolic function in the hypertrophied and failing heart. Circulation 1990; 81(2 suppl): III8-14.
11. Van den Heuvel A, Van Veldhuisen DJ, Blanksma PK, et al. Correlation of myocardial perfusion, as assessed by positron emission tomography, and left ventricular ejection fraction and exercise tolerance in patients with idiopathic dilated cardiomyopathy [abstract]. Circulation 1997; 96(8 suppl): I-69.
12. Van den Heuvel AF, Van Veldhuisen DJ, Blanksma PK, Breekland A, Waalburg W, Crijns HJ. Myocardial blood flow reserve in patients with coronary artery disease as assessed by positron emission tomography: evidence for a disproportional impairment in heart failure [abstract]. Eur Heart J 1997; 18(abstr suppl): 406.
13. Reichek N, Wilson J, St John Sutton M, Plappert TA, Goldberg S, Hirshfeld JW. Noninvasive determination of left ventricular end-systolic stress: validation of the method and initial application. Circulation 1982; 65: 99-108.
14. Phelps ME, Mazziotta JC, Schelbert HR, editors. Positron emission tomography and autoradiography: principles and applications for the brain and the heart. New York: Raven Press, 1986.
15. Blanksma PK, Willemsen AT, Meeder JG, et al. Quantitative myocardial mapping of perfusion and metabolism using parametric polar map displays in cardiac PET. J Nucl Med 1995; 36: 153-8.
16. Hautvast RW, Blanksma PK, De Jongste MJ, et al. Effect of spinal cord stimulation on myocardial blood flow assessed by positron emission tomography in patients with refractory angina pectoris. Am J Cardiol 1996; 77: 462-7.
17. Schelbert HR, Phelps ME, Huang SC, et al. N-13 ammonia as an indicator of myocardial blood flow. Circulation 1981; 63: 1259-72.

18. Dilsizian V, Bonow RO. Current diagnostic techniques of assessing myocardial viability in patients with hibernating and stunned myocardium [published erratum appears in Circulation 1993;87:2070]. Circulation 1993; 87: 1-20.
19. Bonow RO, Dilsizian V, Cuocolo, A, Bacharach SL. Identification of viable myocardium in patients with chronic coronary artery disease and left ventricular dysfunction. Comparison of thallium scintigraphy with reinjection and PET imaging with ^{18}F-fluorodeoxyglucose. Circulation 1991; 83: 26-37 .
20. Armbrecht JJ, Buxton DB, Schelbert HR. Validation of [1-^{11}C] acetate as a tracer for noninvasive assessment of oxidative metabolism with positron emission tomography in normal, ischemic, postischemic, and hyperemic canine myocardium. Circulation 1990; 81: 1594-605.
21. Beanlands RS, Bach DS, Raylman R, et al. Acute effects of dobutamine on myocardial oxygen consumption and cardiac efficiency measured using carbon-11 acetate kinetics in patients with dilated cardiomyopathy. J Am Coll Cardiol 1993; 22: 1389-98.
22. Carpentier A, Chachques JC, Acar C, et al. Dynamic cardiomyoplasty at seven years. J Thorac Cardiovasc Surg 1993; 106: 42-54
23. Van den Berg MP, Brouwer MH, Wijnberg DS, Brügemann J, Van der Maaten JM, Ebels T. De eerste Groningse ervaringen met dynamische cardiomyoplastiek. Ned Tijdschr Geneeskd 1997; 141: 1480-4.
24. Parodi O, DeMaria R, Oltrona L, et al. Myocardial blood flow distribution in patients with ischemic heart disease or dilated cardiomyopathy undergoing heart transplantation. Circulation 1993; 88: 509-22.
25. Neglia D, Parodi O, Gallopin M, et al. Myocardial blood flow response to pacing tachycardia and to dipyridamole infusion in patients with dilated cardiomyopathy without overt heart failure. A quantitative assessment by positron emission tomography. Circulation 1995; 92: 796-804.
26. Inoue T, Sakai Y, Morooka S, et al. Coronary flow reserve in patients with dilated cardiomyopathy. Am Heart J 1993; 125: 93-8.
27. Doi YL, Chikamori T, Tukata J, et al. Prognostic value of thallium-201 perfusion defects in idiopathic dilated cardiomyopathy. Am J Cardiol 1991; 67: 188-93.
28. Maseri A, Crea F, Cianflone D. Myocardial ischemia caused by distal coronary vasoconstriction. Am J Cardiol 1992; 70: 1602-5.
29. Treasure CB, Alexander RW. The dysfunctional endothelium in heart failure. J Am Coll Cardiol 1993; 22 (4 Suppl A): 129A-134A.
30. Dzau VJ. Autocrine and paracrine mechanisms in the pathophysiology of heart failure. Am J Cardiol 1992; 70: 4C-11C.
31. Beanlands RSB, DeKemp RA, Smith S, Johansen H, Ruddy TD. F-18-fluorodeoxyglucose PET imaging alters clinical decision making in patients with impaired ventricular function. Am J Cardiol 1997; 79: 1092-5.
32. Wolpers HG, Burchert W, Van den Hoff J, Weinhardt R, Meyer GJ, Lichtlen PR. Assessment of myocardial viability by use of ^{11}C-acetate and positron emission tomography. Threshold criteria of reversible dysfunction. Circulation 1997; 95: 1417-24.
33. Beanlands RS, Schwaiger M. Changes in myocardial oxygen consumption and efficiency with heart failure therapy measured by ^{11}C acetate PET. Can J Cardiol 1995; 11: 293-300.
34. Opie LH. Effects of regional ischemia on metabolism of glucose and fatty acids. Relative rates of aerobic and anaerobic energy production during myocardial infarction and comparison with effects of anoxia. Circ Res 1976; 38(5 suppl 1): I52-74.

35. Camici P, Ferrannini E, Opie LH. Myocardial metabolism in ischemic heart disease: basic principles and application to imaging by positron emission tomography. Prog Cardiovasc Dis 1989; 32: 217-38.

36. Cannon RO 3rd. Does coronary endothelial dysfunction cause myocardial ischemia in the absence of obstructive coronary artery disease [editorial]. Circulation 1997; 96: 3251-4.

37. Jansson K, Karlberg KE, Nylander E, Karlsson E, Nyquist O, Dahlström U. More favourable haemodynamic effects from metoprolol than from captopril in patients with dilated cardiomyopathy. Eur Heart J 1997; 18: 1115-21.

38. A randomized trial of beta-blockade in heart failure. The Cardiac Insufficiency Bisoprolol Study (CIBIS). CIBIS Investigators and committees. Circulation 1994; 90: 1765-73.

39. Packer M, O'Connor CM, Ghali JK, et al. Effects of amlodipine on morbidity and mortality in severe chronic heart failure. Prospective Randomized Amlodipine Survival Evaluation Study Group. N Engl J Med 1996; 335: 1107-14.

Chapter 17

STUDY OF CARDIAC FUNCTION WITH PET OR SPECT

Guido Germano

Introduction

The measurement and knowledge of myocardial function is extremely important for the diagnostic and prognostic assessment of the cardiac patient. It is well known, for example, that the likelihood of 1-year survival after myocardial infarction is directly and exponentially proportional to the value of the resting left ventricular ejection fraction (LVEF) [1]. Measurement of myocardial function has traditionally been implemented with planar nuclear (first pass, gated blood pool) and planar non-nuclear techniques (echocardiography, contrast ventriculography), as well as, more recently, with tomographic nuclear (gated perfusion SPECT, gated blood pool SPECT, gated PET) and tomographic non-nuclear techniques (cine MRI, cine CT). Of all these techniques, only gated perfusion SPECT and PET offer the opportunity to simultaneously acquire information on both the perfusion and the function of the left ventricle, and to do it in three-dimensional and quantitative fashion. Since it is increasingly being reported that the knowledge of global LVEF provides incremental prognostic value over that of myocardial perfusion alone [2], gated perfusion SPECT and PET are likely to be increasingly utilized in this era of health care cost containment and emphasis on outcomes, and will represent the main focus of this chapter. The myocardial function parameters obtainable from gated perfusion SPECT and gated PET are LVEF, regional (segmental) myocardial wall motion and wall thickening. Before addressing each of them in detail, it is appropriate to briefly describe the acquisition of a gated SPECT or PET study.

Van der Wall et al. (eds.),
Advanced Imaging in Coronary Artery Disease, 273-287.

Gated acquisition

Standard SPECT and PET acquisitions are conceptually different in that SPECT involves acquiring a set of temporally consecutive, two-dimensional projection images parallel to the patient's axis, while PET acquires a set of simultaneous, contiguous two-dimensional "slices" perpendicular to the patient's axis. In practice, the end result is in both cases a three dimensional image set (often reoriented perpendicularly to the left ventricle's long axis[3,4]), whose reconstruction typically involves some filtering (smoothing) of the acquired data[5]. In gated acquisition, multiple three-dimensional image sets are generated, each corresponding to a different interval of the cardiac cycle.

In clinical practice, a gated acquisition is very similar to a non-gated acquisition in terms of injected activity (which is limited by target organ and whole body dose) and acquisition time (which is limited by the patient's ability to remain motionless, as well as by clinical throughput considerations). Counts collected at each acquisition angle (SPECT) or plane (PET) are divided amongst several images (typically 8 to 16), so it is inevitable for gated imaging to produce images of lower statistics, compared to standard imaging. This problem may be compounded by the presence of arrhythmias and heart rate variations, leading to the rejection of beats that cannot be reliably assigned to a specific interval. The relatively low statistical quality of gated images is partially obviated by the use of increased smoothing (lower cutoff filters) compared to standard imaging, before or during reconstruction. However, it is strongly recommended that myocardial perfusion be evaluated from the "ungated" or summed image set, and that this image set contain all counts from the gated acquisition plus all counts rejected (outside the cardiac beat length acceptance window). In other words, counts rejected during a gated acquisition should be accumulated in a "trashbin" frame, complete with their position information, and added to the other frames during creation of the ungated images.

It is the author's opinion that gated SPECT acquisitions can be performed using virtually all non-rapid washout perfusion agents in current clinical use, whether 99^{m}Tc-based agents or ^{201}Tl. Isotope half life limits gated PET to ^{18}F-FDG acquisitions, although gated blood pool PET using ^{15}-O carbon monoxide has been described[6]. Typical doses and acquisition times for gated perfusion SPECT and PET acquisitions are reported in table 1. Shorter acquisitions have been reported[7], but they are not routinely used at this time.

	Gated ^{99m}Tc SPECT	Gated ^{201}Tl SPECT	Gated ^{18}FDG PET
Injected dose [mCi]	25-30	3-3.5	5-10
Time/projection [sec]	25 (50)	35 (70)	N/A
# of projections (180°)	60 (30)	60 (30)	N/A
Total acquisition time [min]	25 (1-head) 12.5 (2-heads 90°) 16.7 (3-heads)	35 (1-head) 17.5 (2-heads 90°) 23.3 (3-heads)	~ 20

Table 1. *Acquisition parameters for gated SPECT and gated PET studies*

Quantitative LVEF measurement

Measurement of the global LVEF from gated SPECT or PET should be implemented by fully exploiting the three-dimensional nature of the tomographic datasets. In essence, this means estimating the location of the left ventricular endocardial surface and the valve plane in the three-dimensional space, followed by straight summation of the volumes of the voxels bound by these two structures. Techniques for the identification of the endocardial surface vary from threshold-based methods [8] to gradient-based approaches [9], to our own algorithm based on artificial intelligence combined with the Gaussian fitting of count profiles normal to the myocardium [10].

In all methods, once the boundaries of the LV cavity have been found for every gating interval, the largest (end-diastolic volume, EDV) and the smallest (end-systolic volume, ESV) volumes are taken to represent the end-diastolic and the end-systolic interval, respectively, and the LVEF is calculated with the standard formula:

$$LVEF = (EDV-ESV)/EDV * 100 \qquad (1)$$

All methods are likely to involve some error in the determination of the endocardial surface. This is a direct consequence of the relatively low resolution of tomographic nuclear images (~10 mm FWHM for PET, ~15 mm FWHM for SPECT) compared to the thickness of the myocardial wall (10-15 mm), as pointed out by Hoffman et al. [11]. Fortunately, the error is likely in the same direction at end-diastole and end-systole, and is therefore expected to be at least partially canceled out when the ratio volumes are taken in the calculation of the LVEF. LVEF values measured by the Cedars-Sinai Medical Center algorithm from gated SPECT images have been validated against first pass [10] and gated blood pool[12] at our institution, and against first pass [13], gated blood pool [14], 2-D echocardiography [15] and contrast ventriculography [16] at other sites (table 2). Validation of the LVEFs obtained applying the same algorithm to gated PET images is currently under way [17].

Author	# patients	"Gold standard"	r
Moriel (1993)	50	Gated blood pool	0.92
Germano (1995)	65	First pass	0.91
Di Leo (1997)	57	Contrast ventriculography	0.85
Everaert (1997)	40	Gated blood pool	0.93
He (1997)	15	First pass	0.87
Zanger (1997)	35	Echocardiography	0.79

Table 2. *Validation of Cedars-Sinai's quantitative gated SPECT LVEFs*

Figures 1 and 2 show the output of the Cedars-Sinai algorithm for a normal and an abnormal gated SPECT study, respectively. Algorithms for the quantitative measurement of LVEF should effectively deal with cases where large perfusion defects are present in the gated images.

This can be done either by precisely segmenting the LV myocardium in the initial phase of the algorithm (so that no thresholding is needed later), and/or by "patching" the defect area using gradient continuity constraints derived from the points immediately surrounding the defect [10].

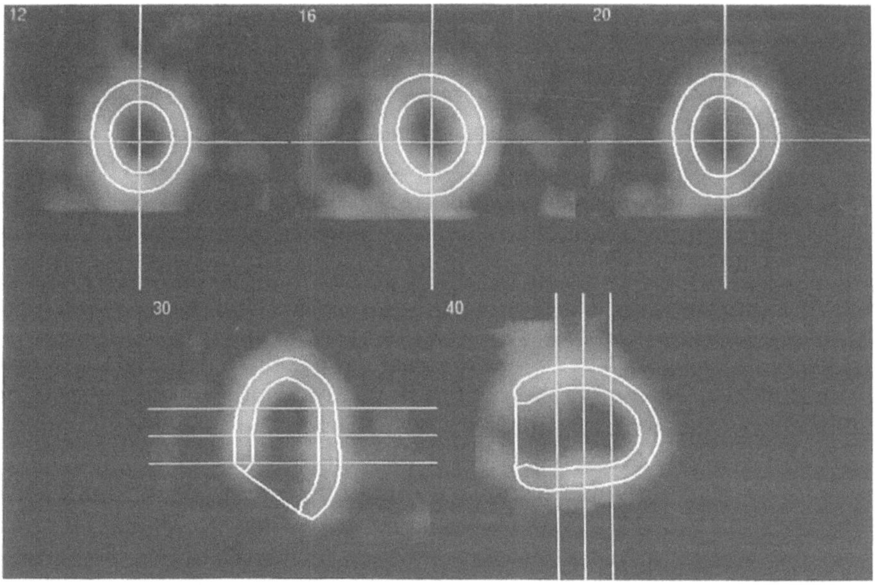

Figure 1. *Myocardial contours overlayed by the quantitative gated SPECT algorithm onto three short axis images (top row, left to right = apical, mid and basal), a mid-horizontal and a mid-vertical long axis image (bottom row) of a normal patient at end-diastole*

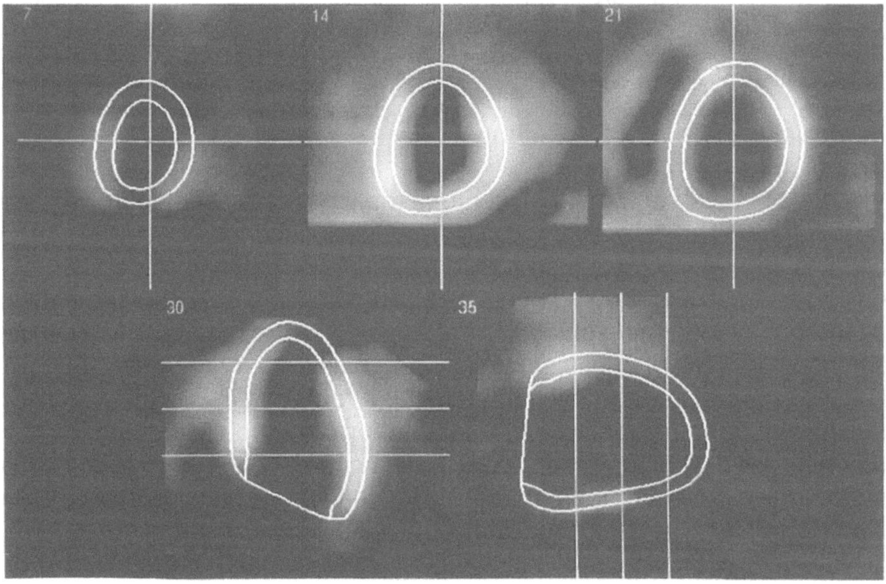

Figure 2. *Myocardial contours overlayed by the quantitative gated SPECT algorithm onto the end-diastolic tomographic images of a patient with severe and extensive left anterior descending coronary artery disease (CAD)*

An interesting question is whether 8- or 16-frames should be employed in gated acquisitions. It essentially depends on how accurately one wants to measure end-systolic volumes, since end-systole occupies a relatively shorter portion of the cardiac cycle compared to end-diastole. An 8-point time-volume curve will have somewhat reduced dynamic range compared to a 16-point curve, and will therefore result in generally lower LVEF values. On the other hand, 8-interval gated images have better count statistics, and it has been demonstrated for gated perfusion SPECT that the decrease in LVEFs is small (3-5 LVEF points) and remarkably uniform over a wide range of LVEFs [10].

It is the author's opinion that 8-frames gating (possibly with a systematic 3-5 LVEF points upward correction of the measured LVEF values) should be preferred for routine clinical use, with 16-frames gating reserved for special applications. In any event, it should not be expected for diastolic function to be accurately measurable from 16-frames gated acquisitions, as higher temporal sampling of the LV cavity volume curve is needed for that purpose. Measurements of absolute end-diastolic and end-systolic volumes are more error-prone than that of LVEF, as explained earlier. Nevertheless, validation of absolute volumes using our algorithm [15] as well as other techniques [18] has been reported for gated SPECT, and a transient ischemic dilation index based on the ratio of ungated post-stress volumes to ungated rest volumes has been demonstrated to be a highly specific and moderately sensitive marker of severe and extensive coronary artery disease [19].

Regional motion and thickening

Visual scoring of segmental myocardial motion and thickening from gated tomographic images is more complex than visual scoring of perfusion, and certainly less standardized. The Cedars-Sinai approach for gated SPECT employs a total of 20 LV segments, including 6 evenly-spaced segments in each of an apical, mid-ventricular and basal short axis slice, and 2 apical segments in a mid-ventricular vertical long axis slice [20]. The gated SPECT images are read in cinematic mode, using a "smoothed" cinematic display routine that performs real time 3-point temporal interpolation of the images (kernel = 0.5, 1, 0.5) to reduce noise. Wall motion is assessed based on the endocardial motion in a 256-tone gray scale display, and it is scored on a 6 point scale (0 = normal, 1 = mild hypokinesia, 2 = moderate hypokinesia, 3 = severe hypokinesia, 4 = akinesia, 5 = dyskinesia) in the 20 segments described above. Wall thickening is scored on a 5 point scale (0 = normal, 1 = mildly impaired, 2 = moderately impaired, 3 = severely impaired thickening, 4 = absent thickening), and it is based on the perceived myocardial wall "brightening" from diastole to systole [21] in the same 20 segments, using both the 256-tone gray scale and a 10-step color scale.

One of the most attractive features of gated nuclear imaging is that the perfusion and function data are acquired simultaneously, and are therefore intrinsically registered. This is a key helping feature in identifying myocardial segments with "mismatches" between perfusion and function. For example, normal thickening in a low-count region of the myocardium can improve the specificity of the perfusion SPECT study by correctly identifying, as an attenuation artefact, what perfusion analysis alone would misdiagnose as coronary artery disease [22].

Quantitative assessment of regional motion and thickening

Although quantitative methods for assessing regional wall motion and wall thickening have been derived for gated SPECT [18, 21, 23-27], and gated PET[28-31], none of these methods are completely automatic and none have reached widespread, practical clinical application. Also, on a practical basis, none of the routine clinical methods allow a truly three-dimensional assessment of regional ventricular function.

Our research group at Cedars-Sinai Medical Center has recently developed a totally automated method for the quantitative measurement of regional myocardial wall motion and thickening from gated SPECT images [32].

This method is similar to that developed and validated with respect to the automatic determination of LVEF [10], and it is based on the identification of three-dimensional endocardial and epicardial surfaces throughout the cardiac cycle. Regional motion is measured as the distance between a given point of the endocardial surface at end-diastole and end-systole. This distance is expressed in absolute terms (mm), and measured perpendicularly to the average mid-myocardial surface between end-diastole and end-systole, a modification of the "centerline" method [33] similar to that previously reported by other investigators [9]. Myocardial thickening is computed as the variation in thickness between end-diastole and end-systole, and expressed as the percent increase from diastolic thickness. Thickness measurements are derived taking into account both the distance between the endocardial and the epicardial surfaces (geometric approach) and the apparent increase in counts from end-diastole and end-systole due to the partial volume effect (count approach) [32].

Correlation of quantitative to visual segmental function was performed by first extracting motion and thickening circumferential profiles from the end-diastolic and end-systolic images of each patient, and combining such profiles in "raw" motion and thickening polar maps similar to those previously described by our group for perfusion analysis [34]. Then, both polar maps were divided into 20 sections corresponding to the same six basal, six mid-ventricular, six apical short axis segments and two apical long axis segments used for visual assessment, and the average quantitative motion and thickening in each section calculated [35]. Unlike standard clinical reading, in which motion and thickening estimates are correlated and combined with perfusion assessment to yield a coherent final interpretation serving a diagnostic or prognostic goal, in this study motion and thickening assessment was conducted independently and with the primary goal of comparing it to the automatic software assessment. Thus, visual scoring of wall motion was based exclusively on endocardial motion, while visual scoring of wall thickening was based on the brightening of the entire myocardium. In the case of perceived absent radionuclide uptake in a segment, that segment was, by definition, defined to be akinetic.

The algorithm has been validated in 79 clinical patients, in all of which it executed successfully (success was defined as the generation of endocardial and epicardial contours that matched the contours visually apparent in the images). Figure 3 compares visual motion scores and quantitative absolute motion in the 79 patients' 1580 individual myocardial segments. In particular, the mean values and the standard deviations of quantitative absolute motion in the 1125, 139, 156, 82, 43 and 35 segments with visual motion scores of 0, 1, 2, 3, 4 and 5, respectively, are displayed. Regression analysis performed on these means shows excellent agreement ($y = 6.57-1.30x$, $r = 0.975$, SEE = 0.61 mm) between visual and quantitative assessment. Figure 4 compares visual thickening scores and quantitative percent thickening in the same 1580 individual myocardial segments. Regression analysis performed on the mean values of quantitative percent thickening in the 1296, 96, 101, 43 and 44 segments with visual thickening scores of 0, 1, 2, 3 and 4, respectively, shows extremely good agreement ($y=37.98-8.90x$, $r=0.951$, SEE.=5.25%) between visual and quantitative assessment.

Figure 5 shows one of the three-dimensional displays used for the assessment of regional motion with our approach. In this display, the endocardial surface's location at end-diastole is presented as a fixed grid, while its location throughout the cardiac cycle is given by a pulsating (cine) shaded surface.

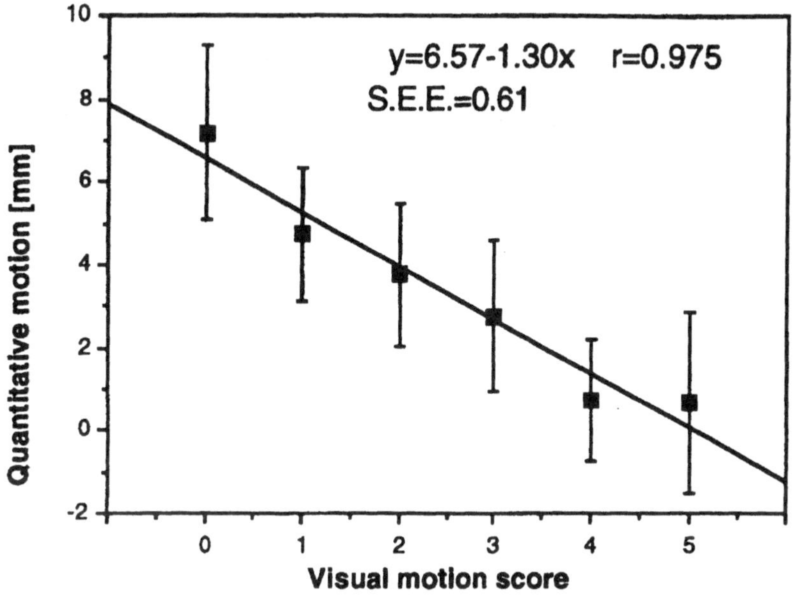

Figure 3. Correlation between visual and quantitative motion in 1580 segments

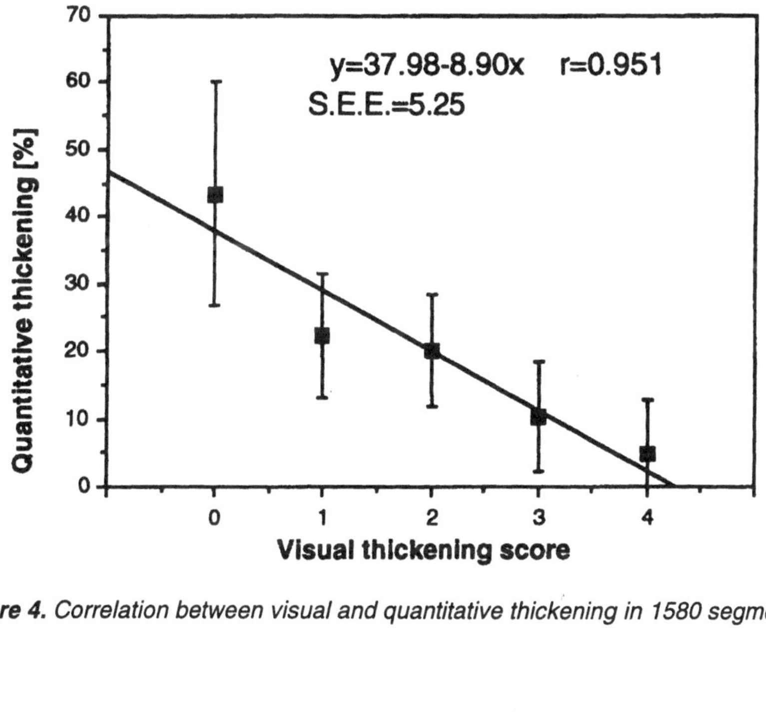

Figure 4. Correlation between visual and quantitative thickening in 1580 segments

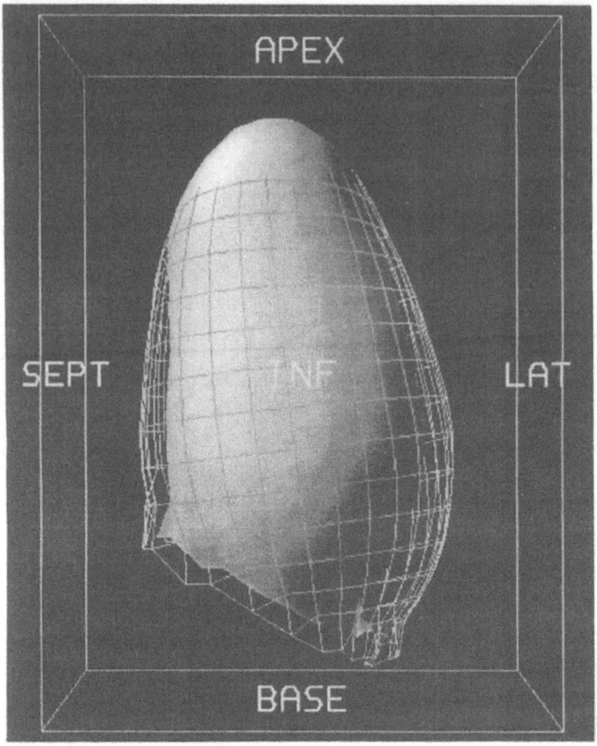

Visual assessment of the displacement of the endocardium from its end-diastolic position is an easy and intuitive way to evaluate endocardial motion, as demonstrated in figure 5 for a patient with severe and extensive left anterior descending coronary artery disease (same patient as in figure 2).

Quantitative measurement of all segmental motion and thickening information can be readily presented in polar map format, as seen in figure 6.

Figure 5. *Three-dimensional display of the LV endocardial surface at end-diastole (grid) and end-systole (shaded surface), for regional myocardial motion assessment of the patient in figure 2. Note the absent motion of the apical region of the LV*

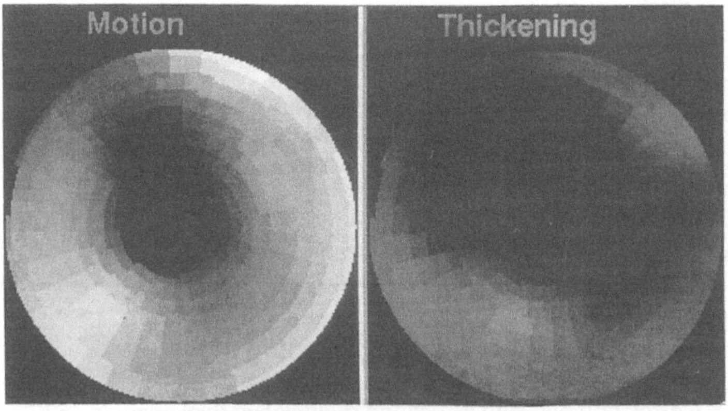

Figure 6. *Motion and thickening polar maps for the patient in figures 2 and 5. Note the generally poor thickening of the LV myocardium, as well as its absent motion at the apex*

Issues in quantitation of regional motion and thickening

Extensive work with a variety of modalities has pointed to the difficulty of correcting for translation and rotation of the heart in the assessment of regional ventricular function [36, 37]. The three-dimensional approach employed by our laboratory includes the translational motion of the heart in its measurement of endocardial motion, but eliminates the inaccuracies deriving from the use of a fixed or floating reference system by adopting a three-dimensional extension of the coordinateless centerline method. Rotation of the heart during systole is not accounted for by our approach, as the author believes that cardiac SPECT or PET images do not have the resolution that would allow to detect and correct differential cardiac torque. It has been demonstrated, however, that this correction has very little effect in the assessment of the basal two thirds of the left ventricle, and its clinical relevance in assessing the distal one third of the left ventricle is uncertain[37].

Also, Cedars-Sinai's quantitative approach utilizes end-diastolic and end-systolic measurements only. Wall motion abnormalities which may occur earlier (or later) than end-systole are therefore not detected by this technique. Figure 3 shows that our automatic algorithm assigned to the 35 dyskinetic segments (visual score = 5) a mean quantitative motion comparable to that of the 43 akinetic segments (visual score = 4), with a larger variance not directly to be ascribed to statistical considerations. It has been demonstrated that dyskinesis, as an example, in patients with myocardial infarction frequently occurs before the end of systole [38]. Modifications of our approach could be made to account for abnormalities not detected at end-systole, but are not part of the present evaluation. This limitation may be exacerbated by the use of only 8 frames per cardiac cycle.

It is reasonable to postulate that normal limits for myocardial wall motion and thickening could be developed similarly to what done for myocardial perfusion [39,40]. However, determination of normal limits and criteria of abnormality would be unlikely to be based solely on absolute measurements of motion and thickening, as demonstrated by the fact that quantitative measurements corresponding to visual scores of 0 are not clearly separated from those corresponding to visual scores >0, in figures 3 and 4. This potential limitation is by no means peculiar to nuclear medicine techniques. Echocardiography faces the same problem, as summarized by Katz et al. "*Normal segmental cavity shrinkage has been reported to vary from 0 percent (i.e., akinesis) to 100 percent and segmental wall thickening to vary from 0 to 150 percent*" [37]. Similarly, magnetic resonance imaging studies have reported a normal thickening range of 18%-100% [41] and overall normal thickening of 48%±28% [42], the latter a value consistent with our average normal thickening value of 43%±17%, shown in figure 4 for visual score =0. Our investigation is, at this stage, only concerned with whether one can measure absolute endocardial motion and myocardial thickening accurately and automatically, the issue of normal limits will be the goal of future research.

Clinical implications

An interesting practical question, especially in a clinical environment without access to quantitative software, is the following: "Is it necessary to evaluate both motion and thickening, or are these two measurements essentially equivalent?" In general, myocardial segments that move normally also thicken normally, and segments that do not move do not thicken. However, there are important exceptions. Post-surgery patients exhibit reduced or paradoxical septal motion in the presence of normal septal thickening. Conversely, patients with small infarcts may display normal motion together with absent thickening, because the small infarcted area is "tethered" by the adjacent normal myocardium. In these cases, evaluating both motion and thickening is, clearly, the key to making a correct diagnosis of regional dysfunction, and it is advisable to never systematically overlook either one of these two important functional indicators. It is not indispensable that assessments of motion and thickening be performed separately, however, as expert visual analysis may combine them in a "hybrid" score of segmental function. Future software development is likely to produce hybrid motion/thickening parametric representations such as generalized functional polar maps, taking a significant step towards complete integration of function and perfusion into a "one-stop" nuclear map for global LV myocardium assessment.

References

1. Risk stratification and survival after myocardial infarction. N Engl J Med 1983;309:331-6.
2. Mahmarian JJ, Mahmarian AC, Marks GF, Pratt CM, Verani MS. Role of adenosine thallium-201 tomography for defining long-term risk in patients after acute myocardial infarction. J Am Coll Cardiol 1995;25:1333-40.
3. Kuhle WG, Porenta G, Huang SC, Phelps ME, Schelbert HR. Issues in the quantitation of reoriented cardiac PET images. J Nucl Med 1992;33:1235-42.
4. Germano G, Kavanagh PB, Su HT, et al. Automatic reorientation of three-dimensional, transaxial myocardial perfusion SPECT images. J Nucl Med 1995;36:1107-14.
5. Germano G, Kavanagh PB, Chen J, et al. Operator-less processing of myocardial perfusion SPECT studies. J Nucl Med 1995;36:2127-32.
6. Miller TR, Wallis JW, Landy BR, Gropler RJ, Sabharwal CL. Measurement of global and regional left ventricular function by cardiac PET. J Nucl Med 1994;35:999-1005.
7. Mazzanti M, Germano G, Kiat H, Friedman J, Berman DS. Fast technetium 99m-labeled sestamibi gated single-photon emission computed tomography for evaluation of myocardial function. J Nucl Cardiol 1996;3:143-9.
8. Nichols K, DePuey EG, Rozanski A. Automation of gated tomographic left ventricular ejection fraction. J Nucl Cardiol 1996;3:475-82.
9. Faber TL, Akers MS, Peshock RM, Corbett JR. Three-dimensional motion and perfusion quantification in gated single-photon emission computed tomograms. J Nucl Med 1991;32:2311-7.
10. Germano G, Kiat H, Kavanagh PB, et al. Automatic quantification of ejection fraction from gated myocardial perfusion SPECT. J Nucl Med 1995;36:2138-47.
11. Hoffman EJ, Huang SC, Phelps ME. Quantitation in positron emission computed tomography: 1. Effect of object size. J Comput Assist Tomogr 1979;3:299-308.
12. Moriel M, Germano G, Kiat H, et al. Automatic measurement of left ventricular ejection fraction by gated SPECT Tc-99m sestamibi: a comparison with radionuclide ventriculography [abstract]. Circulation 1993;88(4 Suppl):I582.
13. He ZX, Mahmarian JJ, Preslar JS, Verani MS. Correlations of left ventricular ejection fractions determined by gated SPECT with thallium and sestamibi and by first-pass radionuclide angiography [abstract]. J Nucl Med 1997;38(5 Suppl):27P.
14. Everaert H, Franken P, Flamen P, Momen A, Bossuyt A. Left ventricular volumes and ejection fraction from gated SPECT myocardial perfusion studies [abstract]. J Nucl Cardiol 1997;4(1 part 2):S102.
15. Zanger D, Bhatnagar A, Hausner E, et al. Automated calculation of ejection fraction from gated Tc-99m sestamibi images - comparison to quantitative echocardiography. J Nucl Cardiol 1997;4(1 part 2):S78.
16. Di Leo C, Bestetti A, Tagliabue L, et al. 99mTc-tetrofosmin gated-SPECT LVEF: correlation with echocardiography and contrastographic ventriculography [abstract]. J Nucl Cardiol 1997;4(1 part 2):S56.
17. Blanksma PK. Personal communication. 1997.
18. Faber TL, Stokely EM, Peshock RM, Corbett JR. A model-based four-dimensional left ventricular surface detector. IEEE Trans Med Imaging 1991;10:321-9.

19. Mazzanti M, Germano G, Kiat H, et al. Identification of severe and extensive coronary artery disease by automatic measurement of transient ischemic dilation of the left ventricle in dual-isotope myocardial perfusion SPECT. J Am Coll Cardiol 1996;27:1612-20.
20. Berman DS, Kiat H, Friedman JD, et al. Separate acquisition rest thallium-201/stress technetium-99m sestamibi dual-isotope myocardial perfusion single-photon emission computed tomography: a clinical validation study. J Am Coll Cardiol 1993;22:1455-64.
21. Cooke CD, Garcia EV, Cullom SJ, Faber TL, Pettigrew RI. Determining the accuracy of calculating systolic wall thickening using a fast Fourier transform approximation: a simulation study based on canine and patient data. J Nucl Med 1994;35:1185-92.
22. DePuey EG, Rozanski A. Using gated technetium-99m-sestamibi SPECT to characterize fixed myocardial defects as infarct or artifact. J Nucl Med 1995;36:952-5.
23. Mochizuki T, Murase K, Fujiwara Y, Tanada S, Hamamoto K, Tauxe WN. Assessment of systolic thickening with thallium-201 ECG-gated single-photon emission computed tomography: a parameter for local left ventricular function. J Nucl Med 1991;32:1496-500.
24. Marcassa C, Marzullo P, Sambuceti G, Parodi O. Prediction of reversible perfusion defects by quantitative analysis of post-exercise electrocardiogram-gated acquisition of technetium-99m 2-methoxyisobutylisonitrile myocardial perfusion scintigraphy. Eur J Nucl Med 1992;19:796-9.
25. Marcassa C, Marzullo P, Parodi O, Sambuceti G, L'Abbate A. A new method for noninvasive quantitation of segmental myocardial wall thickening using technetium-99m 2-methoxy-isobutyl-isonitrile scintigraphy--results in normal subjects. J Nucl Med 1990;31:173-7.
26. Fukuchi K, Uehara T, Morozumi T, et al. Quantification of systolic count increase in technetium-99m-MIBI gated myocardial SPECT. J Nucl Med 1997;38:1067-73.
26. Williams K, Taillon L. Reversible ischemia in severe stress technetium 99m-labeled sestamibi perfusion defects assessed from gated single-photon emission computed tomographic polar map Fourier analysis. J Nucl Cardiol 1995;2:199-206.
28. Bartlett ML, Buvat I, Vaquero JJ, Mok D, Dilsizian V, Bacharach SL. Measurement of myocardial wall thickening from PET/SPECT images: comparison of two methods. J Comput Assist Tomogr 1996;20:473-81.
29. Yamashita K, Tamaki N, Yonekura Y, et al. Quantitative analysis of regional wall motion by gated myocardial positron emission tomography: validation and comparison with left ventriculography. J Nucl Med 1989;30:1775-86.
30. Yamashita K, Tamaki N, Yonekura Y, et al. Regional wall thickening of left ventricle evaluated by gated positron emission tomography in relation to myocardial perfusion and glucose metabolism. J Nucl Med 1991;32:679-85.
31. Buvat I, Bartlett ML, Kitsiou AN, Dilsizian V, Bacharach SL. A "hybrid" method for measuring myocardial wall thickening from gated PET/SPECT images. J Nucl Med 1997;38:324-9.
32. Germano G, Erel J, Lewin H, Kavanagh P, Berman D. Automatic quantitation of regional myocardial wall motion and thickening from gated technetium-99m sestamibi myocardial perfusion single-photon emission computed tomography. J Am Coll Cardiol 1997;30:1360-67.

33. Sheehan FH, Dodge HT, Mathey D, Brown BG, Bolson EL, Mitten S. Application of the centerline method: analysis of change in regional left ventricular wall motion in serial studies. Comput Cardiol, 1983: 97-100.
34. Germano G, Van Train KF, Garcia EV, et al. Quantitation of myocardial perfusion with SPECT: current issues and future trends. In: Zaret BL, Beller G, editors. Nuclear cardiology: state of the art and future directions. St. Louis: Mosby, 1993: 77-88.
35. Germano G, Kavanagh PB, Berman DS. Effect of the number of projections collected on quantitative perfusion and left ventricular ejection fraction measurements from gated myocardial perfusion single-photon emission computed tomographic images. J Nucl Cardiol 1996;3:395-402.
36. Sheehan FH. Principles and practice of contrast ventriculography. In: Skorton DJ, editor. Marcus cardiac imaging : a companion to Braunwald's Heart disease. 2nd ed. Philadelphia: Saunders; 1996: 164-87.
37. Katz AS, Force TL, Folland ED, Aebischer N, Sharma S, Parisi AF. Echocardiographic assessement of ventricular systolic function. In: Skorton DJ, editor. Marcus cardiac imaging : a companion to Braunwald's Heart disease. 2nd ed. Philadelphia: Saunders, 1996: 297-324.
38. Weyman AE, Franklin TD Jr., Hogan RD, et al. Importance of temporal heterogeneity in assessing the contraction abnormalities associated with acute myocardial ischemia. Circulation 1984;70:102-12.
39. Garcia EV, Cooke CD, Van Train KF, et al. Technical aspects of myocardial SPECT imaging with technetium-99m sestamibi. Am J Cardiol 1990;66:23E-31E.
40. Van Train KF, Garcia EV, Maddahi J, et al. Multicenter trial validation for quantitative analysis of same-day rest-stress technetium-99m-sestamibi myocardial tomograms. J Nucl Med 1994;35:609-18.
41. Sechtem U, Sommerhoff BA, Markiewicz W, White RD, Cheitlin MD, Higgins CB. Regional left ventricular wall thickening by magnetic resonance imaging: evaluation in normal persons and patients with global and regional dysfunction. Am J Cardiol 1987;59:145-51.
42. Pflugfelder PW, Sechtem UP, White RD, Higgins CB. Quantification of regional myocardial function by rapid cine MR imaging. AJR Am J Roentgenol 1988;150:523-9.

Chapter 18

MAGNETIC RESONANCE IMAGING OF CARDIAC FUNCTION AND FLOW: PRESENT AND FUTURE

Albert C. van Rossum

Introduction

Soon after its clinical introduction more than a decade ago, it became evident that magnetic resonance (MR) imaging of the heart and vascular system could not only provide excellent depiction of the anatomy but also of function and physiology. Images with high spatial resolution and tissue contrast were obtained without using ionizing radiation and offered a wide field-of-view without restrictions to image plane orientations. The tomographic approach allowed for accurate measurement in three dimensions of heart and vessel structures and quantification of blood flow, in a highly reproducible and operator-independent manner.

However, the imaging procedure was relatively slow. Synchronization of MR acquisitions with the cardiac cycle by means of gating techniques is required in order to avoid image degradation from the continuous motion of the heart and the bloodstream. This again further lengthens the imaging procedure, making MR imaging of the heart less convenient for everyday clinical work. With ongoing progress in technology the speed of acquisition and the image quality have importantly improved. High resolution images of cardiovascular anatomy and dynamic display of cardiac function and blood flow can now routinely be assessed within breath-hold periods of 15 to 20 cardiac cycles. The most advanced MR imaging systems may even provide real-time imaging, avoiding the need for gated acquisitions. These recent developments make MR imaging of the heart more practical and are leading to a gradual increase of its use in daily routine.

Van der Wall et al. (eds.),
Advanced Imaging in Coronary Artery Disease, 289-306.

MR imaging techniques for evaluation of function and flow

Cine MR imaging

Whereas spin-echo imaging is generally used for evaluation of morphology, cine MR imaging is applied for assessment of function [1]. Cine MR imaging is based on the use of gradient-echo techniques, which allow to image with a high temporal resolution and make the blood appear bright. The images are obtained at one or more anatomic levels and at multiple time frames throughout the cardiac cycle. Cinematographical display of these images provides a movie of the dynamics of cardiac structures and of blood flow during the cardiac cycle. Currently, most manufacturers supply their new MR imaging systems with sequences for fast gradient-echo imaging, which make use of short repetition times (TR), short echo times (TE) and k-space segmentation [2]. With these, cine MR images of a single slice can be acquired in 15 to 20 cardiac cycles. For most patients it is feasible to do this in a breath-hold, thus reducing breathing artifacts. The penalty that has to be paid for this rapid imaging is a decrease of the signal-to-noise ratio. However, the loss of signal can be regained using dedicated cardiac surface coils. Application of these coils is nowadays considered a prerequisite for state-of-the-art cardiac MR imaging.

A phenomenon characteristic of gradient-echo cine MR imaging is referred to as intravoxel dephasing. In turbulent flow, changes in magnitude and direction of the velocity of hydrogen nuclei within a single voxel cause attenuation or complete loss of the MR signal. This signal void occurs for example at the proximity of rapidly moving valves or at sites where flow is accelerated and non-uniform. Jets of signal loss therefore are indicative of valvular stenosis or incompetence. The jet area of signal loss is importantly influenced by the length of the TE applied in the gradient-echo sequence and decreases with shorter TE. Consequently, the area of signal loss is at the best a semi-quantitative measure of the severity of valvular defects and is reduced using the fast breath-hold techniques with short TE compared to conventional non-breath-hold cine MR imaging.

Gradient-echo sequences can be modified such, that they may be used for tracking the displacement of noninvasively applied tags in the myocardial wall, for quantification of blood flow velocity, and for measuring myocardial perfusion.

Myocardial tagging

A very precise method of evaluating myocardial function is MR myocardial tissue tagging. The technique consists of applying a series of radiofrequency pulses that precede the standard imaging sequence [3]. These prepulses produce localized regions of altered magnetization which saturate the myocardial tissue. When the magnetic saturation is applied in thin planes perpendicular to the imaging plane, the intersection lines will result in the appearance of dark stripes in the image (figure 1). These tagging lines, which may be produced parallel to each other or in a grid pattern, are now a property of the myocardial and surrounding tissue. By imaging and tracking the tags as a function time, the regional intramural deformation of the myocardium can be observed and quantified [4]. In contrast to traditional noninvasive imaging modalities including echocardiography and standard cine MR imaging, myocardial tagging allows to differentiate between rigid body motion of the heart and true intramural deformation of the myocardium.

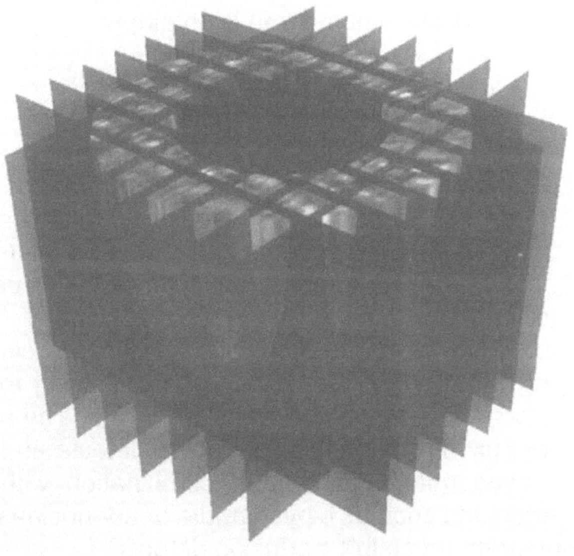

Figure 1. *Schematic illustration of magnetic saturation applied in parallel planes, intersecting the heart. The intersections with the myocardium appear as dark tagging lines in the imaging plane (figure 3).*

Velocity mapping

A well validated approach of quantifying blood flow with MR imaging is the use of a technique based on measuring the phase of the MR signal. Various names are used to describe it, amongst which phase-contrast imaging, phase velocity mapping, and velocity-encoded cine MR imaging. The technique is based on the phenomenon that hydrogen nuclei moving in a gradient magnetic field experience phase-shifts proportional to their velocity[5]. The phase information is determined within each pixel and is used to construct velocity maps. At each point (pixel) on this map the velocity is functionally displayed by using a gray scale and can be read-out numerically[6]. The direction of velocity can be measured in three-dimensions, but routinely it is obtained through-plane with the imaging plane perpendicular to the direction of flow. It is important to set the velocity-sensitivity of the sequence above the expected peak velocity, in order to avoid phase wrapping (aliasing).

In most cases velocity mapping is used to quantify the velocity of flowing blood, but it can also be applied to determine the velocity of the myocardium. Pixelwise integration of velocities (cm/s) distributed over the cross section of a vessel and multiplied with vessel cross-sectional area (cm^2) yields the flow-rate (ml/s). By consecutive temporal integration over the cardiac cycle the stroke volume (ml) is obtained.

First-pass techniques and myocardial perfusion

When fast gradient-echo techniques are applied after bolus injection of a contrast agent, signal intensity changes of the myocardium can be imaged, reflecting the changes in contrast agent concentration related to regional perfusion. From these signal-intensity-versus-time curves several semiquantitative perfusion parameters may be derived [7]. A potential advantage compared to nuclear methods of assessing myocardial perfusion with MR imaging is the high spatial resolution allowing to discriminate between subendocardial and subepicardial perfusion. The approach may be used to detect fixed, irreversible, perfusion defects as in scar tissue resulting from myocardial infarction. In combination with vasodilating pharmacological agents such as dipyridamole or adenosine the technique may also demonstrate reversible perfusion defects.

In order to quantify or at least semi-quantify myocardial perfusion, the changes in signal intensity must be measured with a high temporal resolution. The speed of image acquisition using fast gradient-echo sequences usually is in the order of 250-300 ms, allowing to cover two or three slices in the left ventricular short axis per heart beat with a spatial resolution of ~ $5mm^2$. Trade-offs can be made between spatial resolution, temporal resolution and signal-to-noise ratio. Even faster imaging with echoplanar techniques may prove to be necessary in the near future. Another point of consideration is the type of the MR contrast media to be used. Several arguments favor the use of so called T1-enhancing contrast agents as compared to magnetic susceptibility agents. Gadolinium-DTPA is the classic representative of the former group of agents and is widely available for clinical use. It rapidly diffuses from the blood pool into the interstitium, thereby complicating the quantitative assessment of perfusion. Newly developed T1-enhancing agents that stick to the blood pool may prove advantageous in this respect. Many of the above mentioned aspects are currently subject to investigation [8].

Postprocessing and analysis

A distinct feature of cardiac MR imaging and an important justification of its use, is the potential for highly accurate and reproducible quantification of ventricular function, blood flow and perfusion. This is time-consuming and can only be accomplished successfully in clinical routine with the aid of (semi-) automatic computer programs [9]. To this purpose, dedicated software is required to help defining at consecutive time frames throughout the cardiac cycle contours of endocardial and epicardial borders, displacement of myocardial tags, vessel cross-sections, and regional signal-intensity changes in the myocardium. This step is then followed by automatic calculation of cardiac chamber volumes, myocardial strains, flow in vessels and perfusion parameters. Interpretation of data can be made more comprehensible by presentation of functional images and three-dimensional volume rendering. User friendly software for postprocessing and quantitative analysis is an indispensable adjunct to take maximum advantage of the potential of cardiac MR imaging.

Application of function and flow assessment by MR imaging

Ischemic heart disease

Global ventricular function and mass

Ventricular volumes can be calculated without geometrical assumptions by summation of cavity areas multiplied by the slice thickness of a stack of consecutive short axis cine images encompassing the heart. Stroke volume, ejection fraction and cardiac output are directly derived from end-diastolic and end-systolic images. A less time consuming determination of stroke volume and flow rate of the left and right ventricle is obtained by measuring flow in the ascending aorta and pulmonary artery respectively, using MR velocity mapping. However, the latter does not provide the information on chamber volumes, ejection fraction and regional myocardial function . When both endocardial and epicardial border of the left ventricle are traced, the myocardial volume multiplied by the specific gravity of the myocardium (1.05 g/cm^3) yields left ventricular mass. Many experimental and clinical studies have demonstrated the accuracy of these measurements [2, 10-12].

Regional myocardial function

The high spatial resolution in the order of 1 to 2 mm allows to accurately measure regional systolic wall thickening on cine MR images. In contrast to the analysis of wall motion used in echocardiography, systolic wall thickening is less susceptible to subjective interpretation from the investigator.

Myocardial infarction is characterized by a reduced diastolic wall thickness and lack of systolic wall thickening (figure 2). Baer et al. found that in akinetic myocardial segments, an enddiastolic wall thickness assessed by MR imaging of $\geq$ 5.5 mm had a sensitivity of 72% and a specificity of 89% for predicting viable myocardium [13]. Viability was defined as residual metabolic activity obtained in corresponding segments by FDG-PET of > 50% of uptake in normally contracting segments. Using the functional parameter of systolic wall thickening during administration of low dose dobutamine (10 µg/kg/min) rather than the morphological criterion of enddiastolic wall thickness, the same authors found that a recruitable contractile reserve of $\geq$1 mm was a better predictor of PET-defined viability, with a sensitivity and specificity of 81% and 95% respectively. When at least one of both MRI parameters fulfilled viability criteria, the sensitivity increased to 88% with a minor decrease in specificity (87%).

The detection of stress-induced ischemia has been studied using dobutamine in a dose up to 20 µg/kg/min [14,15]. The reported sensitivities for identifying one-vessel, two-vessel, and three-vessel disease were 88%, 91% and 100% respectively.

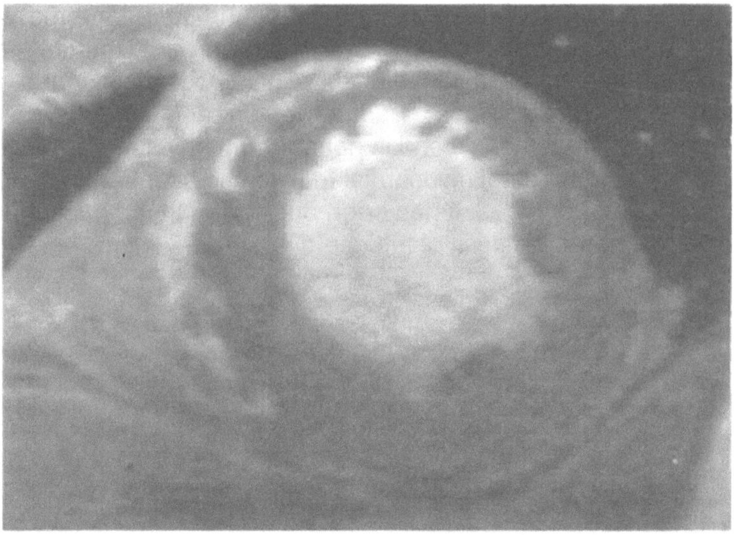

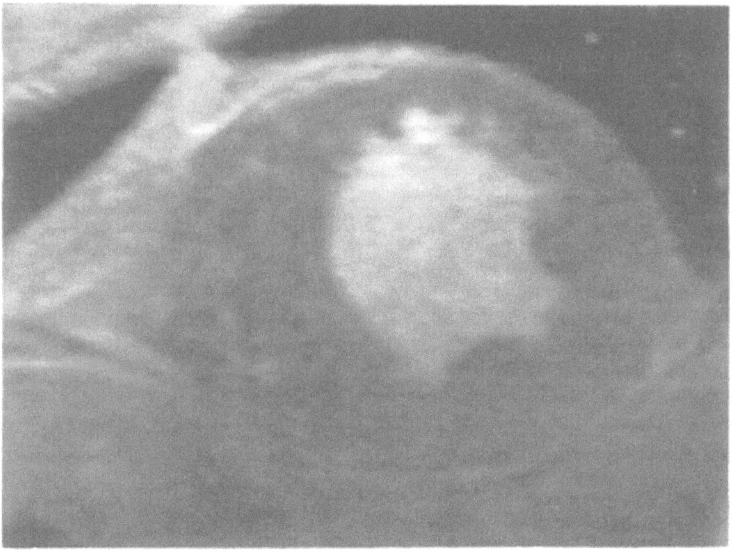

Figure 2. *Breath-hold cine MR images in the midventricular short axis of the left ventricle obtained at diastole* ***(A)*** *and systole* ***(B)****, in a patient with sustained anterior infarction and combined aortic stenosis and insufficiency. The anteroseptal segment demonstrates a reduced wall thickness and thickening, the remaining segments are hypertrophic, and global contraction seems poor. The following global LV functional parameters were calculated: enddiastolic volume 245 ml, endsystolic volume 176 ml, ejection fraction 28%, LV mass 265 grams. (see also figure 6).*

Although the measurement of myocardial thickening on cine MR images is accurate, it is susceptible to errors induced by through-plane motion. The use of myocardial tagging techniques allows to precisely quantify regional intramural deformation avoiding the effect of rigid body motion and through-plane motion on wall thickness measurements. Tagging techniques have been applied in animal models and in patients with myocardial infarction to study differences in regional myocardial function adjacent and remote from the infarct area (figure 3)[16-18]. It has been postulated that these differences may play a role in the process of left ventricular remodeling.

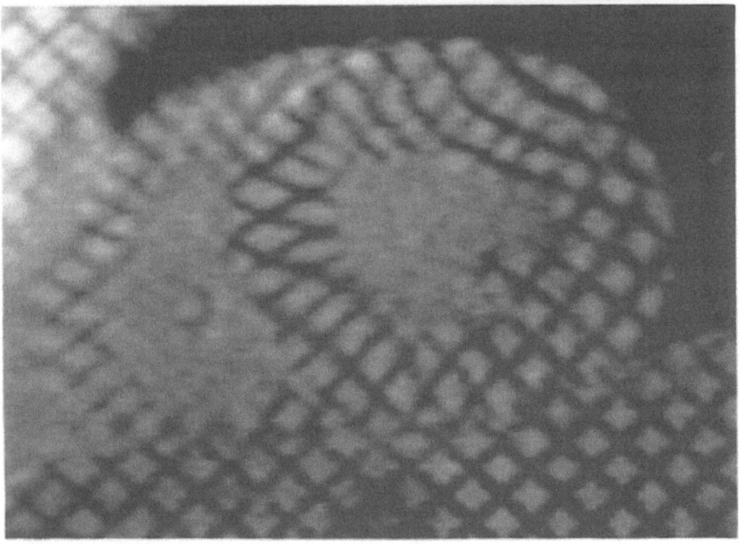

Figure 3. *Cine MR image in the LV short axis using myocardial tagging in a patient with 1 week old posterolateral infarction. In systole the grid of tag-lines shows absence of deformation in the infarct segment.*

Regional myocardial perfusion

Whereas contrast first-pass MR imaging can identify myocardial perfusion abnormalities in healed infarctions[19], assessment of stress-induced hypoperfusion seems a more valuable goal to pursue for clinical use.

Wilke et al. demonstrated a good correlation between MRI assessed myocardial mean transit time and microsphere-assessed myocardial blood flow in dogs, using pharmacologic vasodilation to improve the detection of myocardial ischemia [20]. The slope of the signal-intensity-versus-time curve was also related to myocardial blood flow.

Manning et al. measured peak signal intensity at rest during the first-pass of the paramagnetic contrast agent Gadolinium-DTPA in 20 patients with > 90% stenosis with single vessel coronary artery disease [21]. They found a decrease in peak signal intensity and a lower slope of the signal-intensity-versus-time curve in myocardium perfused by a stenotic vessel. After revascularization, peak signal intensity recovered to normal values in 9/10 patients. The significance of this study is that it indicates the possibility to detect perfusion abnormalities at rest in patients with a critical coronary artery stenosis, normalizing after revascularization.

Several investigators have compared first-pass MR myocardial perfusion imaging with nuclear techniques in patients with coronary artery disease (figure 4)[22-27]. Limitations of these studies included either the use of a suboptimal temporal resolution, single plane acquisition, visual analysis only of a small number of relatively large myocardial segments, and small numbers of patients. In a recent study myocardial perfusion reserve was quantified with multislice first-pass MR imaging in patients with angina and non-significant coronary lesions. A significant correlation was found between the myocardial perfusion reserve and intracoronary Doppler derived flow reserve using adenosine [28]. So far, the role of MR imaging of myocardial perfusion for routine clinical patient management is not determined.

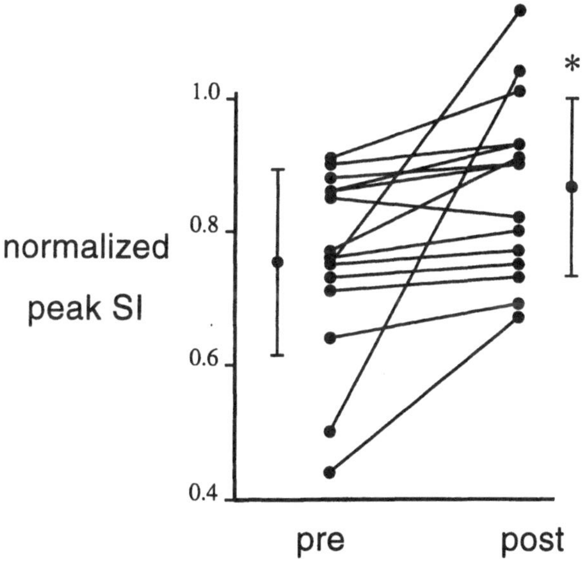

Figure 4. *Gadolinium enhanced first-pass MR imaging was performed in patients before and a few hours after PTCA . In the subendocardium of the area supplied by the stenotic coronary artery, peak contrast enhancement relative to normal myocardium increased in 14 out of 15 patients (from reference 7).*

Coronary artery flow

Fast, k-space segmented gradient-echo sequences, have been used to image coronary arteries [29-32]. However, these techniques still suffer from a lack of accuracy to detect coronary artery lesions in a manner useful for clinical routine [33]. It is expected that the forthcoming use of contrast agents that stick to the blood pool will improve the accuracy.

A different and more functional approach to assess the severity of coronary artery stenoses is by directly measuring coronary flow and coronary flow reserve using MR velocity mapping. This technique was proven to be accurate in large vessels, in vessels with small diameters and in canine coronary arteries[34-36].

Two studies reported initial results in coronary arteries of volunteers, measuring flow in diastole only, during breath-holds of 24 to 32 heartbeats [37,38]. In the study by Edelman et al flow increased fourfold after administration of adenosine. Using dipyridamole an increase of the diastolic flow velocity was found in the left anterior descending coronary artery (LAD) of healthy volunteers of 3.14 ± 0.59[39]. Hundley et al measured volumetric flow at multiple phases of the cardiac cycle in the LAD of patients with coronary artery disease [40]. They found a high correlation between catheterization (intracoronary Doppler) and MR imaging in the determination of coronary flow at rest and adenosine induced flow reserve. Breath-hold flow measurements with MR velocity mapping require a large acquisition window within the cardiac cycle in the order of 100 - 150 ms. This seems to be feasible in the LAD, but is subject to substantial motion artifacts in the more vigorously moving right coronary artery, especially during systole and early diastole. Recently we showed that by use of respiratory gating with navigator echoes the acquisition window can be reduced to 50 ms, thus also allowing phasic flow measurements in the right coronary artery [41,42].

Also the function of coronary artery bypass grafts can be assessed using flow velocity mapping techniques [43]. Volume flow of sequential grafts to three regions was significantly higher than in single grafts, 136 ± 106 ml/min versus 63 ± 41 ml/min respectively. Comparable to MR myocardial perfusion imaging, the current state of MR coronary artery flow mapping is in a developmental stage.

Non-ischemic heart disease

MR imaging of anatomy in concert with imaging of function and flow proved to be valuable in congenital heart disease, pericardial disease, cardiomyopathy and valvular heart disease.

Congenital heart disease

In patients with congenital heart disease MR imaging is helpful in assessing the morphology of cardiac chambers and their relation to the great arteries and veins, in evaluating complex anomalies, and in the follow-up after surgery. Specifically valuable when compared to echocardiography, is cine MR imaging of the right ventricle and pulmonary arteries in cyanotic anomalies and the quantitative determination of intracardiac and systemic-to-pulmonary shunts [44-47]. Shunt calculation can be derived from MR flow velocity mapping in the aorta and pulmonary artery, or by measuring the difference in right and left ventricular stroke volume obtained with the consecutive multislice cine imaging approach [48].

Pericardial and myocardial disease

In patients with thickened pericardium ($\geq$4 mm) measurement of a blunted diastolic flow peak in the vena cava superior or in the pulmonary veins supports a diagnosis of constrictive pericarditis [49,50]. MR tissue tagging using a parallel stripe pattern may be helpful to detect adherence of thickened pericardium to the chest wall and myocardium, and to differentiate thickened pericardial tissue from pericardial effusion.

Left and right ventricular mass can be accurately measured with MR imaging and may be used to monitor the effects of drug therapy in patients with hypertrophic cardiomyopathy or left ventricular hypertrophy. Measuring the volume changes of the ventricles in the early filling phase yields a measure of diastolic function. Determination of strain values using myocardial tagging may also become a useful tool for assessment of diastolic function, provided that tag persistence is long enough to cover the early diastolic phase of the cardiac cycle.

Valvular heart disease

In our experience the evaluation of valvular morphology has improved with the advent of breath-hold cine MR imaging. Bicuspid aortic valve, mitral valve prolapse, anomaly of the tricuspid valve associated with Ebstein's disease can be easily recognized and may be an adjunct to ambiguous echocardiographic findings. Nonetheless, due to its superior temporal resolution, transesophageal echocardiography is the technique of choice for evaluating the rapidly moving vegetations attached to the valves in endocarditis.

Valvular regurgitation or stenosis are readily identified by jets of signal loss proximal or distal to the valves respectively (figure 5). Length and area of the jet are at the best semi-quantitative parameters of the severity of the valvular defect [51]. They depend on hemodynamic and technical factors such as the size or shape of the valve orifice and the length of the TE [52].

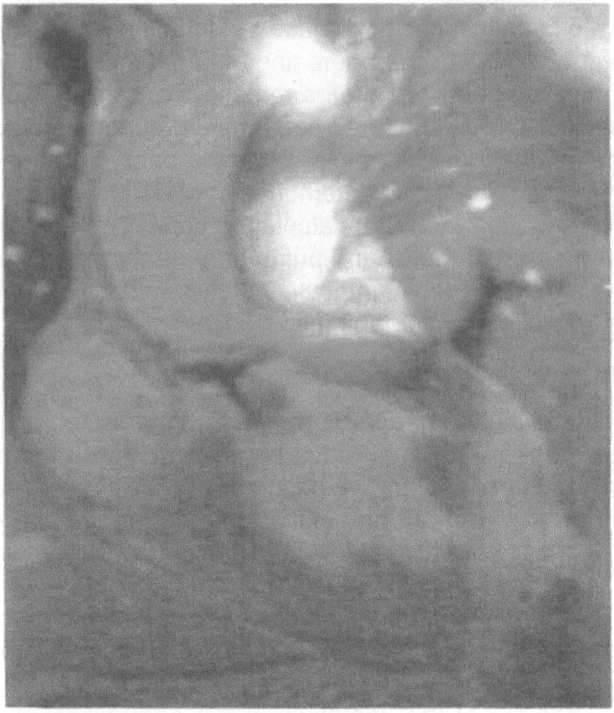

Figure 5. *Same patient as in figure 2. Breath-hold cine MR imaging showed a relatively small diastolic regurgitation jet, although the regurgitation volume was large (see figure 6). This is likely to be caused by the high enddiastolic LV pressure, and by the short TE used in breath-hold sequences.*

MR velocity mapping offers the capability of a quantitative approach of the valvular defect severity. In valvular stenosis the peak velocity can be measured, allowing calculation of the pressure gradient across the stenosis through the modified Bernoulli equation [53]. To do this, it is absolutely necessary to use an MR system with powerful magnetic field gradients and short TE pulse sequences. With accurate positioning of the imaging plane perpendicular to the doming valve leaflets a direct tracing of the orifice area is feasible. Heavily calcified valves however, may lead to overestimation of the orifice area.

From an isolated aortic or mitral regurgitation the regurgitation volume can be calculated as the difference from right and left ventricular stroke volume using the three-dimensional geometric data set [54]. When mitral regurgitation is accompanied by an endsystolic reversal of the pulmonary vein flow measured by MR velocity mapping, this is indicative of severe mitral regurgitation [55]. The aortic regurgitation volume and fraction can also be obtained directly from measurement of the antegrade and retrograde volume flow in the ascending aorta (figure 6) [56,57].

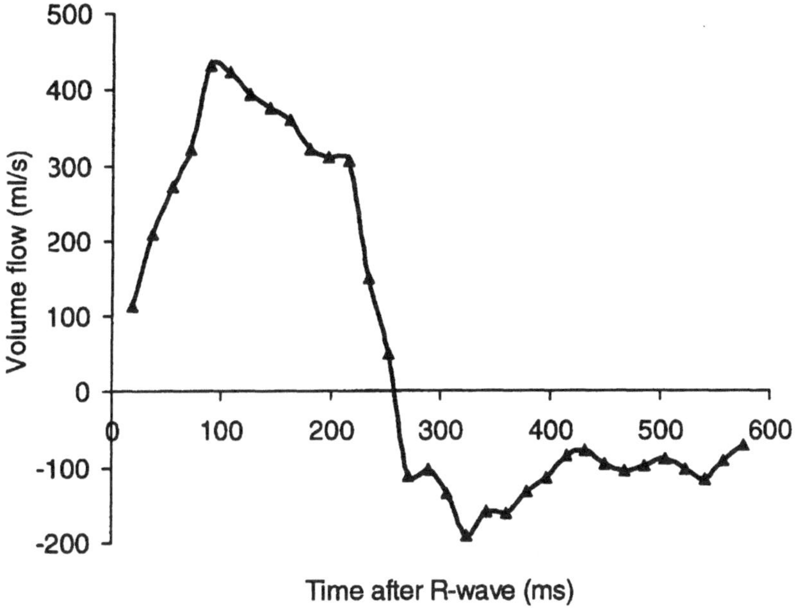

__Figure 6.__ Same patient as in figures 2 and 5. Quantification of aortic flow by cine MR velocity mapping revealed a stroke volume (antegrade integral of the flow curve) of 69.8 ml, similar to the geometrically assessed stroke volume. The regurgitation volume (retrograde integral of the flow curve) was 36.6 ml, yielding a regurgitation fraction of 52%.

This is a simple and rapid approach, yielding accurate information of the volumetric overload of the ventricle which can not be performed with Doppler echocardiography. When combined aortic and mitral regurgitations exist, each of the regurgitation volumes can be calculated by combining the geometrically assessed stroke volume with aortic retrograde flow.

Conclusion

The accuracy of MR imaging to depict cardiac anatomy and quantify cardiac function is by now well established in several fields of heart disease and exceeds that of other noninvasive techniques. The question remains whether such an accuracy and reproducibility is beneficial in daily patient care. Most likely it is, but this still has to be proven in studies that relate the data obtained by MR imaging with patient-outcome. Next, these must be followed by studies of cost-effectiveness.

Progress is required with regard to the evaluation of ischemic heart disease. Although quantification of mechanical function is now routinely applicable, MR techniques for imaging of coronary arteries, measurement of coronary flow, and assessment of myocardial perfusion are still immature and have to be further developed. If combined high resolution imaging of perfusion and function can be achieved, MR imaging will be a most powerful tool in the management of cardiac disease.

References

1. Sechtem U, Pflugfelder PW, White RD, et al. Cine MR imaging: potential for the evaluation of cardiovascular function. AJR Am J Roentgenol. 1987;148:239-46.
2. Sakuma H, Fujita N, Foo TK, et al. Evaluation of left ventricular volume and mass with breath-hold cine MR imaging. Radiology 1993;188:377-80.
3. Axel L, Dougherty L. MR imaging of motion with spatial modulation of magnetization. Radiology 1989;171:841-5.
4. Young AA, Imai H, Chang CN, Axel L. Two-dimensional left ventricular deformation during systole using magnetic resonance imaging with spatial modulation of magnetization [published erratum . appears in Circulation 1994;90-:1585] Circulation 1994;89:740-52.
5. Firmin DN, Nayler GL, Kilner PJ, Longmore DB. The application of phase shifts in NMR for flow measurement. Magn Reson Med 1990; 14:230-41.
6. Van Rossum AC, Sprenger M. Magnetic resonance imaging and quantitation of blood flow. In: van der Wall EE, de Roos A, editors. Magnetic resonance imaging in coronary artery disease. Dordrecht: Kluwer Academic Publishers; 1991.p.49-80.
7. Keijer JT. First-pass magnetic resonance imaging of myocardial perfusion: a quantitative approach [dissertation]. Amsterdam: Vrije Universiteit Amsterdam; 1996.
8. Mühler A. Assessment of myocardial perfusion using contrast-enhanced MR imaging: current status and future developments. MAGMA 1995;3:21-33.
9. Holman ER, Buller VG, de Roos A, et al. Detection and quantification of dysfunctional myocardium by magnetic resonance imaging. A new three-dimensional method for quantitative wall-thickening analysis. Circulation 1997;95:924-31.
10. Van Rossum AC, Visser FC, Sprenger M, van Eenige MJ, Valk J, Roos JP. Evaluation of magnetic resonance imaging for determination of left ventricular ejection fraction and comparison with angiography. Am J Cardiol 1988;62:628-33.
11. Semelka RC, Tomei E, Wagner S, et al. Interstudy reproducibility of dimensional and functional measurements between cine magnetic resonance studies in the morphologically abnormal left ventricle. Am Heart J 1990;119:1367-73.
12. Shapiro EP,Rogers WJ, Beyar R, et al. Determination of left ventricular mass by magnetic resonance imaging in hearts deformed by acute infarction. Circulation 1989;79:706-11.
13. Baer FM, Voth E, Schneider CA, Theissen P, Schicha H, Sechtem U. Comparison of low-dose dobutamine-gradient-echo magnetic resonance imaging and positron emission tomography with [18F]fluorodeoxyglucose in patients with chronic coronary artery disease. A functional and morphological approach to the detection of residual myocardial viability. Circulation 1995;91:1006-15.
14. Pennell DJ, Underwood SR, Manzara CC, et al. Magnetic resonance imaging during dobutamine stress in coronary artery disease. Am J Cardiol 1992;70:34-40.
15. Van Rugge FP, Van der Wall EE, Spanjersberg SJ, et al. Magnetic resonance imaging during dobutamine stress for detection and localization of coronary artery disease. Quantitative wall motion analysis using a modification of the centerline method. Circulation 1994;90:127-38.
16. Kramer CM, Lima JAC, Reichek N, et al. Regional differences in function within noninfarcted myocardium during left ventricular remodeling. Circulation 1993;88:1279-88.

17. Kramer CM, Rogers WJ, Theobald TM, Power TP, Petruolo S, Reichek N. Remote noninfarcted region dysfunction soon after first anterior myocardial infarction. A magnetic resonance tagging study. Circulation 1996;94:660-6.
18. Marcus JT, Götte MJ, Van Rossum AC, et al. Myocardial function in infarcted and remote regions early after infarction in man. Assessment by magnetic resonance tagging and strain analysis. Magn Reson Med 1997;38:803-10.
19. Van Rugge FP, van der Wall EE, van Dijkman PR, Louwerenburg HW, de Roos A, Bruschke AV. Usefulness of ultrafast magnetic resonance imaging in healed myocardial infarction. Am J Cardiol 1992;70:1233-7.
20. Wilke N, Simm C, Zhang J, et al. Contrast-enhanced first-pass myocardial perfusion imaging: correlation between myocardial blood flow in dogs at rest and during hyperemia. Magn Reson Med 1993;29:485-97.
21. Manning WJ, Atkinson DJ, Grossman W, Paulin S, Edelman RR. First-pass nuclear magnetic resonance imaging studies using gadolinium-DTPA in patients with coronary artery disease. J Am Coll Cardiol 1991;18:959-65.
22. Schaefer S, Van Tyen R, Saloner D. Evaluation of myocardial perfusion abnormalities with gadolinium-enhanced snapshot MR-imaging in humans. Work in progress. Radiology 1992;185:795-801.
23. Klein MA, Collier BD, Hellman RS, Bamrah VS. Detection of chronic coronary artery disease: value of pharmacologically stressed, dynamically enhanced turbo-fast low-angle shot MR images. Am J Roentgenol 1993;161:257-63.
24. Eichenberger AC, Schuiki E, Koechli VD, Amann FW, McKinnon GC, Von Schulthess GK. Ischemic heart disease: Assessment with Gadolinium-enhanced ultrafast MR imaging and dipyridamole stress. J Magn Reson Imaging 1994;4:425-31.
25. Walsh EG, Doyle M, Lawson M, Blackwell GG, Pokost GM. Multislice first-pass myocardial perfusion imaging on a conventional clinical scanner. Magn Reson Med 1995;34:39-47.
26. Keijer JT, Bax JJ, van Rossum AC, Visser FC, Visser CA. Myocardial perfusion imaging: clinical experience and recent progress in radionuclide scintigraphy and magnetic resonance imaging. Int J Card Imaging 1997;13:415-31.
27. Lauerma K, Virtanen KS, Sipilä LM, Hekali P, Aronen HJ. Multislice MRI in assessment of myocardial perfusion in patients with single-vessel, proximal left anterior descending coronary artery disease before and after revascularization. Circulation 1997;96:2859-67.
28. Wilke N, Jerosch-Herold M, Wang Y, et al. Myocardial perfusion reserve: assessment with multisection, quantitative, first-pass MR imaging. Radiology 1997;204:373-84.
29. Manning WJ, Li W, Edelman RR. A preliminary report comparing magnetic resonance coronary angiography with conventional angiography [published erratum appears in N Engl J Med 1993;330:152]. N Engl J Med 1993; 328:828-32.
30. Duerinckx AJ, Urman MK. Two-dimensional coronary MR angiography: analysis of initial clinical results. Radiology 1994; 193:731-8.
31. Pennell DJ, Keegan J, Firmin DN, Gatehouse PD, Underwood SR, Longmore DB. Magnetic resonance imaging of coronary arteries: technique and preliminary results. Br Heart J 1993; 70:315-26.
32. Post JC, Van Rossum AC, Hofman MB, Valk J, Visser CA. Three-dimensional respiratory gated MR angiography of coronary arteries: comparison with conventional coronary angiography. AJR Am J Roentgenol 1996;166:1399-404.

33. Post JC, van Rossum AC, Hofman MB, De Cock CC, Valk J, Visser CA. Clinical utility of two-dimensional magnetic resonance angiography in detecting coronary artery disease. Eur Heart J 1997; 18:426-33.
34. Van Rossum AC, Sprenger M, Visser FC, Peels KH, Valk J, Roos JP. An in vivo validation of quantitative blood flow imaging in arteries and veins using magnetic resonance phase-shift techniques. Eur Heart J 1991; 12:117-26.
35. Hofman MB, Visser FC, Van Rossum AC, Vink QM, Sprenger M, Westerhof N. In vivo validation of magnetic resonance volume flow measurements with limited spatial resolution in small vessels. Magn Reson Med 1995; 33:778-84.
36. Clarke GD, Eckels R, Chaney C, et al. Measurement of absolute epicardial coronary artery flow and flow reserve with breath-hold cine phase-contrast magnetic resonance imaging. Circulation 1995; 91:2627-34.
37. Edelman RR, Manning WJ, Gervino E, Li W. Flow velocity quantification in human coronary arteries with fast, breath-Hold MR Angiography. J Magn Reson Imaging 1993; 3:699-703.
38. Keegan J, Firmin D, Gatehouse P, Longmore D. The application of breath hold phase velocity mapping techniques to the measurement of coronary artery blood flow velocity: phantom data and initial in vivo results. Magn Reson Med 1994; 31:526-36.
39. Sakuma H, Blake LM, Amidon TM, et al. Coronary flow reserve: noninvasive measurements in humans with breath-hold velocity-encoded cine MR imaging. Radiology 1996;198:745-50.
40. Hundley WG, Lange RA, Clarke GD, et al. Assessment of coronary arterial flow and flow reserve in humans with magnetic resonance imaging. Circulation 1996;93:1502-8.
41. Hofman MBM, Van Rosssum AC, Sprenger M, Westerhof N. Assessment of flow in the right human coronary artery by magnetic resonance phase contrast velocity measurements: effects of cardiac and respiratory motion. Magn Reson Med 1996;35:521-31.
42. Post JC. Magnetic resonance coronary angiography: a clinical evaluation [dissertation]. Amsterdam: Vrije Universiteit Amsterdam, 1997.
43. Galjee MA, van Rossum AC, Doesburg T, van Eenige MJ, Visser CA. Value of magnetic resonance imaging in assessing patency and function of coronary artery bypass grafts. An angiographically controlled study. Circulation 1996;93:660-6.
44. Kersting-Sommerhoff BA, Diethelm L, Stanger P, et al. Evaluation of complex congenital ventricular anomalies with magnetic resonance imaging. Am Heart J 1990;120:133-42.
45. Martinez JE, Mohiaddin RH, Kilner PJ, et al. Obstruction in extracardiac ventriculopulmonary conduits: value of nuclear magnetic resonance imaging with velocity mapping and Doppler echocardiography. J Am Coll Cardiol 1992;20:338-44.
46. Hirsch R, Kilner PJ, Connelly MS, Redington AN, St John Sutton MG, Somerville J. Diagnosis in adolescents and adults with congenital heart disease. Prospective assessment of individual and combined roles of magnetic resonance imaging and transesophageal echocardiography. Circulation 1994;90:2937-51.
47. Helbing WA, Rebergen SA, Maliepaard C, et al. Quantification of right ventricular functin with magnetic resonance imaging in children with normal hearts and with congenital heart disease. Am Heart J 1995;130:828-37.

48. Hundley WG, Li HF, Lange RA, et al. Assessment of left-to-right intracardiac shunting by velocity-encoded, phase-difference magnetic resonance imaging. A comparison with oximetric and indicator dilution techniques. Circulation 1995;91:2955-60.

49. Masui T, Finck S, Higgins CB. Constrictive pericarditis and restrictive cardiomyopathy: evaluation with MR imaging. Radiology 1992;182:369-73.

49. Mohiaddin RH, Wann SL, Underwood R, Firmin DN, Rees S, Longmore DB. Vena caval flow: assessment with cine MR velocity mapping. Radiology 1990;177:537-41.

51. Wagner S, Auffermann W, Buser P, et al. Diagnostic accuracy and estimation of the severity of valvular regurgitation from the signal void on cine magnetic resonance images. Am Heart J 1989;118:760-7.

52. Suzuki J, Caputo GR, Kondo C, Higgins CB. Cine MR imaging of valvular heart disease: display and imaging parameters affect the size of the signal void caused by valvular regurgitation. AJR Am J Roentgenol 1990;155:723-7.

53. Kilner PJ, Manzara CC, Mohiaddin RH, et al. Magnetic resonance jet velocity mapping in mitral and aortic valve stenosis. Circulation 1993;87:1239-48.

54. Sechtem U, Pflugfelder PW, Cassidy MM, et al. Mitral or aortic regurgitation: quantification of regurgitant volumes with cine MR imaging. Radiology 1988;167:425-30.

55. Galjee MA, Van Rossum AC, Van Eenige MJ, et al. Magnetic resonance imaging of the pulmonary venous flow pattern in mitral regurgitation. Independence of the investigated vein. Eur Heart J 1995;16:1675-85.

56. Sondergaard L, Lindvig K, Hildebrandt P, et al. Quantification of aortic regurgitation by magnetic resonance velocity mapping. Am Hear J 1993;125:1081-90.

57. Globits S, Blake L, Bourne M, et al. Assessment of hemodynamic effects of angiotensin-converting enzyme inhibitor therapy in chronic aortic regurgitation by using velocity encoded cine magnetic resonance imaging. Am Heart J 1996;131:289-93.

Chapter 19

DEVELOPMENT OF LIGANDS FOR RECEPTOR IMAGING

Philip H. Elsinga, Aren van Waarde, Ton J. Visser and Willem Vaalburg

Introduction

The noninvasive characterization of the cardiac nervous system by positron emission tomography (PET) may provide important pathophysiological information in various cardiac diseases. Changes in numbers of neurotransmitter receptors have been associated with myocardial ischemia and infarction, congestive heart failure, cardiomyopathy, as well as diabetes or thyroid-induced heart muscle disease. Knowledge on these receptor densities is based on post mortem or biopsy material. With PET it is possible to investigate the whole heart in vivo. A prerequisite for imaging of the cardiac nervous system is the availability of appropriate radioligands, which includes its radiolabeling and evaluation in animals and human volunteers. This chapter gives an overview of the process of development of a radioligand for the β-adrenergic receptor, which is illustrative for the development of radioligands in general.

Cardiac β-adrenoceptors

It is now generally accepted that the β-adrenoceptor density is altered in various pathophysiological conditions, including hypertension [1], heart failure, myocardial ischemia, hypertrophic (HCM) and dilated cardiomyopathy (DCM)[2]. A suitable procedure for *in vivo* visualization and quantitation of cardiac β-adrenoceptors by PET would be of great clinical interest.

Van der Wall et al. (eds.),
Advanced Imaging in Coronary Artery Disease, 307-319.

Myocardial β-adrenergic receptors play an important role in the regulation of the heart rate (positive chronotropic effect) and the myocardial contractility (positive inotropic effect) [2]. β-Adrenoceptors are present in the atria as well as the ventricles. Most available data about β-adrenoceptors are obtained from cardiac transplant donors. In humans, the average β-adrenoceptor density (B_{max}) in ventricles and atria is 70-100 fmol/mg protein.

The β-adrenoceptor was initially subdivided into β_1- and β_2-subtypes [3]. Recently a β_3-subtype has been cloned [4]. The relative proportion of the β_1- and β_2-subtypes is usually determined by radioligand competition studies with subtype-selective β-adrenoceptor antagonists. Consequently the receptor density (B_{max}) and affinity constant (K_D) are obtained using Scatchard plots[5,6] or by iterative computer analysis [7]. In the human heart the ratio of the β_1/β_2-subtypes is about 80/20, whereas in the lungs this ratio is 30/70.

Heart failure is defined as the inability of the heart to supply peripheral organs with sufficient amounts of blood for their metabolic requirements. In addition to several pathophysiological processes, the sympathetic nervous system is activated as a compensatory mechanism. After prolonged activation of the β-adrenoceptors by increased levels of catecholamines, desensitization occurs, which is associated with a decreased β-adrenoceptor density and/or a decreased ability to activate adenylate cyclase.

In various forms of heart failure, the β-adrenoceptor density is reduced [2,8,9]. The loss of receptors can be global (the β_1 and β_2 subtypes being equally affected) [2] or subtype-selective (the number of β_1 adrenoceptors being lowered whereas that of β_2-adrenoceptors is relatively unchanged) [8,9]. In dilated cardiomyopathy (DCM) the ratio of β_1/β_2-adrenoceptors is shifted from 80/20 to about 60/40 with a B_{max} of 30-50 fmol/mg protein in end-stage DCM [2]. In other forms like ischemic cardiomyopathy and mitral valve disease the ratio of the subtypes remains unchanged, while the B_{max} is reduced to about 30-40 fmol/mg protein. In vivo, little information is available about the time course of the alterations and the spatial distribution of the β-adrenoceptor population within the heart and the influence of therapy.

PET-ligands for β-adrenoceptors

A positron emitting radiotracer should meet certain criteria in order to be a suitable receptor ligand for PET. The ligand-β-adrenoceptor interaction must be the major mechanism underlying accumulation of radioactivity in target tissue. Other mechanisms like non-specific binding, binding to non β-adrenoceptor binding sites or accumulation of radiolabeled metabolites in the region of interest should contribute as little as possible. Some generally accepted criteria for a radiotracer are [10,11]:

1) *High affinity.* Radioligands should bind with high affinity to β-adrenoceptors (dissociation constant $K_D<10^{-9}M$). The ratio of the concentrations of bound and free ligand is an important parameter and is maximally equal to B_{max}/K_D for a single class of sites. The binding potential B_{max}/K_D should be >10 for obtaining an adequate contrast in PET-images [11].
2) *High specificity.* Radioligands should bind to only one receptor (sub)type.
3) *Saturability,* which can provide information on the receptor density in various tissues and the apparent affinity of the radioligand for these sites.
4) *Stereoselectivity.* Interaction with receptors is stereoselective. In the case of β-adrenoceptors the (S)-isomer antagonists is the biologically active compound. Nonspecific binding or binding to non-adrenergic binding sites is usually not stereospecific.
5) *Distribution related to the physiological response.* A radioligand should only bind to functional receptors and not to internalized receptors inside the cell membrane. In this respect the lipophilicity plays an important role. Lipophilic PET-ligands will bind to both internalized and externalized (functional) receptors, while hydrophilic ligands only bind to cell surface receptors.
6) *The radioligand must be non-toxic at the applied dosages.* When a dual injection protocol for receptor quantification is used, a carrier amount of 'cold' ligand is injected. In this case, a more stringent toxicological examination is necessary than for a non-carrier-added injection.

Several positron emitting β-ligands have been prepared and evaluated for imaging purposes, such as carbon-11 labeled CGP 20712A [12], metoprolol, propranolol, atenolol [13] and pindolol [14]. With the exception of pindolol, all these radioligands failed to image cardiac β-adrenoceptors, because either the affinity was too low or showed high non-specific binding.

At this moment, four potent PET-ligands are available for the visualization of β-adrenoceptors, i.e. (S)-[^{11}C]CGP 12177, (S)-[^{18}F]fluorocarazolol, (S)-[^{11}C]carazolol and (S)-[^{11}C]CGP 12388. The chemical structures are shown in figure 1 and important ligand characteristics in table 1. A major drawback of these tracers is the lack of selectivity for either the β_1 or the β_2-subtype. The radioligands are in different stages of evaluation. In the next paragraphs the status of each tracer will be discussed.

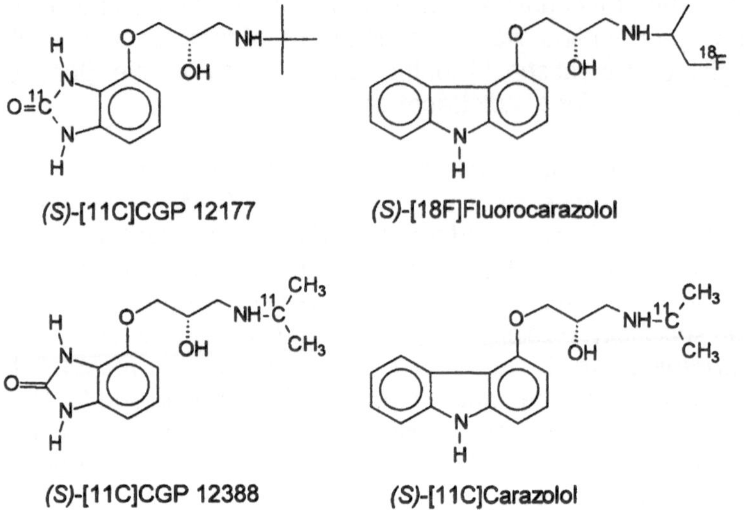

Figure 1. *Chemical structures of potent β-adrenoceptor radioligands for PET*

	CGP 12177	F-carazolol	Carazolol	CGP 12388
K_D (β_1) (nM)	0.33	0.41	0.059	Sub-nM
K_D (β_2) (nM)	0.90	0.10	0.023	Sub-nM
Log P	-0.50	2.20	1.36	-0.64
Half-life (min)	20.4	109.8	20.4	20.4
S.A. (Tbq/mmol)	0.37-18.5 variable	>74	22-30	22-30
Yield (Gbq, EOS)	8	0.37	1.85	1.85
Total/NS (10')	3.2	2.9	1.5	4.4
Total/NS (60')	7.1	4.9	3.6	7.2
Metabolites (60')				
Plasma (% native)	67 $\pm$ 8	2	72 $\pm$ 4	61 $\pm$ 9
Heart (% native)	>90	83 $\pm$ 4	-	94 $\pm$ 2

Table 1. *Characteristics of (S)-[^{11}C]CGP 12177, (S)-[^{18}F]fluorocarazolol, (S)-[^{11}C]carazolol and (S)-[^{11}C]CGP 12388. K_D=affinity constant. LogP= the logarithm of the octanol/water partition coefficient. S.A. = specific activity. Total/NS (NS=non-specific binding) values are obtained from PET-images of rats of the right lung*

(S)-[^{11}C]CGP 12177

(S)-[^{11}C]CGP 12177 is an established radioligand producing excellent PET-images of the human heart. (S)-[^{11}C]CGP 12177 has been used to determine cardiac β-adrenoceptor density in dogs [15] and humans [16,17]. Using a two-injection protocol (high and low specific activity), the B_{max} can be calculated with a graphical method [18] (figure 2). Due to its hydrophilic character (S)-[^{11}C]CGP 12177 binds only to functional receptors at the cell surface and not to internalized receptors. The radioligand is slowly metabolized. Except for its (subtype) selectivity, (S)-[^{11}C]CGP 12177 meets all criteria for a suitable PET-receptor ligand.

$$(B'_{max} - C^*(T_1 - \varepsilon))\left[1 - e^{\left(\frac{D_1^* + D_1}{D_0^*}\right)\log\left(\frac{B'_{max} - C_0^*}{B'_{max}}\right)}\right] - C_1^*\left(\frac{D_1 + D_1^*}{D_1^*}\right) = 0$$

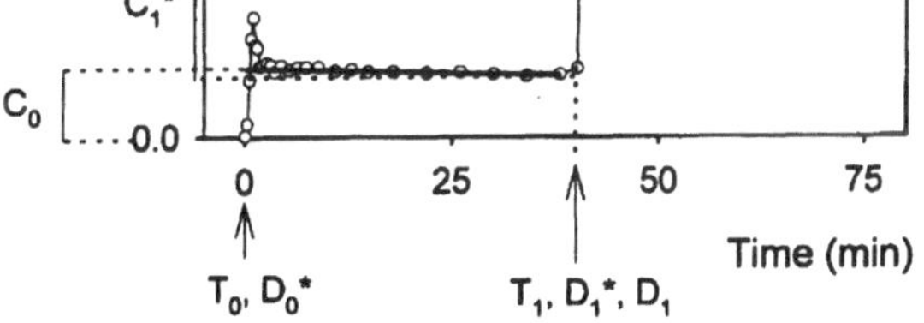

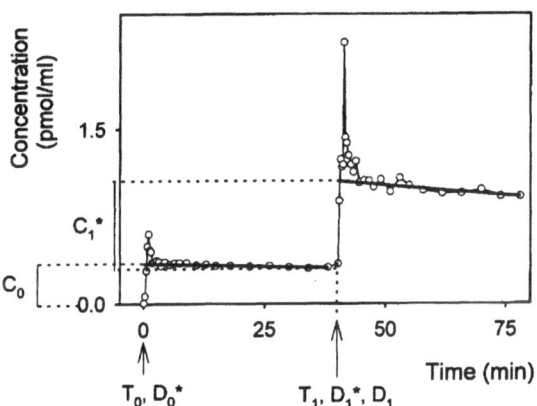

__Figure 2.__ A typical example of a time activity curve after a dual injection of (S)-[^{11}C]CGP 12177. The equation for the calculation of the β-adrenoceptor density B_{max}, as developed by Delforge [15]. B_{max} = β-adrenoceptor density; C^* $(T_1\text{-}\epsilon)$= concentration of labeled ligand just before the second injection; D_0^*, D_1^* = dose of radioligand in the first and second injection respectively; D_1 = dose of non-labeled in the second injection; C_0^* and C_1^* = estimated concentration of bound immediately after the first and second injection, respectively.

(S)-[^{11}C]CGP 12177 is produced by reaction of [^{11}C]phosgene with the appropriate (S)-diamine precursor in high radiochemical yields [19-21]. Several groups reported low and variable specific activities. The troublesome and laborious radiolabeling via [^{11}C]phosgene is an important drawback to apply [^{11}C]CGP 12177 for clinical studies and prevents widespread use of this radioligand.

(S)-[^{18}F]Fluorocarazolol and (S)-[^{11}C]carazolol

(S)-[^{18}F]Fluorocarazolol and (S)-[^{11}C]carazolol are non-subtype selective, lipophilic radioligands with high affinity for the β-adrenoceptor. (S)-[^{18}F]fluorocarazolol passed the blood-brain-barrier, which enables the possibility to investigate cerebral β-adrenoceptors [22].

The use of fluorine-18 has advantages of higher specific activity and a longer half life, which enables prolonged PET-studies. A general labeling method using [^{18}F]fluoroacetone to introduce ^{18}F in the isopropyl group was applied to carazolol [23,24]. (S)-[^{11}C]Carazolol is produced in an analogous way from [^{11}C]acetone [25].

(S)-[^{11}C]Carazolol has been evaluated by Berridge and coworkers in mice and pigs [26]. The pig heart was clearly visualized. Specific binding to β-adrenoceptors was demonstrated by injection of the bioactive (S)-[^{11}C]-isomer, followed by a second injection of the (R)-isomer, which only binds non-specifically.

Specific binding to β-adrenoceptors of (S)-[^{18}F]Fluorocarazolol was demonstrated either by injection by the (S)-isomer, followed by a second injection of the R-isomer [23] and by blocking experiments in rats with several subtype selective and non-selective β-adrenoceptor antagonists [27] and in vivo saturation experiments [28]. The experiments showed, that (S)-[^{18}F]fluorocarazolol was blocked according to the proper pharmacology and that B_{max}-values were in good agreement with the literature data.

Metabolite analysis of (S)-[^{18}F]fluorocarazolol showed a rapid appearance of polar metabolites in plasma, while at 60 min post injection 92% and 82% of the total radioactivity in lung and heart was unmetabolized (S)-[^{18}F]fluorocarazolol[24]. In a PET-study with male Wistar rats and lambs, the lungs were clearly visualized and the pulmonary uptake was strongly decreased (>90%) after pre-treatment of the animals with propranolol. The heart could not be visualized. However, PET-images in humans clearly showed the lung, heart [29] (figure 3) and specific brain areas, like frontal cortex and caudate nucleus [22]. The myocardium/plasma ratio increased to a plateau value of 18, which was reached at 45-50 min post injection. Uptake in heart was strongly inhibited after ingestion of pindolol. The myocardial uptake was reduced to 39% at 60 min post injection.

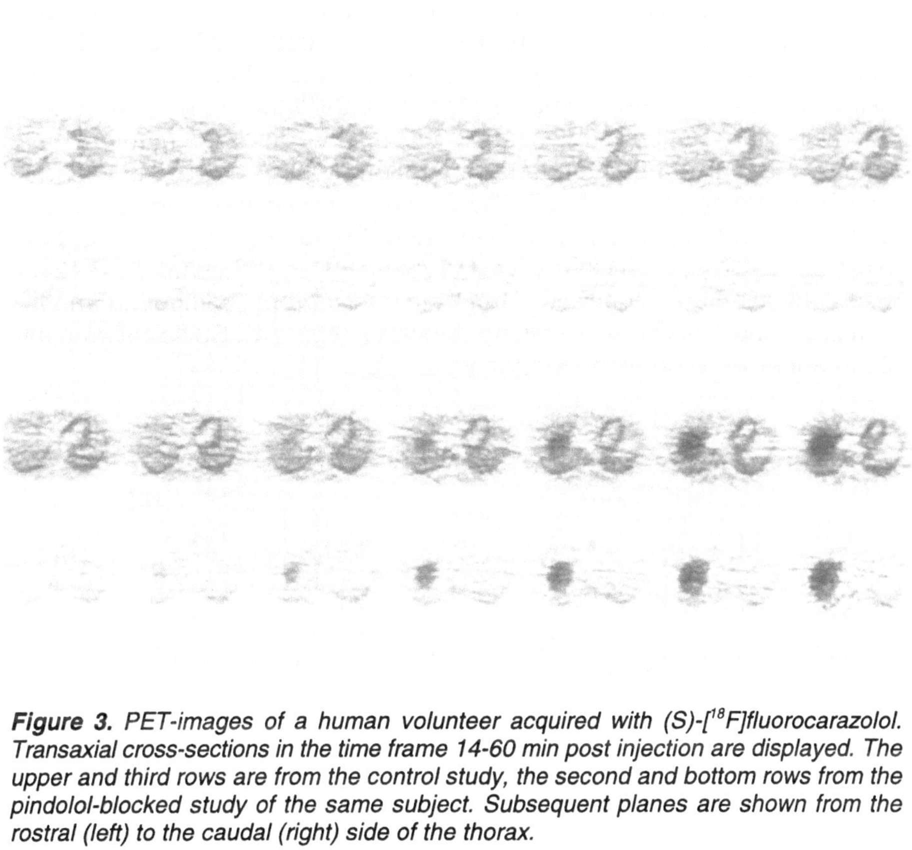

Figure 3. *PET-images of a human volunteer acquired with (S)-[^{18}F]fluorocarazolol. Transaxial cross-sections in the time frame 14-60 min post injection are displayed. The upper and third rows are from the control study, the second and bottom rows from the pindolol-blocked study of the same subject. Subsequent planes are shown from the rostral (left) to the caudal (right) side of the thorax.*

The human PET-studies as described above have been performed with non-carrier-added (S)-[^{18}F]fluorocarazolol and for this purpose an acute toxicity study in mice was carried out. (S)-[^{18}F]fluorocarazolol passed this toxicity test. In order to determine the receptor density in humans by a dual-injection protocol using pharmacological dosages, more extensive toxicity studies were carried out. Unfavorable toxicity data did us decide to stop human studies with (S)-[^{18}F]fluorocarazolol.

(S)-[^{11}C]CGP 12388

Because of the problems involved in routine production of (S)-[^{11}C]CGP 12177, it was worthwhile to develop another hydrophilic ß-adrenoceptor PET-ligand for clinical use. (S)-CGP 12388 was selected as a suitable candidate. CGP 12388 is the isopropyl analogue of CGP 12177 (t-butyl group). *In vitro* experiments have indicated that racemic CGP 12388 is an almost equally potent antagonist as racemic CGP 12177 (isoprenaline antagonism, isolated guinea pig heart, chronotropy: ED_{50} CGP 12388: 0.0025 µg/mL, CGP 12177: 0.0017 µg/mL, *unpublished results of Ciba-Geigy*). (S)-CGP 12388 can be labeled using 2-[^{11}C]acetone via a one-pot procedure. This synthetic procedure is less troublesome and therefore more suitable for clinical use than the preparation of (S)-[^{11}C]CGP 12177 from [^{11}C]phosgene. In addition the [^{18}F]labeled analogue of (S)-CGP 12388 was prepared. A general labeling method using [^{18}F]fluoroacetone was applied to (S)-CGP 12388. Both (S)-[^{11}C]CGP 12388 and (S)-[^{18}F]fluoro-CGP 12388 were conveniently synthesized [30] from the desisopropyl compound and the corresponding radiolabeled acetone derivative (figure 4). Sufficient amounts of the tracer were obtained for patient studies.

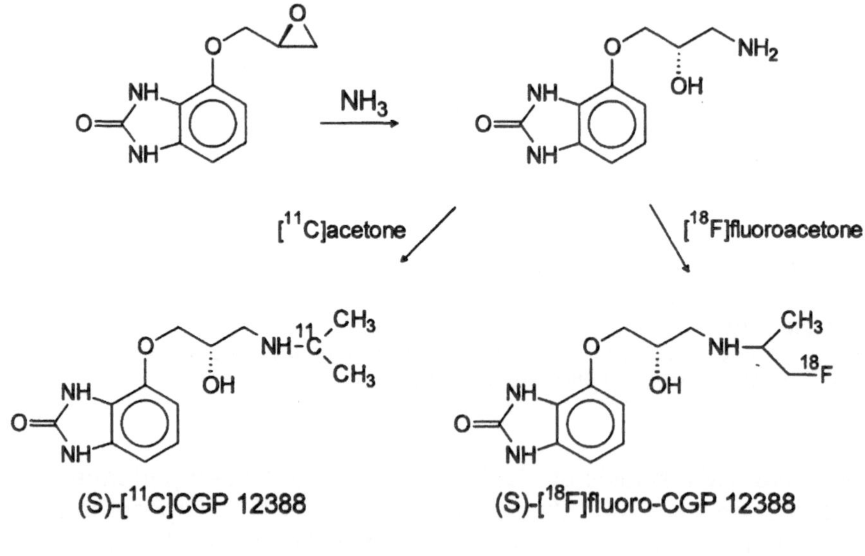

Figure 4. *Synthesis of (S)-[^{11}C]CGP 12388 and (S)-[^{18}F]fluoro-CGP 12388.*

Specific binding of (S)-[^{11}C]CGP 12388 and (S)-[^{18}F]fluoro-CGP 12388 to ß-adrenoceptors was demonstrated in rats. (S)-[^{11}C]CGP 12388 is superior to the [^{18}F]-analogue as the uptake values in lung, heart and spleen are higher. Non-specific binding is similar for both compounds. The differences in biodistribution can be explained from the fluorine substitution in the isopropyl group. In previous studies with fluorinated metoprolol and carazolol it was shown that fluorine substitution resulted in a 4-5 fold loss in affinity for ß-adrenoceptors [24,31]. The K_D for (S)-[^{18}F]fluoro-CGP 12388 is expected to exceed 1 nM, which is considered to be the maximal K_D for a suitable PET-ligand for the visualization of ß-adrenoceptors in the heart [11]. Additional evidence for receptor binding of (S)_[^{11}C]CGP 12388 was acquired from blocking experiments with the subtype selective β-adrenoceptor antagonists CGP 20712A (β_1-selective) and ICI 118,551 (β_2-selective) [32]. Cardiac uptake could be inhibited by CGP 20712A, but not by ICI 118,551. Metabolism of (S)-[^{11}C]CGP 12388 was similar to (S)-[^{11}C]CGP 12177 [32]. The fraction of plasma radioactivity representing parent compound decreased from 99.9% at time zero to 60.6 "8.8% at t=40 min. Radiochromatograms of tissue extracts made 60 min post injection indicated that the heart contains mainly native (S)-[^{11}C]CGP 12388.

Due to its easy preparation and comparable *in vivo* behavior with (S)-[^{11}C]CGP 12177 and (S)-[^{18}F]fluorocarazolol, (S)-[^{11}C]CGP 12388 seems a very promising tracer for visualization and quantification of ß-adrenoceptors. Evaluation in humans should prove its suitability in clinical PET.

Comparison of radioligands

A comparison between the biodistribution data of the CGP 12388 analogues, [^{11}C]CGP 12177 and [^{18}F]fluorocarazolol is shown in table 2. At 10 min post injection total/non-specific binding of (S)-[^{11}C]CGP 12388 in lung (6.9) and heart (3.5) is comparable with that of (S)-[^{11}C]CGP 12177 (lung 7.2, heart 4.9). The ratios for the [^{18}F]analogue are twofold lower. Comparison of data at 60 min post injection with (S)-[^{18}F]fluorocarazolol results in higher total/non-specific binding ratios for lung (13.8) and heart (4.3) as compared to (S)-[^{11}C]CGP 12388 (lung 9.5, heart 2.7). The higher ratios for (S)-[^{18}F]fluorocarazolol may be explained by its higher affinity and lipophilicity.

In PET-studies of rats the lungs were clearly visualized with both radiolabeled CGP 12388 analogs, while the heart was not visible. Similar images have been obtained with (S)-[^{18}F]fluorocarazolol. After treatment with propranolol the lungs were no longer visible.

In lung tissue, the ratio total/non-specific binding at 60 min post injection for (S)-[^{11}C]CGP 12388 was 7.2. Experiments with (S)-[^{11}C]CGP 12177 showed a similar ratio of total/non-specific binding, while after injection of (S)-[^{18}F]fluorocarazolol a ratio of 4.9 was observed.

		10 min post injection			
		[^{11}C]CGP 12388	[^{18}F]CGP 12388	[^{3}H]CGP 12177	[^{18}F]FCR
Heart	con	2.52±0.38	1.98±0.57	4.57±1.43	n.d.
	prop	0.72±0.18	1.09±0.25	0.94±0.16	
Lung	con	8.65±1.00	4.29±0.45	16.5±2.7	n.d
	prop	1.26±0.56	1.37±0.41	2.3±0.3	
		60 min post injection			
		[^{11}C]CGP 12388	[^{18}F]CGP 12388	[^{3}H]CGP 12177	[^{18}F]FCR
Heart	con	2.03±0.83	1.09±0.30	n.d.	2.68±0.16
	prop	0.76±0.23	0.46±0.19		0.62±0.11
Lung	con	8.38±2.62	3.66±0.54	n.d	15.9±2.74
	prop	0.88±0.16	0.59±0.14		1.15±0.30

Table 2. *Comparison between CGP 12388-analogues, [^{3}H]CGP 12177* and [^{18}F]fluorocarazolol Uptake values expressed as DAR. N=4 in each group. Mean ± SD con = control group, prop = propranolol blocked group. n.d.= not determined.[^{18}F]FCR is (S)-1'-[^{18}F]fluorocarazolol. *Administered mass of [^{3}H]CGP 12177 was similar to those of the other ligands.*

Future

So far, the optimal β-adrenoceptor ligand for PET is still a matter of research. The development of a β_1-subtype selective radioligand would be a great improvement. For this purpose [^{11}C]CGP 20712A [12] and HX-CH 44 BS [33] have been synthesized. [^{11}C]CGP 20712A showed very high non-specific binding. The affinity constant of HX-CH 44 BS exceeds 1 nM [34]. Therefore images made with this radioligand can be expected to show poor signal to noise ratios. In the near future we will focus on the evaluation of (S)-[^{11}C]CGP 12388 in humans as an alternative for (S)-[^{11}C]CGP 12177. If the human studies are successful, a high affinity and easily to prepare radioligand will come available for clinical PET.

References

1. Michel MC, Brodde OE, Insel PA. Peripheral adrenergic receptors in hypertension. Hypertension 1990;16: 107-20.
2. Brodde OE. Beta$_1$- and beta$_2$-adrenoceptors in the human heart: properties, function, and alterations in chronic heart failure. Pharmacol Rev 1991; 43: 203-42.
3. Lands AM, Arnold A, McAuliff P, Luduena FP, Brown TG Jr. Differentiation of receptor systems activated by sympathomimetic amines. Nature 1967;214: 597-8.
4. Watson S, Abbott A. TiPS receptor nomenclature supplement. Trends Pharmacol. Sci 1990; Suppl:1-30.
5. Scatchard G. The attraction of proteins for small molecules and ions. Ann NY Acad. Sci. 1949;51: 660 72.
6. Barnett DB, Rugg EL, Nahorski SR. Direct evidence of two types of beta-adrenoceptor binding site in lung tissue. Nature 1978;273: 166-8.
7. Minneman KP, Hegstrand LR, Molinoff PB. Simultaneous determination of beta-1 and beta-2 adrenergic receptors in tissues containing both receptor subtypes. Mol Pharmacol 1979;16: 34-46.
8. Bristow MR, Ginsburg R, Umans V, et al. Beta$_1$- and beta$_2$-adrenergic-receptor subpopulations in nonfailing and failing human ventricular myocardium: coupling of both receptor subtypes to muscle contraction and selective beta$_1$-receptor down-regulation in heart failure. Circ Res 1986;59:297-309.
9. Michel MC, Pingsmann A, Beckeringh JJ, Zerkowski HR, Doetsch N, Brodde OE. Selective regulation of beta$_1$- and beta$_2$-adrenoreceptors in the human heart by chronic β-adrenoreceptor antagonist treatment. Br J Pharmacol 1988;94: 685-92.
10. Eckelman WC. The application of receptor theory to receptor binding and enzyme-binding oncologic radiopharmaceuticals. Nucl Med Biol1994; 21: 759-69.
11. Van Waarde A, Elsinga PH, Anthonio RL, et al. Study of cardiac receptor ligands by positron emission tomography. In: Van der Wall EE, Blanksma PH, Niemeyer MG, Paans AM, editors. Cardiac positron emission tomography. Dordrecht: Kluwer Academic Publishers; 1995:171-82.
12. Elsinga PH, van Waarde A, Visser GM, Vaalburg W. Synthesis and preliminary evaluation of (R,S)-1-[2((carbamoyl-4-hydroxy)phenoxy)-ethylamino]-3-[4(1-[^{11}C]-methyl-4-trifluoromethyl-2-imidazolyl)phenoxy]-2-propanol ([^{11}C]CGP 20712A) as a selective beta-1 adrenoceptor ligand for PET. Nucl Med Biol 1994;21: 211-7.
13. Antoni G, Ulin J, Långström B. Synthesis of the ^{11}C-labelled beta-adrenergic receptor ligands atenolol, metoprolol and propranolol. Appl Radiat Isot 1989; 40: 561-4.
14. Prenant C, Sastre J, Crouzel C, Syrota A. Synthesis of [^{11}C]pindolol. J Label Compd Radiopharm 1987;24: 227-32.
15. Delforge J, Syrota A, Lançon JP, et al. Cardiac beta-adrenergic receptor density measured in vivo using PET, CGP 12177 and a new graphical method [published erratum appear in J Nucl Med 1994;32:739-48]. J Nucl Med 1991;32:739-48.

16. Merlet P, Delforge J, Syrota A, et al. Positron emission tomography with ^{11}C CGP-12177 to assess beta-adrenergic receptor concentration in idiopathic dilated cardiomyopathy. Circulation 1993;87: 1169-78.
17. Lefroy DC, De Silva R, Choudhury L, et al. Diffuse reduction of myocardial beta-adrenoceptors in hypertrophic cardiomyopathy: a study with positron emission tomography. J Am Coll Cardiol 1993;22: 1653-60.
18. Delforge J, Nakajima K, Syrota A, et al. PET investigation of beta-adrenergic receptors using CGP 12177 [abstract]. J Nucl Med 1989;30: 825.
19. Boullais C, Crouzel C, Syrota A. Synthesis of 4-(3-t-butylamino-2-hydroxy-propoxy)-benzimidazol-2[^{11}C]-one (CGP 12177). J Label Compd Radiopharm 1985;23: 565-7.
20. Brady F, Luthra SK, Tochon-Danguy H-J, et al. Asymmetric synthesis of a precursor for the automated radiosynthesis of *S*-(3'-t-butylamino-2'-hydroxypropoxy)-benzimidazol-2-[^{11}C]one (*S*-[^{11}C]CGP 12177) as a preferred radioligand for beta-adrenergic receptors. Appl Radiat Isot 1991;42: 620-8.
21. Aigbirhio F, Pike VW, Francotte E, et al. *S*-[1-(2,3-Diaminophenoxy)]-3'-(N-t-butylamino)propan-2'-ol - Simplified asymmetric synthesis with CD and chiral HPLC analysis. Tetrahedron Asymmetry 1992;3: 539-44.
22. Van Waarde A, Visser TJ, Elsinga PH, et al. Imaging beta-adrenoceptors in the human brain with (*S*)-1'-[^{18}F]fluorocarazolol. J Nucl Med 1997;38:934-9.
23. Zheng L, Berridge MS, Ernsberger P. Synthesis, binding properties and ^{18}F labeling of fluorocarazolol, a high affinity beta-adrenergic receptor antagonist. J Med Chem 1994;37:3219-30.
24. Elsinga PH, Vos MG, Van Waarde A, et al. (S,S)- and (S,R)-1'-[^{18}F]fluorocarazolol, ligands for the visualization of pulmonary beta-adrenergic receptors with PET. Nucl Med Biol 1996;23:159-67.
25. Berridge MS, Cassidy EH, Terris AH, Vesselle JM Preparation and in vivo binding of [^{11}C]carazolol; a radiotracer for the beta-adrenergic receptor. Int J Rad Appl Instrum B 1992;19:563-9.
26. Berridge MS, Nelson AD, Zheng L, Leisure GP, Miraldi F. Specific beta-adrenergic receptor binding of carazolol measured with PET. J Nucl Med 1994; 35: 1665-76.
27. Van Waarde A, Elsinga PH, Brodde OE, Visser GM, Vaalburg W. Myocardial and pulmonary uptake of *S*-1'-[^{18}F]fluorocarazolol in intact rats reflects radioligand binding to beta-adrenoceptors. Eur J Pharmacol 1995;272: 159-68.
28. Doze P, Van Waarde A, Elsinga PH, Van Loenen-Weemaes AM, Willemsen AT, Vaalburg W. Validation of S-1=-[18F]fluorocarazolol for in vivo imaging and quantification of cerebral β-adrenoceptors. J Cereb Blood Flow Metab. Submitted.
29. Visser TI, Van Waarde A, Van der Mark TW, et al. Characterization of pulmonary and myocardial beta-adrenoceptors with S-1:-[fluorine-18]fluorocarazolol. J Nucl Med 1997;38:169-74.
30. Elsinga PH, Van Waarde A, Jaeggi KA, Schreiber G, Heldoorn M, Vaalburg W. Synthesis and evaluation of (*S*)-4-(3-(2=-[^{11}C]-isopropylamino)-2-hydroxypropoxy)-2H-benzimidazol-2-one ((*S*)-[^{11}C]-CGP 12388) and (*S*)-4-(3-(1=-[^{18}F]-fluoroisopropylamino)-2-hydroxypropoxy)-2H-benzimidazol-2-one ((*S*)-[^{18}F]fluoro-CGP 12388) for visualization of beta-adrenoceptors with positron emission tomography. J Med Chem 1997;40:3829-35.
31. De Groot TJ, Van Waarde A, Elsinga PH, Visser GM, Brodde OE, Vaalburg W. Synthesis and evaluation of 1'-[^{18}F]fluorometoprolol as a potential tracer for the visualization of beta-adrenoceptors with PET. Nucl Med Biol 1993;20: 637-42.

32. Van Waarde A, Elsinga PH, Doze P, Heldoorn M, Jaeggi KA, Vaalburg W. A novel beta-adrenoceptor ligand for PET: evaluation in experimental animals. Eur J Pharmacol. In press 1998.
33. Dolle F, Valette H, Hinnen S, Escargueil C, Crouzel C. Carbon-11 labeling and in vivo characterization of a highly selective cardiac β1-adrenoceptor antagonist. Proceedings of the 12th Int Symp radiopharm Chem, Uppsala, Sweden, June 1997; 603-4.
34. Daemmgen JW, Engelhardt G, Pelzer H. Pharmacological properties of an extremely selective beta1-adrenoceptor antagonist, 2-[4-[3-(tert-butylamino)-2-hydroxypropoxy]phenyl]-3-methyl-6-methoxy-4(3H)-quinazoline ([+/-] HX-CH 44 BS). Arzneimittelforschung 1985;35:383-90.

Chapter 20

SURGICAL TREATMENT OF HEART FAILURE

René M.H.J. Brouwer, Maarten P. van den Berg, Eduard L. Mooyaard

Introduction

Heart failure is defined as cardiac pumping dysfunction with circulatory and neurohormonal responses and develops as a consequence of cardiac disease[1]. Ischemic heart disease accounts for more than 60% of all cases with heart failure. In a substantial number of cases the aetiology is unknown and the term idiopathic cardiomyopathy is used. The importance of valvular disease and hypertension as a cause of heart failure has declined steadily[2]. Heart failure has become one of the most prevalent cardiovascular disorders and represents a significant clinical and financial burden in the Western World [3]. The prevalence is expected to increase further, predominantly due to aging of the population, higher survival rates after acute myocardial infarction and longer survival of persons with heart disease. Furthermore, simulation models predict a transition from acute to chronic cardiovascular disease due to a significant increase in age adjusted ischemic heart disease in the Netherlands by 2010, that is largely attributable to heart failure [4]. The prevalence in the general population ranges from 1.0 to 5.0 individuals per 1000 with a steep increase to 30 to 130 individuals per 1000 for those aged over 65 years [5,6]. Between 1980 and 1992, the annual number of hospital admissions in the Netherlands increased almost by 70%, and in 1989 the health care costs were Dfl 436 million or 1% of the national health care budget [6]. In the US it is estimated that 3 million individuals are afflicted by heart failure and nearly 500,000 new cases are diagnosed each year. In 1989 the associated health care cost were more than $8 billion [7].

Van der Wall et al. (eds.),
Advanced Imaging in Coronary Artery Disease, 321-333.

The prognosis of heart failure remains bad despite improvements in pharmacological treatments. The Framingham Study clearly showed that once heart failure has developed, only 25% of the men and 37% of women were alive after 5 years [8,9]. In other words, approximately 50% of patients die within 3 years of presentation. Although heart transplantation (Htx) has proven efficacious with a 5 year survival of 60-70%, the limited number of donors makes it applicable to only a small proportion of patients [10,11]. Because of the increasing demand for Htx in the setting of a relatively fixed supply of donor hearts, the waiting time for patients has increased and often exceeds 6 months, or even 1 year [10]. Currently 25% of the patients on the waiting lists die due to circulatory decompensation or sudden death. However, as the waiting lists expands, priority is awarded solely on the basis of the waiting time of patients, who now usually undergo Htx after they have already survived a major period of jeopardy.

Paradoxically, the survival benefit decreases from Htx for these patients as the waiting lists lengthens: for patients already surviving more than 6 months without Htx, actuarial survival over the next 12 months is as high or even higher as the 1 year survival after Htx [11]. Thus, the expected improvement in survival after Htx is negligible over the subsequent year for patients waiting for more than 6 months. Therefore, one may argue that Htx should be reserved for the most critically-ill patients in which the survival benefit of transplantation is expected to be maximal [12]. In other words, stable patients should be re-evaluated to determine whether transplantation is still indicated or should be selected for alternative surgical treatment for heart failure, such as the dynamic cardiomyoplasty or the volume reduction of the left ventricle for end-stage heart failure [13-15].

Dynamic Cardiomyoplasty

The dynamic cardiomyoplasty (DCMP) is rapidly gaining popularity as an alternative surgical treatment for chronic congestive heart failure due to ischemic or idiopathic dilated cardiomyopathy. Its primary objectives are 1) to improve symptoms of congestive heart failure and 2) to retard the progressive ventricular dilatation. The biophysical basis for the DCMP is that electrical stimulation of a skeletal muscle can increase its resistance to fatigue by converting fast-twitch type II fibers to fatigue-resistant slow-twitch type I fibers. This means that, using an electrical stimulation training protocol to increase the number of impulses in the burst stepwise over several weeks, the skeletal muscle undergoes changes in myosin ATPase, force development characteristics and becomes resistant to fatigue [16,17].

The DCMP procedure, normally performed on the beating heart without cardio- pulmonary bypass, consists of a ventricular assist with the left or right latissimus dorsi muscle (LDM) [13]. After meticulous mobilization of the LDM to avoid any injury of the neurovascular pedicle, intramuscular electrodes are implanted near the trifurcation of the thoracodorsal nerve. Then, trial stimulation ensures that strong contraction of the whole muscle can be elicited. Next, a segment of the second or third rib is removed so that the LDM and the electrodes can be placed into the pleural space. The proximal insertion of the LDM to the humerus is transsected and reattached to the chest wall. The patient is turned to the supine position. After the sternotomy is carried out, the heart is exposed and epicardial sensing electrodes are placed. The LDM is retrieved from the pleural cavity and wrapped around both ventricles. Most commonly, a posterior wrap or clockwise rotation is used for predominant left ventricular failure. The positioning of the LDM is carried out using the 'flap sliding technique': two long clamps hold two stay sutures placed on the leading edge of the LDM; posterior displacement of the clamps allows the free edge of the LDM to slide below the apex and the left ventricle without mobilisation of the heart. Finally, the sensing and stimulating electrodes are connected to a synchronised burst stimulator (Transform® Cardiomyostimulator, model 4710, Medtronic, Minneapolis, USA) that is programmed to sense R waves and fire burst stimuli so that the LDM will contract in synchrony with cardiac systole (figure 1).

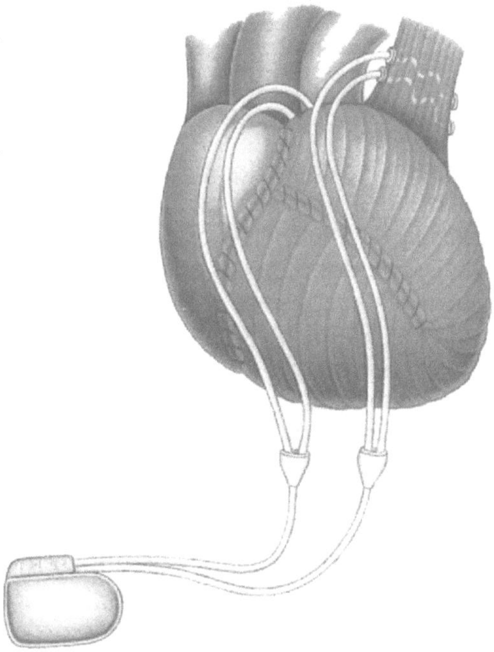

Figure 1. *The LDM is mobilized and intramuscular electrodes are implanted near the trifurcation of the thoracodorsal nerve supplying this muscle. A segment of the second or third rib is removed so that the LDM and the electrodes can be placed into the pleural space. Epicardial sensing electrodes are placed on the right ventricle. The LDM is retreived from the pleural space and wrapped around the left ventricle and part of the right ventricle.The sensing and stimulated electrodes are connected to a synchronized stimulator that is programmed to sense R waves and fire burst stimuli so that the LDM will contract in synchrony with cardiac systole.*

After 2 weeks without stimulation (the time necessary for the LDM to adhere to the heart), progressive sequential stimulation is undertaken which after 10 weeks culminates to full stimulation with trains of impulses and maximum pulses amplitude A 2:1 mode is used to prevent overstimulation and muscle damage. Doppler-echocardiography serves to assess the proper timing of stimulation since the LDM should contract only after mitral valve closure (figure 2).

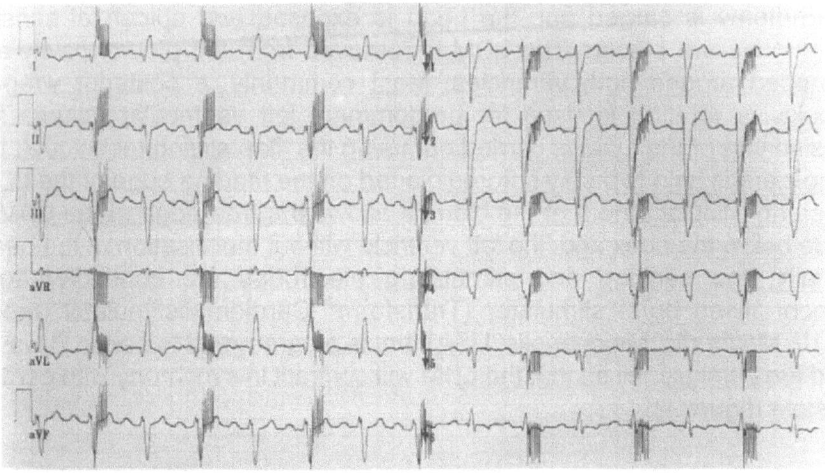

Figure 2. *Electrocardiogram of a patient after the DCMP procedure. In a 2:1 mode, 6 burst spikes can be identified after the QRS complex.*

The current indication for dynamic cardiomyoplasty include patients at high risk of dying due to severe cardiomyopathies. In fact, this indication does not essentially differ from Htx criteria. Therefore, patients for this procedure are normally screened based on factors that have been related to mortality in patients with congestive heart failure. These include parameters relating to New York Heart Association (NYHA) class III or IV, cardiac pump dysfunction, such as left ventricular (LV) ejection fraction less than 25%, peak oxygen consumption (VO_2 - max) during exercise below 16 ml/min/kg and high ventricular filling pressures [18]. On the other hand, patients submitted to DCMP need to be stable enough on medication to withstand a waiting period of 10 weeks before effective skeletal muscle flap adaptation occurs. Therefore patients on intravenous inotropic drugs, persistent NYHA class IV, but also severe mitral valvular incompetence and malignant arrhythmias are considered unsuitable for DCMP (table 1) [14].

The long-term results of the DCMP are encouraging. The freedom from death after 7 years varies from 42 to 70% and is comparable with the long-term results of the Htx [10,11,19,20]. Moreover it compares favorably with the 20% survival at 3 years in medically treated patients [3]. Clinically, functional improvement can be noticed with an increase in exercise capacity, reduction in the need for drugs, and reduction of the number of episodes of hospitalisation for congestive heart failure. In the majority of patients daily activities, mental health and quality of interactions improve remarkably. Additional advantages of the DMP compared to Htx are:

1) no waiting list
2) no rejection treatment
3) the possibility for Htx
4) lower costs than Htx [13,14,18-21].

Permanent NYHA class IV
LV ejection fraction < 15%
Hypertrophied, restrictive cardiomyopathies
Severe biventricular failure
Severe mitral valvar incompetence
Atrial fibrillation
Severe pulmonary hypertension
LV end-diastolic diameter > 75 mm
LV end-diastolic pressure > 45 mm Hg
Severe respiratory insufficiency
Neurovascular disease
Cachexia

Table 1. *Contraindications for dynamic cardiomyoplasty* [14]
LV= left ventricular

The functional improvement results from enhanced heart function due to several mechanisms. First, the efficiency of DCMP depends on the mechanical characteristics of the heart and LDM and the amount of wrapping.

The power of the transformed LDM is identical to the power developed by the heart during the systolic contraction [22]. However, only a portion of this force is used since only a part of the LDM can be wrapped around the heart. The larger the heart, the lesser its efficiency. Second, the wrapped LDM, which acts like a girdle, reduces LV wall stress, prevents further dilatation of the heart and restores the LV pressure-volume relation [23].

Positron emission tomography (PET)-imaging allows for quantitative assessment of the perfusion and metabolism of the myocardium, and has gained widespread acceptance as a diagnostic tool in patients with ischemic heart disease. Therefore, PET- imaging might a be a means to investigate the effect of DCMP on the myocardium, which is otherwise hard to establish. The basic principle of the PET-imaging is that myocardial blood flow is determined with radio labeled ammonia ($^{13}NH_3$) and myocardial metabolism is assessed using radio labeled glucose (FDG). Perfusion reserve can be determined as the ratio between maximal blood flow after pharmacological provocation (for instance with dipyridamole) and basal blood flow. Areas with hypoperfusion and low FDG uptake ('mismatch defect') reflect chronic ischemia. Finally, radio labeled acetate (carbon-11 acetate) is used for aerobic metabolism assessment, both in the basal state and after inotropic stimulation [24-27]. In Groningen (AZG), DCMP patients underwent a protocol consisting of 3 images: an image prior to the operation, and an image 3 and 6 months postoperatively. Preliminary findings in these patients suggest that DCMP does not have a major impact on myocardial metabolism, however, perfusion reserve would appear to increase after DCMP (figure 3). The latter finding might be compatible with the presumed reducing effect of DCMP on left ventricular wall stress.

Finally, the outcome of the DCMP is influenced by specific preoperative and intraoperative variables. Multivariate analysis has produced NYHA class IV, atrial fibrillation, and poor right ventricular ejection fraction (RVEF) as incremental risk factors for death. Survival analysis performed on all patients in the combined world experiences, revealed that significant higher operative mortality in the NYHA Class IV patients as compared to NYHA Class III. A patient with atrial fibrillation has a risk 6 times higher than a similar patient in normal sinus rhythm at time of the operation. The reason for this phenomenon is the loss of the atria kick and its associated impairment of ventricular filling. DCMP is designed to augment systolic function and does this at the expense of impaired diastolic filling. Therefore DCMP is contraindicated in the absence of the atria kick. Likewise, each 10% decrease in RVEF would lead to an increase in relative risk by almost 1.5 times. Poor RVEF in fact represents end-stage biventricular failure unamenable to correction by a muscle wrap which assists only the left ventricle[28-30].

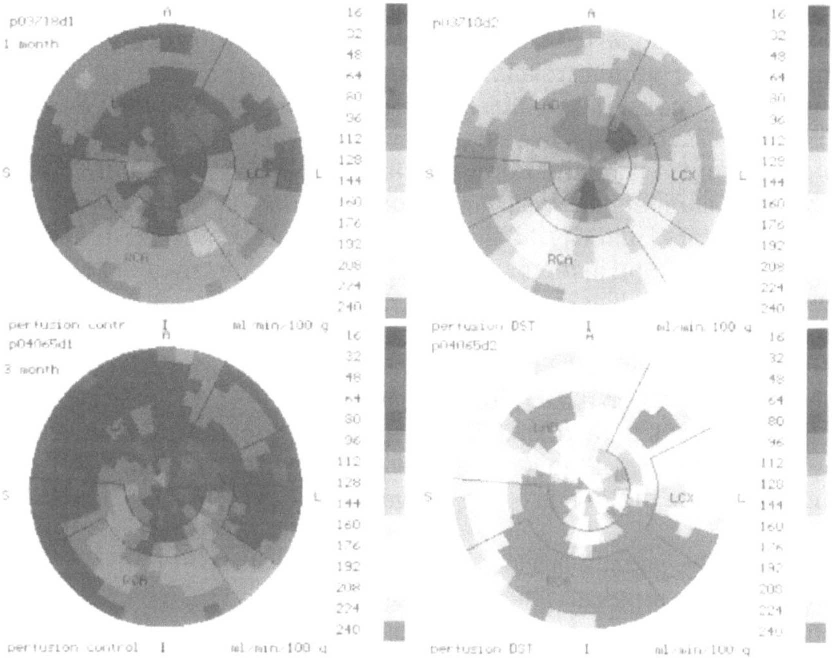

Figure 3. *Polar map displays of positron emission tomography myocardial perfusion in a patient who underwent a DCMP. Myocardial perfusion is displayed in a color scale as shown to the right of the polar map, in such a way that the apex is located in the center of the map and the basis of the heart at the periphery. In the maps the perfusion areas of the major coronary vessels are displayed. In the upper panels the results are shown as obtained 1 month after surgery, in the lower panels the results obtained 3 months after surgery. At left resting perfusion is shown, at right perfusion after dipyridamole infusion. It can be seen that the increase in perfusion after dipyridamole infusion (perfusion reserve) is larger after 3 months than it is shortly after surgery.*

(See also Colour Plates, p.341)

In conclusion, DCMP is a relative new and promising surgical technique for end-stage heart failure. The indication for operation has shifted to a much earlier stage than in the past, that is before the onset of incremental risk factors, such as right ventricular and mitral valvular incompetence and atrial fibrillation. Still much has to be learned about the refinement of the patient selection, the mechanism underlying this technique, and the discrepancy between the subjective and objective results. PET-imaging could fulfil an important role in the search for these answers.

Volume Reduction of the Left Ventricle (Batista Procedure)

Observations of hearts in different mammalian species suggest that heart mass is proportional to body weight and radius of the left ventricle. In order to maintain a normal relationship, an increase in radius will lead to an increase in mass. When the radius increases without changes in mass, dilatation will occur and eventually heart failure. Moreover heart volume and pressure are analogous to muscle length and tension. Furthermore, the average circumferential wall stress (force per unit of cross-sectional area of wall) is related directly to the product of intraventricular pressure and internal radius and inversely to wall thickness, expressed in the Laplace's law: $A = Pa/2h$, where P = intraventricular pressure, a = radius at the endocardial surface, and h = wall thickness. Thus, an increase in the radius leads to increased wall stress, increased myocardial oxygen consumption and consequently to a decrease in stroke volume. So theoretically, there are different options to reverse this process: 1) to decrease of the wall tension by medical therapy 2) to increase the LV mass for example with DCMP or 3) to decrease the radius of the left ventricle.

Most recently, volume reduction of the left ventricle has been introduced as an alternative surgical option for end-stage dilated cardiomyopathy [15,31,32]. This unconventional operation involves surgical resection of a wedge-shape piece of ventricular muscle and results in a reduction in the radius of the left ventricle to its normal size. With the removal of a 3-cm section of the left ventricle, the diameter of the left ventricle is reduced by 1-cm. Similarly, to reduce the internal diameter from 8 to 5-cm, a section of 9-cm has to be excised. According to Laplace's law, the wall stress reduces and the cardiac performance improves instantaneously [33]. Initially the mitral valve apparatus was preserved, however the distance between the anterior and posterior papillary muscle limits the amount of muscle resection. Therefore, mitral valve replacement and excision of the papillary muscle complex should be performed routinely [34].

Patient selection appears to play a major role in operative mortality and selection of lower risk patients (elective rather than salvage) appears to decrease operative mortality. There is some evidence that patients with ischemic cardiomyopathy appear to fare less well than those with a non-ischemic aetiology. Therefore, the best candidates for operation are elective patients with idiopathic dilated cardiomyopathy (NYHA III-IV) with or without valvular involvement, a left ventricle end-diastolic diameter (LVED) > 7cm, and in whom all other treatment options have been exhausted (end-stage heart failure). Generally, the operation is reserved for those too old for Htx or who are excluded for some other reason. However, individual physicians feel that the best patients are those who are candidates for Htx, and that the patient be informed that if the operation is unsuccessful, Htx may still be an option. With careful selection, recent data suggest that short-term results are acceptable with a 1 year survival of 90% with a significant improvement in the NYHA classification [34]. Still significant issues remain regarding not only the surgical techniques e.g. amount of ventricular muscle to be resected, but also the occurrence of sudden death and LV redilatation.

Magnetic resonance imaging (MRI) plays an increasing important role in imaging of the cardiac anatomy [35,36]. The signal void of fast flowing blood produces an excellent delineation of the cardiac wall providing exquisite anatomical detail of the cardiac chambers. Until recently, the acquisition time was relatively long, which resulted in moving-artefacts due to respiratory motion, but new fast MRI pulse sequences are now available. It is possible to obtain chine MRI imaging during one breath-hold. In these gradient images the blood has a high signal intensity compared to the cardiac wall, the so-called 'white blood' images. When multiple short axis sections are made through the left ventricle, end-diastolic and end-systolic dimensions and the ejection fraction of the left ventricle can be determined. Recent studies show that the cine MRI is an effective technique for measuring cardiac function. Also LV mass as well as changes of wall thickness during the cardiac cycle can be easily assessed. MRI therefore makes it possible to depict areas of impaired relaxation and contraction of the cardiac wall. The combination of excellent anatomical detail and determination of cardiac function makes cine MRI an effective tool in the preoperative evaluation of patients with cardiac dysfunction (figure 4). In the preoperative work up for the volume reduction of the left ventricle, the extent of diseased cardiac wall can be determined. Moreover MRI is capable to reproduce the same cross sections in the postoperative period to monitor the effects of the volume reduction.

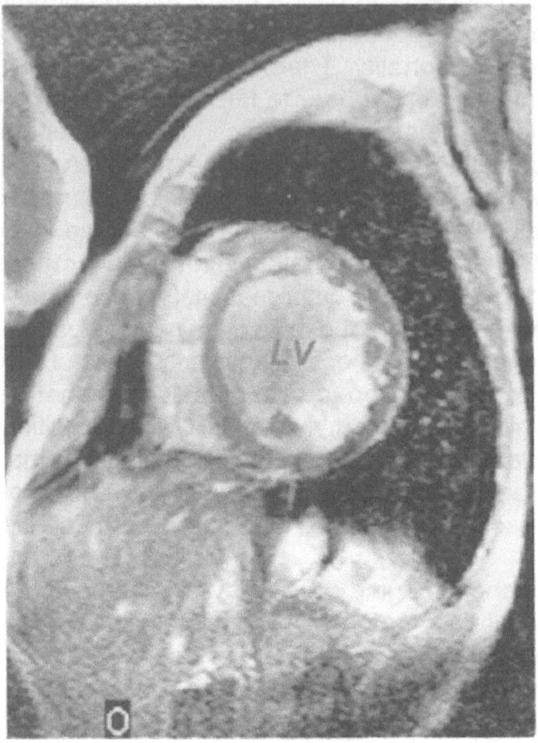

Figure 4. Short axis MRI view for determination of left ventricle (LV) dimension, function, mass and volume.

Conclusion

Heart failure is one of the most prevalent cardiovascular disorders and the prevalence will continue to increase. The prognosis of heart failure is poor with a mortality rate of 6 to 7 times that of the general population with a mortality one year following the onset of heart failure of 30%. The demand for Htx outruns the supply despite all measures to increase the donor pool. Moreover, Htx is the last therapeutic option for a patient with end-stage heart failure. Therefore the development of new surgical techniques for heart failure as an alternative for Htx should be stimulated. Dynamic cardiomyoplasty and the volume reduction of the left ventricle according to Batista might fulfil this goal and initial data on the short- and mid-term results are favorable. With the use of the PET and MRI a better selection of patients and understanding of the mechanisms of these alternative surgical techniques can be achieved.

References

1. Dutch heart failure consensus meeting 1994. Hart Bull 1994;25:254-304.
2. Ghali JK, Kay R, Shelton B, et al. Contemporary etiologies of left ventricular dysfunction and/or heart failure and their influence on prognosis [abstract]. Circulation 1992:86(4 suppl 1):I598.
3. Kannel WB. Epidemiology and prevention of cardiac failure: Framingham Study insights.Eur Heart J 1987;8 Suppl F: 23-6.
4. Bonneux L, Barendregt JJ, Meeter K, Bonsel GJ, van der Maas PJ. Estimating clinical morbidity due to ischemic heart disease and congestive heart failure: the future rise of heart failure. Am J Public Health 1994;84:20-8.
5. Lamberts H, Brouwer HJ, Mohrs J. Reason for encounter-, episode- and process-oriented standard output: from the Transition Project. Amsterdam : Department.of General Practice/Family Medicine, University of Amsterdam, 1991.
6. Van de Lisdonk EH, van den Bosch WJHM, Huygen FJA, Lagro-Jansen ALM, editors. Ziekten in de huisartspraktijk. Utrecht: Bunge, 1990.
7. Mosterd A. Epidemiology of heart failure. [dissertation]. Utrecht: S.N., 1997.
8. Ho KK, Anderson KM, Kannel WB, Grossman W, Levy D. Survival after the onset of congestive heart failure in Framingham Heart Study subjects. Circulation 1993;88:107-15.
9. Koopmanschap MA, van Roijen L, Bonneux L. Kosten van ziekten in Nederland. Herz. ed. Rotterdam: Instituut Maatschappelijke Gezondheidszorg, Erasmus Universiteit Rotterdam, 1991.
10. Sarris GE, Moore KA, Schroeder JS, et al. Cardiac transplantation: the Stanford experience in the cyclosporine era. J Thorac Cardiovasc Surg 1994;108:240-52.
11. Stevenson LW, Hamilton MA, Tillisch IH, et al. Decreasing survival benefit from cardiac transplantation for outpatients as the waiting list lengthens. J Am Coll Cardiol 1991;18:919-25.
12. Brouwer MH, Bams JL, Van den Berg MP, Van Veldhuisen DJ, Ebels T. Succesvolle harttransplantatie bij langdurige beademde patiënten. Ned Tijdschr Geneeskd 1996;140:2353-5.
13. Carpentier A, Chachques JC, Acar C, et al. Dynamic cardiomyoplasty at seven years. J Thorac Cardiovasc Surg 1993;106:42-54.
14. Carpentier A, Chachques JC, Carteaux JP. Dynamic cardiomyoplasty at eleven years. In: Carpentier A, Chachques JC, Grandjean P, editors: Cardiac bioassist. New York: Futura, 1997:3-23.
15. Batista RJ, Santos JL, Takeshita N, Bochinno L, Lima PN, Cunha MA. Partial left ventriculectomy to improve left ventricular function in end-stage heart disease [published erratum appears in J Card Surg 1997;12:ix]. J Card Surg 1996;11:96-8.
16. Salmons S, Jarvis JC. Skeletal muscle as an adaptive contractile biomaterial for cardiac assistance: fundamental considerations. Proceedings of the 14th Annual Conference of the IEEE Engineering in Medicine and Biology Society, Paris, France, 1992, 2798-9.
17. Salmons S, Sreter FA. Significance of impulse activity in the transformation of skeletal muscle type. Nature 1976;263:30-4.
18. Moreira LF, Bocchi EA, Stolf NAG, Bellotti G, Jatene AD. Long-term results of cardiomyoplasty in dilated cardiomyopathy. In: Carpentier A, Chachques JC, Grandjean P, editors. Cardiac bioassist. New York: Futura, 1997:25-35.

19. Van den Berg MP, Brouwer MH, Wijnberg DS, Brügemann J, Van der Maaten JM, Ebels T. De eerste Groningse ervaringen met dynamische cardiomyoplastiek. Ned Tijdschr Geneeskd 1997;141:1480-4.
20. Odim JN, Burgess JH, Chiu RC. Range of responses to dynamic cardiomyoplasty in dilated cardiomyopathy patients. In: Carpentier A, Chachques JC, Grandjean P, editors. Cardiac bioassist. New York: Futura, 1997:97-108.
21. Lee KF, Dignan RJ, Parmar JM, et al. Effects of dynamic cardiomyoplasty on left ventricular performance and myocardial mechanics in dilated cardiomyopathy. J Thorac Cardiovasc Surg 1991;102:124-31.
22. Salmons S, Jarvis JC. Cardiomyoplasty: a look at the fundamentals. In: Carpentier A, Chachques JC, Grandjean PA, editors. Cardiomyoplasty. Mount Kisco, New York: Futura, 1991:3-17.
23. Lorusso R, Sandrelli L, Borghetti V, Schreuder J, Alfieri O. Longterm myocardial assistance by a wrapped skeletal muscle. A clinical experience. In: Carpentier A, Chachques JC, Grandjean P, editors. Cardiac bioassist. New York: Futura, 1997:57-65.
24. Schelbert HR, Phelps ME, Huang SC, et al. N-13 ammonia as an indicator of myocardial blood flow. Circulation 1981;63:1259-72.
25. Tillisch J, Brunken R, Marshall R, et al. Reversibility of cardiac wall-motion abnormalities predicted by positron emission tomography. N Engl J Med 1986;314:884-8.
26. Buxton DB, Nienaber CA, Luxen A ,et al. Noninvasive quantification of regional myocardial oxygen consumption in vivo with (1-^{11}C) acetate and dynamic positron emission tomography. Circulation 1989;79:134-42.
27. Gambhir SS, Schwaiger M, Huan SC, et al. Simple noninvasive quantification method for measuring myocardial glucose utilization in humans employing positron emission tomography and fluorine-18 deoxyglucose.J Nucl Med 1989;30:359-66.
28. Furnary AP, Magovern JA, Christlieb IY, Orie JE, Simpson KA, Magovern GJ. Clinical cardiomyoplasty: preoperative factors associated with outcome. Ann Thorac Surg 1992;54:1139-43.
29. Corin WJ, George DT, Sink JD, Santamore WP. Dynamic cardiomyoplasty acutely impairs left ventricular diastolic function. J Thorac Cardiovasc Surg 1992;104:1662-71.
30. Medtronic Cardiomyoplasty Phase I Study Group. Phase I Clinical results through October 1991, prepared by Medtronic CAS Venture, April 1992.
31. McCarthy M. Batista procedure proves its value in the USA. Lancet 1997;349:855.
32. Angelini GD, Prynn S, Mehta D, et al. Left ventricular- volume reduction for end-stage heart failure [letter]. Lancet 1997;350:489.
33. Dickstein ML, Spotnitz HM, Rose EA, Burkhoff D. Heart reduction surgery: an analysis of the impact on cardiac function. J Thorac Cardiovasc Surg 1997;113:1032-40.
34. Batista RJ, Verde J, Nery P, et al. Partial left ventriculectomy to treat end-stage heart disease. Ann Thorac Surg 1997;64:634-8.
35. Baldy C, Douek P, Croisille P, Magnin IE, Revel D, Amiel M. Automated myocardial edge detection from breath-hold-cine MR images: Evaluation of left ventricular volumes and mass. Magn Reson Imaging 1994;12:589.

36. Cranney GB, Lotan CS, Dean L, Baxley W, Bouchard A, Pohost GM. Left ventricular volume measurement using cardiac axis nuclear magnetic resonance imaging. Validating by calibrated ventricular angiography. Circulation 1990;82:154-63.

Colour Plates

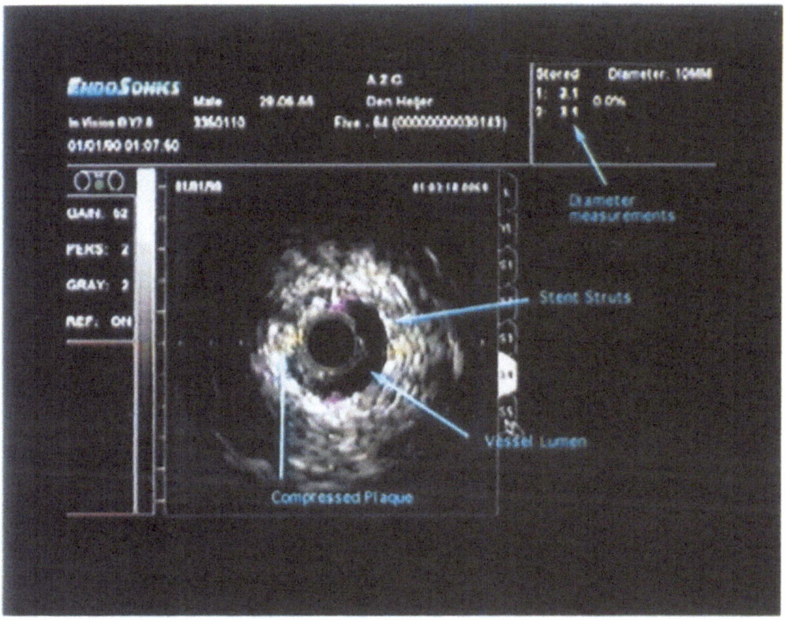

Figure 1, p. 18, Chapter 2.

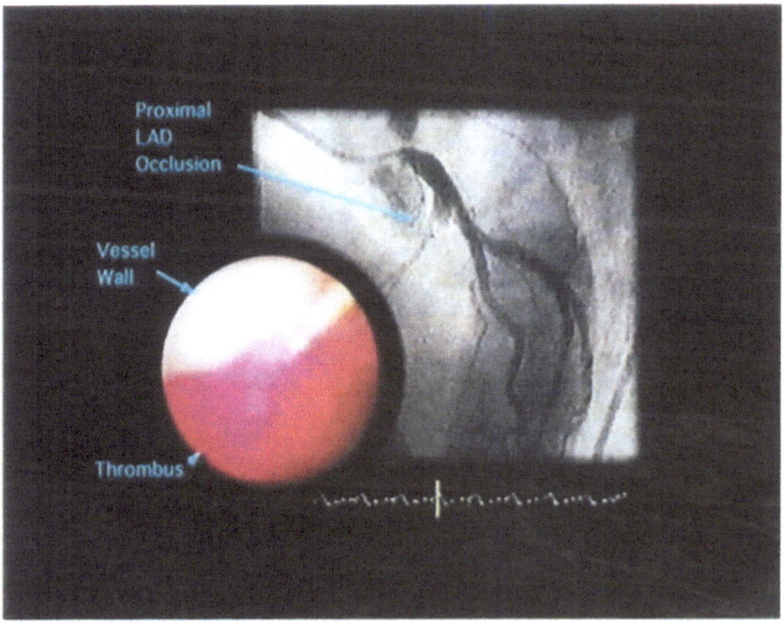

Figure 2, p. 21, Chapter 2.

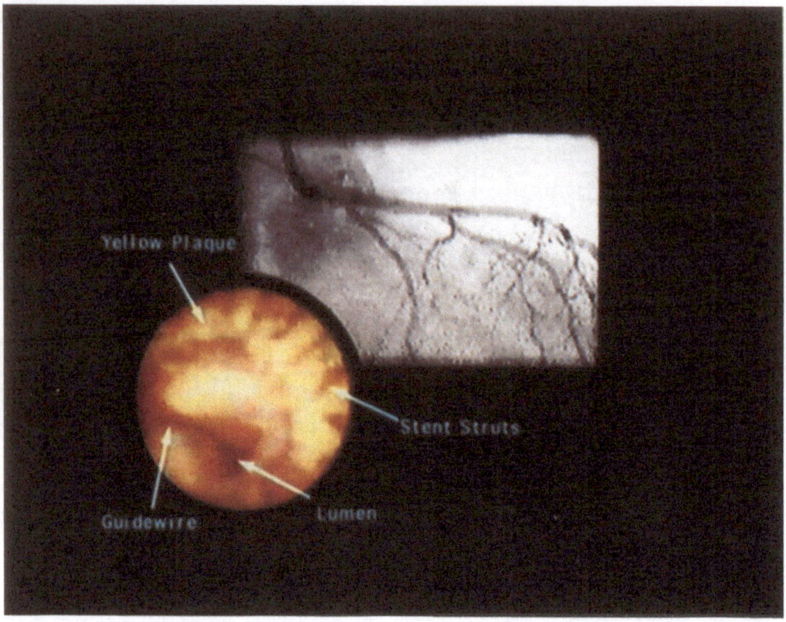

Figure 3, p. 23, Chapter 2

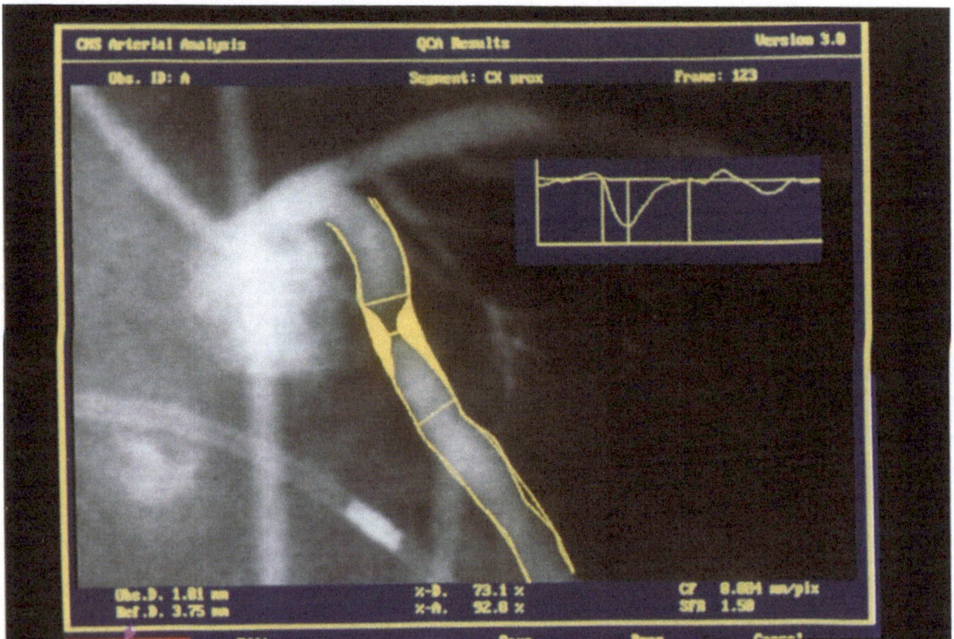

Figure 1, p. 80, Chapter 5.

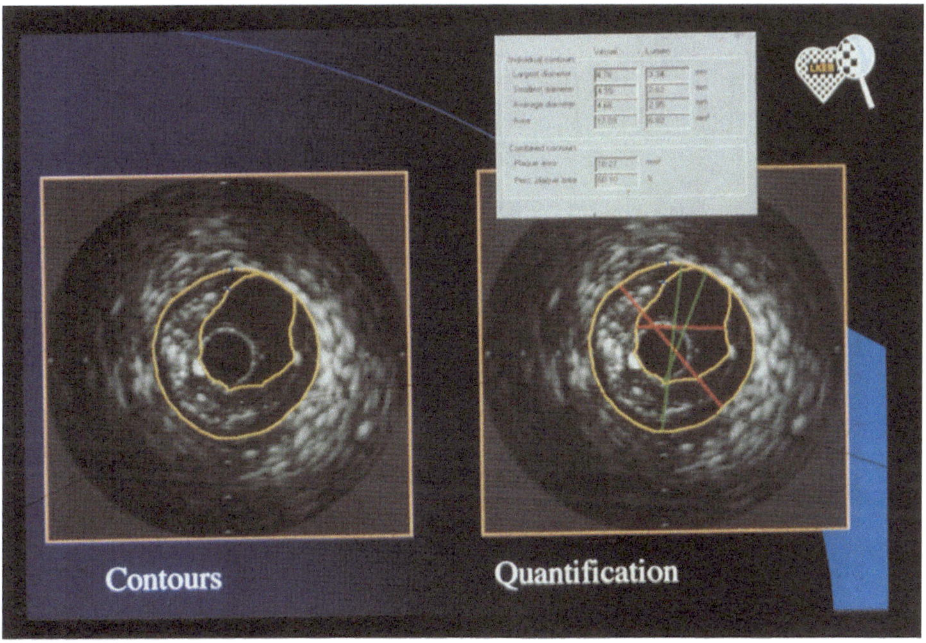

Figure 2, p. 82, Chapter 5.

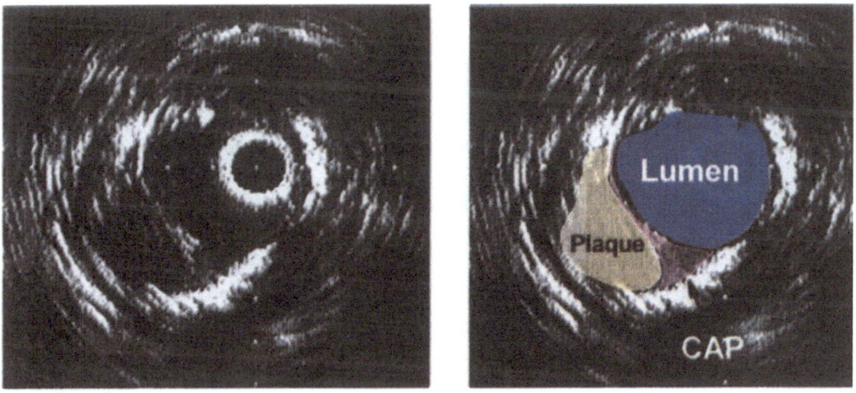

Figure 3, p. 83, Chapter 5.

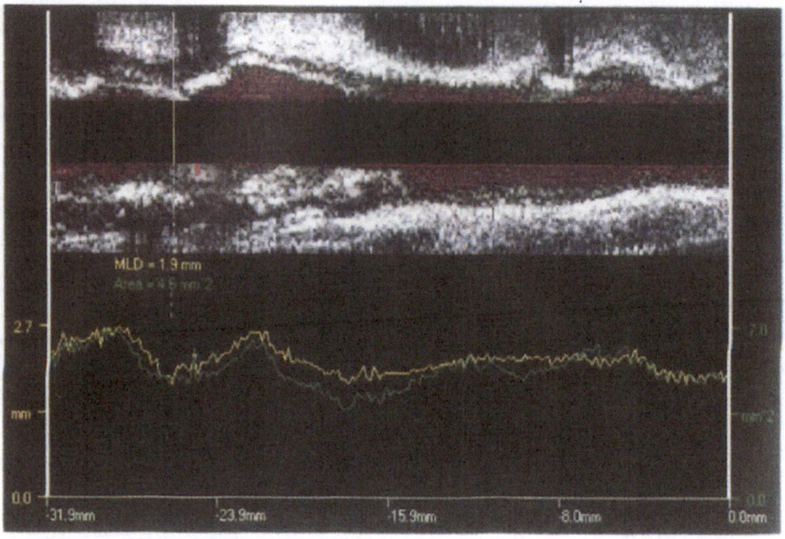

Figure 8, p. 88, Chapter 5.

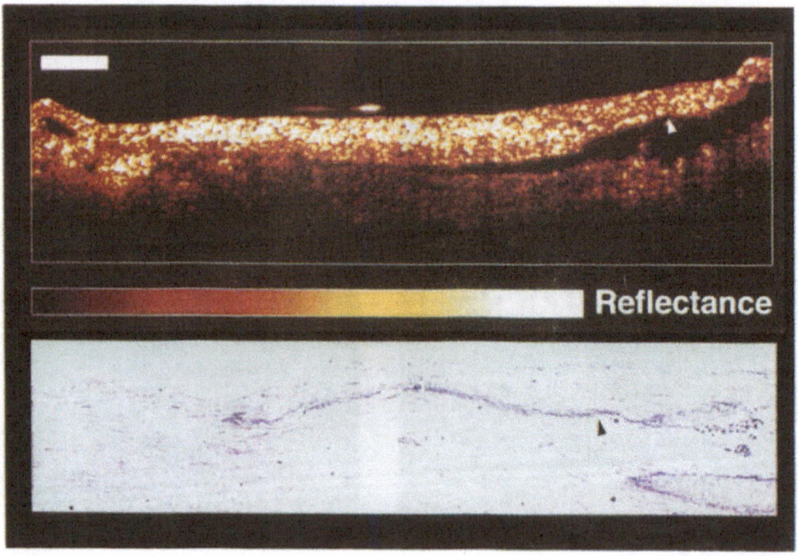

Figure 9, p. 89, Chapter 5.

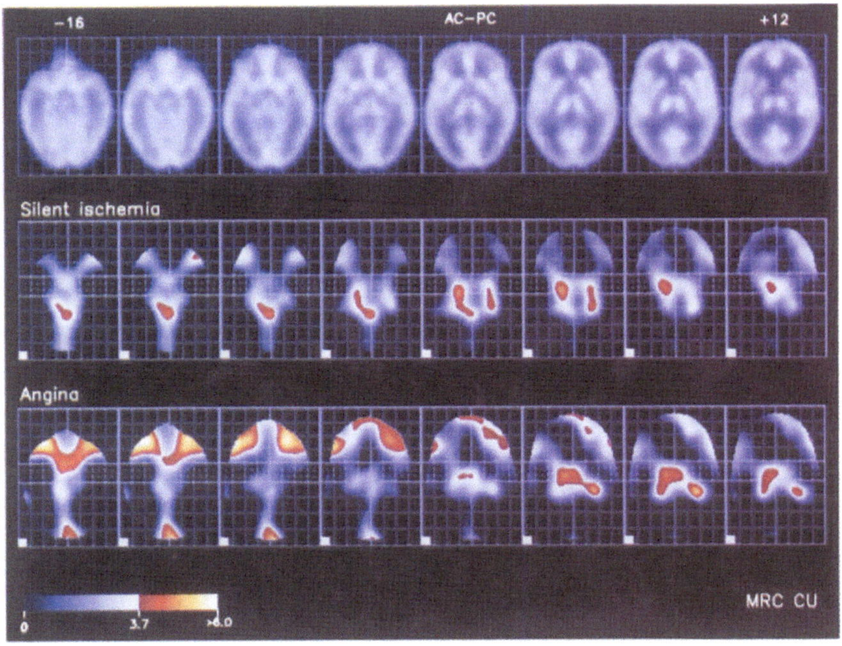

Figure 1, p. 159, Chapter 9.

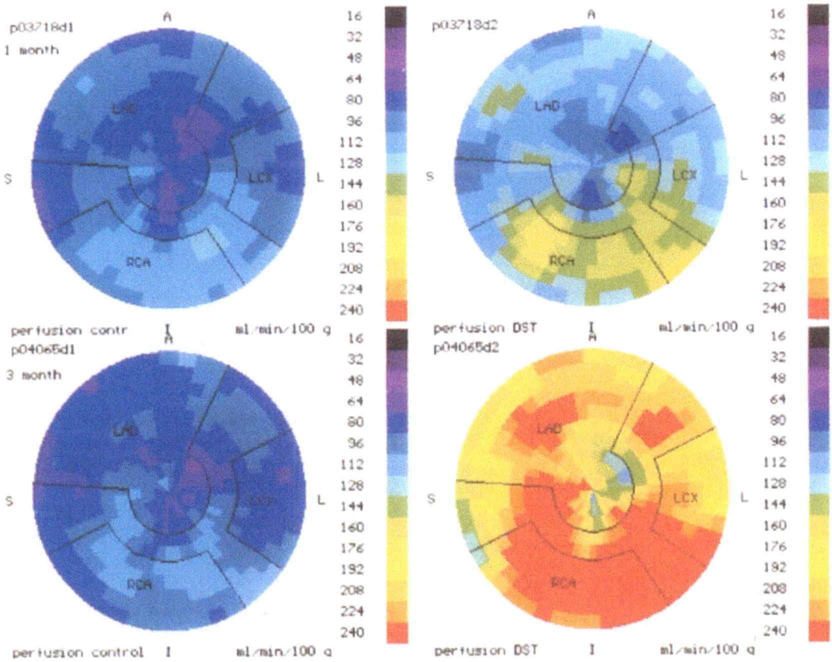

INDEX

Developments in Cardiovascular Medicine

71. E. Aliot and R. Lazzara (eds.): *Ventricular Tachycardias.* From Mechanism to Therapy. 1987 ISBN 0-89838-881-3
72. A. Schneeweiss and G. Schettler: *Cardiovascular Drug Therapoy in the Elderly.* 1988 ISBN 0-89838-883-X
73. J.V. Chapman and A. Sgalambro (eds.): *Basic Concepts in Doppler Echocardiography.* Methods of Clinical Applications based on a Multi-modality Doppler Approach. 1987 ISBN 0-89838-888-0
74. S. Chien, J. Dormandy, E. Ernst and A. Matrai (eds.): *Clinical Hemorheology.* Applications in Cardiovascular and Hematological Disease, Diabetes, Surgery and Gynecology. 1987 ISBN 0-89838-807-4
75. J. Morganroth and E.N. Moore (eds.): *Congestive Heart Failure.* Proceedings of the 7th Annual Symposium on New Drugs and Devices, held in Philadelphia, Pa., U.S.A. (1986). 1987 ISBN 0-89838-955-0
76. F.H. Messerli (ed.): *Cardiovascular Disease in the Elderly.* 2nd ed. 1988 ISBN 0-89838-962-3
77. P.H. Heintzen and J.H. Bürsch (eds.): *Progress in Digital Angiocardiography.* 1988 ISBN 0-89838-965-8
78. M.M. Scheinman (ed.): *Catheter Ablation of Cardiac Arrhythmias.* Basic Bioelectrical Effects and Clinical Indications. 1988 ISBN 0-89838-967-4
79. J.A.E. Spaan, A.V.G. Bruschke and A.C. Gittenberger-De Groot (eds.): *Coronary Circulation.* From Basic Mechanisms to Clinical Implications. 1987 ISBN 0-89838-978-X
80. C. Visser, G. Kan and R.S. Meltzer (eds.): *Echocardiography in Coronary Artery Disease.* 1988 ISBN 0-89838-979-8
81. A. Bayés de Luna, A. Betriu and G. Permanyer (eds.): *Therapeutics in Cardiology.* 1988 ISBN 0-89838-981-X
82. D.M. Mirvis (ed.): *Body Surface Electrocardiographic Mapping.* 1988 ISBN 0-89838-983-6
83. M.A. Konstam and J.M. Isner (eds.): *The Right Ventricle.* 1988 ISBN 0-89838-987-9
84. C.T. Kappagoda and P.V. Greenwood (eds.): *Long-term Management of Patients after Myocardial Infarction.* 1988 ISBN 0-89838-352-8
85. W.H. Gaasch and H.J. Levine (eds.): *Chronic Aortic Regurgitation.* 1988 ISBN 0-89838-364-1
86. P.K. Singal (ed.): *Oxygen Radicals in the Pathophysiology of Heart Disease.* 1988 ISBN 0-89838-375-7
87. J.H.C. Reiber and P.W. Serruys (eds.): *New Developments in Quantitative Coronary Arteriography.* 1988 ISBN 0-89838-377-3
88. J. Morganroth and E.N. Moore (eds.): *Silent Myocardial Ischemia.* Proceedings of the 8th Annual Symposium on New Drugs and Devices (1987). 1988 ISBN 0-89838-380-3
89. H.E.D.J. ter Keurs and M.I.M. Noble (eds.): *Starling's Law of the Heart Revisted.* 1988 ISBN 0-89838-382-X
90. N. Sperelakis (ed.): *Physiology and Pathophysiology of the Heart.* Rev. ed. 1988 3rd, revised edition, 1994: see below under Volume 151
91. J.W. de Jong (ed.): *Myocardial Energy Metabolism.* 1988 ISBN 0-89838-394-3
92. V. Hombach, H.H. Hilger and H.L. Kennedy (eds.): *Electrocardiography and Cardiac Drug Therapy.* Proceedings of an International Symposium, held in Cologne, F.R.G. (1987). 1988 ISBN 0-89838-395-1
93. H. Iwata, J.B. Lombardini and T. Segawa (eds.): *Taurine and the Heart.* 1988 ISBN 0-89838-396-X
94. M.R. Rosen and Y. Palti (eds.): *Lethal Arrhythmias Resulting from Myocardial Ischemia and Infarction.* Proceedings of the 2nd Rappaport Symposium, held in Haifa, Israel (1988). 1988 ISBN 0-89838-401-X
95. M. Iwase and I. Sotobata: *Clinical Echocardiography.* With a Foreword by M.P. Spencer. 1989 ISBN 0-7923-0004-1

Developments in Cardiovascular Medicine

96. I. Cikes (ed.): *Echocardiography in Cardiac Interventions.* 1989 ISBN 0-7923-0088-2
97. E. Rapaport (ed.): *Early Interventions in Acute Myocardial Infarction.* 1989 ISBN 0-7923-0175-7
98. M.E. Safar and F. Fouad-Tarazi (eds.): *The Heart in Hypertension.* A Tribute to Robert C. Tarazi (1925-1986). 1989 ISBN 0-7923-0197-8
99. S. Meerbaum and R. Meltzer (eds.): *Myocardial Contrast Two-dimensional Echocardiography.* 1989 ISBN 0-7923-0205-2
100. J. Morganroth and E.N. Moore (eds.): *Risk/Benefit Analysis for the Use and Approval of Thrombolytic, Antiarrhythmic, and Hypolipidemic Agents.* Proceedings of the 9th Annual Symposium on New Drugs and Devices (1988). 1989 ISBN 0-7923-0294-X
101. P.W. Serruys, R. Simon and K.J. Beatt (eds.): *PTCA - An Investigational Tool and a Non-operative Treatment of Acute Ischemia.* 1990 ISBN 0-7923-0346-6
102. I.S. Anand, P.I. Wahi and N.S. Dhalla (eds.): *Pathophysiology and Pharmacology of Heart Disease.* 1989 ISBN 0-7923-0367-9
103. G.S. Abela (ed.): *Lasers in Cardiovascular Medicine and Surgery.* Fundamentals and Technique. 1990 ISBN 0-7923-0440-3
104. H.M. Piper (ed.): *Pathophysiology of Severe Ischemic Myocardial Injury.* 1990 ISBN 0-7923-0459-4
105. S.M. Teague (ed.): *Stress Doppler Echocardiography.* 1990 ISBN 0-7923-0499-3
106. P.R. Saxena, D.I. Wallis, W. Wouters and P. Bevan (eds.): *Cardiovascular Pharmacology of 5-Hydroxytryptamine.* Prospective Therapeutic Applications. 1990 ISBN 0-7923-0502-7
107. A.P. Shepherd and P.A. Öberg (eds.): *Laser-Doppler Blood Flowmetry.* 1990 ISBN 0-7923-0508-6
108. J. Soler-Soler, G. Permanyer-Miralda and J. Sagristà-Sauleda (eds.): *Pericardial Disease.* New Insights and Old Dilemmas. 1990 ISBN 0-7923-0510-8
109. J.P.M. Hamer: *Practical Echocardiography in the Adult.* With Doppler and Color-Doppler Flow Imaging. 1990 ISBN 0-7923-0670-8
110. A. Bayés de Luna, P. Brugada, J. Cosin Aguilar and F. Navarro Lopez (eds.): *Sudden Cardiac Death.* 1991 ISBN 0-7923-0716-X
111. E. Andries and R. Stroobandt (eds.): *Hemodynamics in Daily Practice.* 1991 ISBN 0-7923-0725-9
112. J. Morganroth and E.N. Moore (eds.): *Use and Approval of Antihypertensive Agents and Surrogate Endpoints for the Approval of Drugs affecting Antiarrhythmic Heart Failure and Hypolipidemia.* Proceedings of the 10th Annual Symposium on New Drugs and Devices (1989). 1990 ISBN 0-7923-0756-9
113. S. Iliceto, P. Rizzon and J.R.T.C. Roelandt (eds.): *Ultrasound in Coronary Artery Disease.* Present Role and Future Perspectives. 1990 ISBN 0-7923-0784-4
114. J.V. Chapman and G.R. Sutherland (eds.): *The Noninvasive Evaluation of Hemodynamics in Congenital Heart Disease.* Doppler Ultrasound Applications in the Adult and Pediatric Patient with Congenital Heart Disease. 1990 ISBN 0-7923-0836-0
115. G.T. Meester and F. Pinciroli (eds.): *Databases for Cardiology.* 1991 ISBN 0-7923-0886-7
116. B. Korecky and N.S. Dhalla (eds.): *Subcellular Basis of Contractile Failure.* 1990 ISBN 0-7923-0890-5
117. J.H.C. Reiber and P.W. Serruys (eds.): *Quantitative Coronary Arteriography.* 1991 ISBN 0-7923-0913-8
118. E. van der Wall and A. de Roos (eds.): *Magnetic Resonance Imaging in Coronary Artery Disease.* 1991 ISBN 0-7923-0940-5
119. V. Hombach, M. Kochs and A.J. Camm (eds.): *Interventional Techniques in Cardiovascular Medicine.* 1991 ISBN 0-7923-0956-1
120. R. Vos: *Drugs Looking for Diseases.* Innovative Drug Research and the Development of the Beta Blockers and the Calcium Antagonists. 1991 ISBN 0-7923-0968-5

Developments in Cardiovascular Medicine

121. S. Sideman, R. Beyar and A.G. Kleber (eds.): *Cardiac Electrophysiology, Circulation, and Transport.* Proceedings of the 7th Henry Goldberg Workshop (Berne, Switzerland, 1990). 1991 ISBN 0-7923-1145-0
122. D.M. Bers: *Excitation-Contraction Coupling and Cardiac Contractile Force.* 1991 ISBN 0-7923-1186-8
123. A.-M. Salmasi and A.N. Nicolaides (eds.): *Occult Atherosclerotic Disease.* Diagnosis, Assessment and Management. 1991 ISBN 0-7923-1188-4
124. J.A.E. Spaan: *Coronary Blood Flow.* Mechanics, Distribution, and Control. 1991 ISBN 0-7923-1210-4
125. R.W. Stout (ed.): *Diabetes and Atherosclerosis.* 1991 ISBN 0-7923-1310-0
126. A.G. Herman (ed.): *Antithrombotics.* Pathophysiological Rationale for Pharmacological Interventions. 1991 ISBN 0-7923-1413-1
127. N.H.J. Pijls: *Maximal Myocardial Perfusion as a Measure of the Functional Significance of Coronary Arteriogram.* From a Pathoanatomic to a Pathophysiologic Interpretation of the Coronary Arteriogram. 1991 ISBN 0-7923-1430-1
128. J.H.C. Reiber and E.E. v.d. Wall (eds.): *Cardiovascular Nuclear Medicine and MRI.* Quantitation and Clinical Applications. 1992 ISBN 0-7923-1467-0
129. E. Andries, P. Brugada and R. Stroobrandt (eds.): *How to Face 'the Faces' of Cardiac Pacing.* 1992 ISBN 0-7923-1528-6
130. M. Nagano, S. Mochizuki and N.S. Dhalla (eds.): *Cardiovascular Disease in Diabetes.* 1992 ISBN 0-7923-1554-5
131. P.W. Serruys, B.H. Strauss and S.B. King III (eds.): *Restenosis after Intervention with New Mechanical Devices.* 1992 ISBN 0-7923-1555-3
132. P.J. Walter (ed.): *Quality of Life after Open Heart Surgery.* 1992 ISBN 0-7923-1580-4
133. E.E. van der Wall, H. Sochor, A. Righetti and M.G. Niemeyer (eds.): *What's new in Cardiac Imaging?* SPECT, PET and MRI. 1992 ISBN 0-7923-1615-0
134. P. Hanrath, R. Uebis and W. Krebs (eds.): *Cardiovascular Imaging by Ultrasound.* 1992 ISBN 0-7923-1755-6
135. F.H. Messerli (ed.): *Cardiovascular Disease in the Elderly.* 3rd ed. 1992 ISBN 0-7923-1859-5
136. J. Hess and G.R. Sutherland (eds.): *Congenital Heart Disease in Adolescents and Adults.* 1992 ISBN 0-7923-1862-5
137. J.H.C. Reiber and P.W. Serruys (eds.): *Advances in Quantitative Coronary Arteriography.* 1993 ISBN 0-7923-1863-3
138. A.-M. Salmasi and A.S. Iskandrian (eds.): *Cardiac Output and Regional Flow in Health and Disease.* 1993 ISBN 0-7923-1911-7
139. J.H. Kingma, N.M. van Hemel and K.I. Lie (eds.): *Atrial Fibrillation, a Treatable Disease?* 1992 ISBN 0-7923-2008-5
140. B. Ostadel and N.S. Dhalla (eds.): *Heart Function in Health and Disease.* Proceedings of the Cardiovascular Program (Prague, Czechoslovakia, 1991). 1992 ISBN 0-7923-2052-2
141. D. Noble and Y.E. Earm (eds.): *Ionic Channels and Effect of Taurine on the Heart.* Proceedings of an International Symposium (Seoul, Korea , 1992). 1993 ISBN 0-7923-2199-5
142. H.M. Piper and C.J. Preusse (eds.): *Ischemia-reperfusion in Cardiac Surgery.* 1993 ISBN 0-7923-2241-X
143. J. Roelandt, E.J. Gussenhoven and N. Bom (eds.): *Intravascular Ultrasound.* 1993 ISBN 0-7923-2301-7
144. M.E. Safar and M.F. O'Rourke (eds.): *The Arterial System in Hypertension.* 1993 ISBN 0-7923-2343-2
145. P.W. Serruys, D.P. Foley and P.J. de Feyter (eds.): *Quantitative Coronary Angiography in Clinical Practice.* With a Foreword by Spencer B. King III. 1994 ISBN 0-7923-2368-8

Developments in Cardiovascular Medicine

146. J. Candell-Riera and D. Ortega-Alcalde (eds.): *Nuclear Cardiology in Everyday Practice.* 1994 ISBN 0-7923-2374-2
147. P. Cummins (ed.): *Growth Factors and the Cardiovascular System.* 1993 ISBN 0-7923-2401-3
148. K. Przyklenk, R.A. Kloner and D.M. Yellon (eds.): *Ischemic Preconditioning: The Concept of Endogenous Cardioprotection.* 1993 ISBN 0-7923-2410-2
149. T.H. Marwick: *Stress Echocardiography.* Its Role in the Diagnosis and Evaluation of Coronary Artery Disease. 1994 ISBN 0-7923-2579-6
150. W.H. van Gilst and K.I. Lie (eds.): *Neurohumoral Regulation of Coronary Flow.* Role of the Endothelium. 1993 ISBN 0-7923-2588-5
151. N. Sperelakis (ed.): *Physiology and Pathophysiology of the Heart.* 3rd rev. ed. 1994 ISBN 0-7923-2612-1
152. J.C. Kaski (ed.): *Angina Pectoris with Normal Coronary Arteries: Syndrome X.* 1994 ISBN 0-7923-2651-2
153. D.R. Gross: *Animal Models in Cardiovascular Research.* 2nd rev. ed. 1994 ISBN 0-7923-2712-8
154. A.S. Iskandrian and E.E. van der Wall (eds.): *Myocardial Viability.* Detection and Clinical Relevance. 1994 ISBN 0-7923-2813-2
155. J.H.C. Reiber and P.W. Serruys (eds.): *Progress in Quantitative Coronary Arteriography.* 1994 ISBN 0-7923-2814-0
156. U. Goldbourt, U. de Faire and K. Berg (eds.): *Genetic Factors in Coronary Heart Disease.* 1994 ISBN 0-7923-2752-7
157. G. Leonetti and C. Cuspidi (eds.): *Hypertension in the Elderly.* 1994 ISBN 0-7923-2852-3
158. D. Ardissino, S. Savonitto and L.H. Opie (eds.): *Drug Evaluation in Angina Pectoris.* 1994 ISBN 0-7923-2897-3
159. G. Bkaily (ed.): *Membrane Physiopathology.* 1994 ISBN 0-7923-3062-5
160. R.C. Becker (ed.): *The Modern Era of Coronary Thrombolysis.* 1994 ISBN 0-7923-3063-3
161. P.J. Walter (ed.): *Coronary Bypass Surgery in the Elderly.* Ethical, Economical and Quality of Life Aspects. With a foreword by N.K. Wenger. 1995 ISBN 0-7923-3188-5
162. J.W. de Jong and R. Ferrari (eds.), *The Carnitine System.* A New Therapeutical Approach to Cardiovascular Diseases. 1995 ISBN 0-7923-3318-7
163. C.A. Neill and E.B. Clark: *The Developing Heart: A 'History' of Pediatric Cardiology.* 1995 ISBN 0-7923-3375-6
164. N. Sperelakis: *Electrogenesis of Biopotentials in the Cardiovascular System.* 1995 ISBN 0-7923-3398-5
165. M. Schwaiger (ed.): *Cardiac Positron Emission Tomography.* 1995 ISBN 0-7923-3417-5
166. E.E. van der Wall, P.K. Blanksma, M.G. Niemeyer and A.M.J. Paans (eds.): *Cardiac Positron Emission Tomography.* Viability, Perfusion, Receptors and Cardiomyopathy. 1995 ISBN 0-7923-3472-8
167. P.K. Singal, I.M.C. Dixon, R.E. Beamish and N.S. Dhalla (eds.): *Mechanism of Heart Failure.* 1995 ISBN 0-7923-3490-6
168. N.S. Dhalla, P.K. Singal, N. Takeda and R.E. Beamish (eds.): *Pathophysiology of Heart Failure.* 1995 ISBN 0-7923-3571-6
169. N.S. Dhalla, G.N. Pierce, V. Panagia and R.E. Beamish (eds.): *Heart Hypertrophy and Failure.* 1995 ISBN 0-7923-3572-4
170. S.N. Willich and J.E. Muller (eds.): *Triggering of Acute Coronary Syndromes.* Implications for Prevention. 1995 ISBN 0-7923-3605-4
171. E.E. van der Wall, T.H. Marwick and J.H.C. Reiber (eds.): *Advances in Imaging Techniques in Ischemic Heart Disease.* 1995 ISBN 0-7923-3620-8
172. B. Swynghedauw: *Molecular Cardiology for the Cardiologist.* 1995 ISBN 0-7923-3622-4

Developments in Cardiovascular Medicine

173. C.A. Nienaber and U. Sechtem (eds.): *Imaging and Intervention in Cardiology.* 1996 ISBN 0-7923-3649-6
174. G. Assmann (ed.): *HDL Deficiency and Atherosclerosis.* 1995 ISBN 0-7923-8888-7
175. N.M. van Hemel, F.H.M. Wittkampf and H. Ector (eds.): *The Pacemaker Clinic of the 90's.* Essentials in Brady-Pacing. 1995 ISBN 0-7923-3688-7
176. N. Wilke (ed.): *Advanced Cardiovascular MRI of the Heart and Great Vessels.* Forthcoming. ISBN 0-7923-3720-4
177. M. LeWinter, H. Suga and M.W. Watkins (eds.): *Cardiac Energetics: From Emax to Pressure-volume Area.* 1995 ISBN 0-7923-3721-2
178. R.J. Siegel (ed.): *Ultrasound Angioplasty.* 1995 ISBN 0-7923-3722-0
179. D.M. Yellon and G.J. Gross (eds.): *Myocardial Protection and the K_{ATP} Channel.* 1995 ISBN 0-7923-3791-3
180. A.V.G. Bruschke, J.H.C. Reiber, K.I. Lie and H.J.J. Wellens (eds.): *Lipid Lowering Therapy and Progression of Coronary Atherosclerosis.* 1996 ISBN 0-7923-3807-3
181. A.-S.A. Abd-Eyattah and A.S. Wechsler (eds.): *Purines and Myocardial Protection.* 1995 ISBN 0-7923-3831-6
182. M. Morad, S. Ebashi, W. Trautwein and Y. Kurachi (eds.): *Molecular Physiology and Pharmacology of Cardiac Ion Channels and Transporters.* 1996 ISBN 0-7923-3913-4
183. M.A. Oto (ed.): *Practice and Progress in Cardiac Pacing and Electrophysiology.* 1996 ISBN 0-7923-3950-9
184. W.H. Birkenhäger (ed.): *Practical Management of Hypertension.* Second Edition. 1996 ISBN 0-7923-3952-5
185. J.C. Chatham, J.R. Forder and J.H. McNeill (eds.): *The Heart in Diabetes.* 1996 ISBN 0-7923-4052-3
186. J.H.C. Reiber and E.E. van der Wall (eds.): *Cardiovascular Imaging.* 1996 ISBN 0-7923-4109-0
187. A-M. Salmasi and A. Strano (eds.): *Angiology in Practice.* 1996 ISBN 0-7923-4143-0
188. M.W. Kroll and M.H. Lehmann (eds.): *Implantable Cardioverter Defibrillator Therapy: The Engineering – Clinical Interface.* 1996 ISBN 0-7923-4300-X
189. K.L. March (ed.): *Gene Transfer in the Cardiovascular System.* Experimental Approaches and Therapeutic Implications. 1996 ISBN 0-7923-9859-9
190. L. Klein (ed.): *Coronary Stenosis Morphology: Analysis and Implication.* 1997 ISBN 0-7923-9867-X
191. J.E. Pérez and R.M. Lang (eds.): *Echocardiography and Cardiovascular Function: Tools for the Next Decade.* 1997 ISBN 0-7923-9884-X
192. A.A. Knowlton (ed.): *Heat Shock Proteins and the Cardiovascular System.* 1997 ISBN 0-7923-9910-2
193. R.C. Becker (ed.): *The Textbook of Coronary Thrombosis and Thrombolysis.* 1997 ISBN 0-7923-9923-4
194. R.M. Mentzer, Jr., M. Kitakaze, J.M. Downey and M. Hori (eds.): *Adenosine, Cardioprotection and Its Clinical Application.* 1997 ISBN 0-7923-9954-4
195. N.H.J. Pijls and B. De Bruyne: *Coronary Pressure.* 1997 ISBN 0-7923-4672-6
196. I. Graham, H. Refsum, I.H. Rosenberg and P.M. Ueland (eds.): *Homocysteine Metabolism: from Basic Science to Clinical Medicine.* 1997 ISBN 0-7923-9983-8
197. E.E. van der Wall, V. Manger Cats and J. Baan (eds.): *Vascular Medicine – From Endothelium to Myocardium.* 1997 ISBN 0-7923-4740-4
198. A. Lafont and E. Topol (eds.): *Arterial Remodeling.* A Critical Factor in Restenosis. 1997 ISBN 0-7923-8008-8
199. M. Mercuri, D.D. McPherson, H. Bassiouny and S. Glagov (eds.): Non-Invasive Imaging of Atherosclerosis. 1997 ISBN 0-7923-8036-3
200. W.C. De Mello and M.J. Janse (eds.): *Heart Cell Communication in Health and Disease.* 1997 ISBN 0-7923-8052-5

Developments in Cardiovascular Medicine

201. P.E. Vardas (ed.): *Cardiac Arrhythmias Pacing and Electrophysiology.* The Expert View. 1998 ISBN 0-7923-4908-3
202. E.E. van der Wall, P.K. Blanksma, M.G. Niemeyer, W. Vaalburg and H.J.G.M. Crijns (eds.): *Advanced Imaging in Coronary Artery Disease.* PET, SPECT, MRI, IVUS, EBCT. 1998 ISBN 0-7923-5083-9

Previous volumes are still available

KLUWER ACADEMIC PUBLISHERS – DORDRECHT / BOSTON / LONDON